Traditional Chinese Medicine Is an Intangible Science

My Medical Practice and Reflections of TCM

Traditional Chinese Medicine Is an Intangible Science

My Medical Practice and Reflections of TCM

Boxin Guo

Boxin Chinese Medicine, China

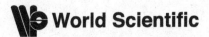

World Scientific

NEW JERSEY · LONDON · SINGAPORE · BEIJING · SHANGHAI · HONG KONG · TAIPEI · CHENNAI · TOKYO

Published by

World Scientific Publishing Co. Pte. Ltd.
5 Toh Tuck Link, Singapore 596224
USA office: 27 Warren Street, Suite 401-402, Hackensack, NJ 07601
UK office: 57 Shelton Street, Covent Garden, London WC2H 9HE

Library of Congress Cataloging-in-Publication Data
Names: Guo, Boxin, author.
Title: Traditional Chinese medicine is an intangible science : my medical practice and
 reflections of TCM / by Boxin Guo.
Other titles: Zhong yi shi wu xing de ke xue. English
Description: New Jersey : World Scientific, 2018. | Translation of Zhong yi shi wu xing de ke xue,
 originally published in Chinese by China Renmin University Press, 2013.
Identifiers: LCCN 2018014015 | ISBN 9789813239296 (hardcover : alk. paper)
Subjects: | MESH: Medicine, Chinese Traditional | Philosophy, Medical | Essays
Classification: LCC R601 | NLM WB 55.C4 | DDC 610.951--dc23
LC record available at https://lccn.loc.gov/2018014015

British Library Cataloguing-in-Publication Data
A catalogue record for this book is available from the British Library.

B&R Book Program

《中医是无形的科学》
Copyright © Guo Boxin
Published in Chinese by China Renmin University Press in 2013
English translation rights arranged with China Renmin University Press

Copyright © 2018 by World Scientific Publishing Co. Pte. Ltd.

For any available supplementary material, please visit
http://www.worldscientific.com/worldscibooks/10.1142/10965#t=suppl

Desk Editor: Ling Xiao 萧玲

Typeset by Stallion Press
Email: enquiries@stallionpress.com

Printed in Singapore

Contents

Foreword to the Chinese edition

Lǐ Kě (李可)

This book is about correcting the wrong diagnostic and therapeutic thoughts of Traditional Chinese Medicine (TCM) doctors.

When there is something wrong with a doctor's physical health, he will harm no one but suffer himself. When there is something wrong with a doctor's thought, it is guilty for him to diagnose and treat patients with this incorrect thought, especially when he does not realize it or conceals this thought for the fear of being criticized, he will make the patient's condition worse and irreversible.

I therefore recommend my peers, the Traditional Chinese Medicine practitioners, to read this book carefully. Recollecting your medical careers after reading this book, you may feel that everything has changed. Just as an old Chinese proverb goes, 'To err is human, to correct, divine.' If you've made mistakes in your medical careers, you correct them. Then you will still be the highly competent doctor.

Traditional Chinese Medicine (TCM) is the unique life science created by the Chinese civilization. It is the collective wisdom of Chinese wise men dating back as far as 5,000 years. *Shennong's Classic of Materia Mdica* (*Shén nóng Běn cǎo jīng,* 神农本草经), which was compiled by generations of people based on the theory of *Book of Changes* (*Yì jīng,* 易经), the masterpiece of Chinese culture, summarizes and elaborates the experience of prescribing Chinese medicinals. Based on the theory of *Book of Changes* (*Yì jīng,* 易经) again, *Huangdi's Internal Classic* (*Huáng dì nèi jīng,* 黄帝内经), which was accomplished in the Warring States

Period, constructs the theoretical framework of ancient TCM. In the Spring & Warring States Period, Qín Yuèrén (秦越人, well-known as Biǎn Què) further developed TCM in *Classic of Difficulties* (*Nàn jīng,* 难经). In the late Eastern Han Dynasty, Zhāng Zhòngjǐng (张仲景), based on the thoughts of *Huangdi's Internal Classic* (*Huáng dì nèi jīng,* 黄帝内经) and *Classic of Difficulties* (*Nàn jīng,* 难经), as well as the advanced thoughts of many famous medical ancestors, wrote *Treatise on Cold Damage Diseases and Miscellaneous Diseases* (*Shāng hán zá bìng lùn,* 伤寒杂病论). This book set up the integrated system of TCM from theory to clinical practice. TCM is also known as Qi-Huang theory. This is the course of development of Traditional Chinese Medicine.

The four great classics mentioned above are the core of TCM. *Treatise on Cold Damage Diseases* (*Shāng hán lùn,* 伤寒论) is the top one among the classics, because the syndrome differentiation of the six meridians formulated by Zhāng Zhòngjǐng (张仲景) is the living soul of TCM. Historically, when we follow the classics, TCM flourishes, otherwise it declines. Therefore, the judgment of a doctor's medical skills can only rely on the core theory of *Treatise on Cold Damage Diseases* (*Shāng hán lùn,* 伤寒论). Back to the classics is the only way to further develop TCM. I hope the book could help us get rid of the wrong diagnostic and therapeutic thoughts of TCM and put things right. I also expect that the book could move on from the classics and forge the future for TCM. May the book bring a new life to the ancient Traditional Chinese Medicine. As a result, I wrote the preface with pleasure.

June 21, 2012
Lingshi, Shanxi

Preface to the English edition

Traditional Chinese medicine is a unique science for human life, innovated by the Chinese nationality. Meanwhile, it is also a treasure enabling the Chinese nationality to defeat illness for thousands of years. Currently, there has been growing passion on traditional Chinese medicine worldwide, with more and more people recognizing and accepting this science. However, when referring to how to study and apply traditional Chinese medicine well, it requires a clear recognition on what kind of science it is, which is a significant premise. Under this premise, learners can have a specific goal in learning traditional Chinese medicine, from which they can avoid detours and master the essence of curing diseases as soon as possible. Therefore, they can help to solve the world's medical problems one by one.

According to this recognition, based on my own examples on treatment of diseases, I have systematically illustrated what kind of science the traditional Chinese medicine is in this book. It aims at providing answers to the relevant confusion and doubt in people's minds and carrying forward traditional Chinese medicine to bring benefit to all mankind.

Boxin Guo
New Zealand,
February 28, 2018

Preface to the Chinese edition

Having been a medical practitioner for about 40 years, I am an old man now. The contents of the book are the practices and the reflections of my medical career for decades. I expect that the book will let more and more people know what Traditional Chinese Medicine is and what a treasure it is. I also expect that the book will inspire and benefit the TCM learners. That is the reason why I wrote this book.

After finishing the draft version, I presented it to Lǐ Kě (李可), my mentor. Although he was ill, he gladly wrote the preface. Meanwhile, he recommended my book to Zhū Liángchūn (朱良春), the mogul in TCM circle. Although Zhu was bed-ridden because of a waist injury, he still wrote an inscription for the book with good grace. As a learner who has been receiving education from them for many years, I am indebted to these two venerable elders for their encouragements.

Xiè Yībīng (谢一兵), deputy Editor-in-Chief of Shanxi Science and Technology Publishing House, and Zhōu Guāngróng (周光荣), desk editor for the book, had solicited contributions from me over 10 years ago. However, I was too busy with medical practice to write anything at that time. I really appreciate their recognition and encouragement when I was writing the book. Through their strenuous efforts in the edition and publication, finally, the book has been accomplished.

I express my gratitude to my wife, Huáng Yún (黄云). For a long time, she has never hesitated to encourage and help me learn TCM. When I was writing this book, she helped me revise the manuscript so carefully that she weighed every single word and sentence, just as *The Book of*

Poetry (Shī Jīng) describes, 'I have not leisure to lie down even undressed.' Without her endeavors, I can never finish the writing.

I express my gratitude to the civil Traditional Chinese Medicine practitioner, Ān Tiěniú (安铁牛), because he not only shares his clinical experience with me selflessly, but also exchanges his understanding of Tao-like Chinese medical knowledge with me. He inspired and helped me a lot while I was writing the book.

I express my gratitude to Táng Qián (唐虔). Although he was fully occupied with business, he kept a watchful eye on my writing and provided many valuable suggestions on it.

I sincerely express my gratitude to all the people who helped me.

For my knowledge is limited and the time between writing and publication was relatively short, it is inevitable to find faults or errors in this book. If readers find any of them, please forgive me and let me know.

Guō Bóxìn (郭博信)
at the end of 2012

Acknowledgments

I would like to extend my deepest gratitude to my wife, Yun Huang, for her support and insights throughout the process of writing. Her continued support guided me towards the right path. Without her encouragement, I would not have been able to finish this book.

My sincere appreciation also extends to Mr. Pingwei Zhang and Ms. Yun Zhou for their contributions to the publication of this book.

I would also like to extend my appreciation to my step-daughter Xiaozhou Shen for her assistance in the medical case arrangements and proofreading work.

Special appreciation also goes to the translation team, namely Marcia Zhang, Hao Wang, Guanrao Nie and Yu Zhong for their professional and hard work in translating such a highly specialized book.

Note on Prescriptions

The prescriptions in this book are for reference only. Readers are advised not to blindly follow the prescriptions in this book because the dosages were differentially prescribed by the author with the particular experience of syndrome differentiation and treatment.

Traditional Chinese Medicine (TCM) is an intangible science

— The discussion on scientific attributes of TCM by taking the example of curing a tumor on the tip of the tongue

In the 1980s, I met a male patient around 40 years old. Now I can only remember that he was introduced as a director general of Heshun County. There was a tumor as big as the size of a longan on the tip of his tongue, hanging out of the mouth every day. He suffered a lot for almost a year, which caused trouble for his eating and speaking.

He had sought for help from many experts from many large-scaled modern hospitals in Beijing and Shanghai. All the experts agreed that the only solution was the resection of the tongue tumor. He had no choice but to come to me for help. After feeling his pulse, I found that the pulse was surging and rapid on both hands, especially at his left Cun position. Meanwhile, his tongue color was deep red. There is a saying in TCM that 'The tongue is the sprout of the heart', which means the heart functions in governing the vessels or in controlling the mind can be analyzed through the color and shape of the tongue. The symptoms and the manifestations of pulse and tongue revealed that he suffered the syndrome of intense heat in the heart meridian, and the tumor was caused by the accumulation of heat in the tip of his tongue. In the TCM system, there is an internal and external relationship between the heart and the small intestine, so I composed modified *Daochi San* (*Redness Removing Powder*) to remove heart heat through the small intestine.

Here were the ingredients of the formula:

Shengdihuang (*Radix Rehmanniae Recens*) 60g
Yuanshen (*Radix Scrophulariae*) 30g
Mutong (*Caulis Akebiae*) 15g
Shenggancaoshao (*Radix Glycyrrhizae*) 20g
Sharen (*Fructus Amomi*) 5g
Zhuye (*Herba Lophatheri*) 6g
Shengjiang (*Rhizoma Zingiberis Recens*) 3 slices

All these medicinals should be decocted with water for oral administration.

After composing the formula, I exhorted him that the tumor was a kind of chronic disease and he should have a long treatment period of taking dozens of doses of the prescription. The confusion could be read from his triste face. He sighed and said: "there is no other good idea, I'll try it whatever!" To my surprise, only a month later, he unexpectedly came to me with pleasure, showing me his tongue that the tumor had disappeared! He felt grateful and told me excitedly that 30 doses of the prescription had all been taken since then and the medicinals worked immediately.

Although the tongue is located in the mouth, a branch of the heart meridian ascends along the tongue. According to *Prescriptions Worth a Thousand Gold Pieces · Treatise on Heart and Meridian* (*Qiān jīn fāng · Xīn zàng mài lùn*, 千金方 · 心脏脉论), 'Tongue is the governor of heart. That's the reason of heart qi circulating through tongue.' Therefore, in Traditional Chinese Medicine, there are sayings such as, 'the heart opens into the tongue', 'the tongue is the sprout of the heart'. Considering its functions in nourishing yin and clearing heat, I chose *Daochi San* (*Redness Removing Powder*) as the basic prescription. I added *Yuanshen* (*Radix Scrophulariae*) into the formula to clear away pathogenic heat located in the upper energizer and to keep downward flowing of pathogenic heat. Adding pungent-warm medicinals such as *Sharen* (*Fructus Amomi*), *Shengjiang* (*Rhizoma Zingiberis Recens*) was to neutralize the harm of sweet-cold medicinals for the purpose of protecting stomach qi.

It is always said that TCM is an empirical medical science. In my opinion, such saying has both sides. I consider it right because experience plays a key role in the diagnosis and treatment of disease. That is the reason why people always seek elderly TCM doctors. It does not mean a young doctor cannot cure patients. But the older the doctor is, the more experience he will get. Experience determines the diagnostic and therapeutic level of a TCM doctor. If a doctor has no experience, he will be unable to treat diseases and to save lives. There are thousands of theories of medical science, but doctoring a patient back to health is the absolute principle. Numerous people have accumulated extremely rich experience of TCM in previous thousands of years. The experience is precious. Without experience, no illness can be cured. Experience is contained with truth and real science. When learning TCM, besides learning the therapeutic and diagnostic principles, we spend most hours on learning experiences of the seniors in curing diseases. Only after absorbing the experiences of the seniors can we fundamentally understand the principles of the diagnosis and treatment. No one is willing to see a doctor who can just talk about the theories of TCM, but has no experience in the diagnosis and treatment. I consider it wrong because TCM is not merely a simple empirical medical science, but a medical science which contains a unique and complete theoretical system. Only when TCM experience is applied under the guidance of TCM theory can TCM treatment achieve peculiar curative effect.

For example, *Daochi San* (*Redness-Removing Powder*) is recorded in the book of *Key to Medicines and Syndromes of Children's Diseases* (*Xiǎo ér yào zhèng zhí jué*, 小儿药证直诀) which was written by Qián Yǐ (钱乙, 1032–1113), a famous pediatrician during the Northern Song Dynasty. He invented this prescription. The original only records: 'This formula is used to treat the child in the syndrome of heat in heart meridian. The symptoms can be observed when the child is sleeping, such as the temperature of the breath from his mouth is high, lying his face down while sleeping, convulsion and gritting teeth. As the pathogenic heat is in the heart meridian so there is feverish sensation in the chest. In this occasion, the child can hardly talk, and is eager to touch cold things, so he lies his face down while sleeping. Under such circumstance, weighing an equal amount of *Shengdihuang* (*Radix Rehmanniae Recens*), *Mutong* (*Caulis Akebiae*) and *Shenggancao* (*Radix Glycyrrhizae*) and powdering them. Each time, 3 qian (1 qian ~ 3 grams) of these medicinals should be decocted with proper amount of *Zhuye* (*Herba Lophatheri*) and water until half done for oral administration. Then the child should take the warm decoction after the meal.' This formula does not mention the tumor treatment, but the treatment of intense heat in the heart meridian of the child. I composed the formula based on *Daochi San* (*Redness-Removing Powder*) because I was guided by the basic theory of 'the heart opens into the tongue', 'the tongue is the sprout of the heart' and, the therapeutic theory of 'treating heat with cold'. How to explain such issue through the aspect of western medical theory? There's no such concept in the modern human anatomy. Strictly speaking, modern human anatomy should be called as corpse anatomy. Modern human anatomy emphasizes the tangible aspect of human body, while TCM focuses on life phenomena of the living person which cannot be observed on corpses. In short, TCM observes the intangible aspect of human body.

Some people always criticize that TCM lacks knowledge of anatomy, but that is a great misunderstanding. The research object of medical science is the human being. No matter what category it is in, medical science at least should understand the human body structure, just as the saying goes, 'anatomy is the basis and starting point of medical treatment arts' which is recorded in *On the Fabric of the Human Body* written in 1543 by Andreas Vesalius who is praised as the founder of modern human anatomy. Both TCM and Western Medicine are included.

Miraculous·the Circulation of Qi and Blood of Meridians (*Líng shū·Jīng shuǐ*, 灵枢·经水), which has a history of over 2,000 years, records, 'For living human being, we can measure the skin and muscle by using fingers to detect different parts of the body from the exterior. For dead body, we can observe the body via anatomy.' The book also in detail introduces the positions, sizes and weights of five zang-organs (heart, lung, spleen, liver, and kidney), six fu-organs (gallbladder, stomach, large intestine, small intestine, bladder, and triple energizer) and extraordinary fu-organs (brain, marrow, bone, vessel, gallbladder, and uterus). It is obvious that TCM is less careful than modern human anatomy in observing the structure of human body.

However, it is the earliest book which records the human anatomy. According to the experts, what the book records is 1,500 years earlier than western anatomy, so it is believed that the first book about human anatomy was written by a Chinese.

Just like our attitude towards our Chinese 'four great inventions', we are only proud that we have the earliest inventions. But western people are proud that the development of western sciences has far exceeded our 'four great inventions'.

Similarly, although only having a history of 200 years, Western Medicine has gradually gone deep in anatomy along with organs, tissues, cells, and molecules, far surpassing TCM. Therefore, people now only learn human body anatomy of Western Medicine, and no one learns the anatomy knowledge of TCM.

It seems that TCM has not made any progress in human body anatomy since 2,000 years ago. However, our ancestors crossed the tangible part of human body and focused on the intangible part, namely, the relationship between the human being and nature, the relationship among the functions of body organs and their mutual relationships. In terms of zang-fu organs, our ancestors invented *Zang Xiang* (the visceral manifestation theory).

Xiang (manifestation) means something is one of the different ways in which it can appear. The clinical application of *Zang Xiang* can be found in the book of *Miraculous·Zang-fu Organs Are the Root* (*Líng shū·Běn zàng*, 灵枢·本藏), 'by observing a person's external manifestation, we can predict the situations of his internal organs and further find out the cause of his illness.'

Miraculous·Inspecting Exterior to Predict Interior (*Líng shū·Wài chuǎi*, 灵枢·外揣) calls this diagnostic method as 'inspecting exterior to predict interior', which means inspecting external manifestation of the human to predict the internal causes.

All the theories of TCM, including not only *Zang Xiang* (the visceral manifestation theory), but also yin-yang, five elements (wu-xing), meridian and collateral, qi, blood, fluid and spirit, are all the results of 'inspecting exterior to predict interior'. These results were achieved by our ancestors with their extraordinary wisdom and keen eyesight. Our ancestors presented the results in TCM way and turned them into a unique language which is TCM terminology. Only those who have deep learning of TCM can understand what the language means, that is to say, only people in the TCM circle could understand this language.

It is not because TCM cannot see the tangible part of human body, but because that TCM only focuses on the intangible part. For example, in

Miraculous (*Líng shū jīng,* 灵枢经), a large amount of texts are about the position, size, dimension, image, name of 365 bones of human skeleton. However, TCM emphasizes the kidney governing bones and considers that bone diseases should be treated from the kidney. The 'kidney governing bones' is intangible. In TCM, medicinals for tonifying the kidney are also applied during treatment of bone fracture patients, so as to facilitate healing the fracture.

I am not an orthopedist of TCM and I am unable to set a fracture. If a patient who only has fractures without dislocations, or a patient who has bone dislocations but has been treated by an orthopedist, the patient's broken bone will be healed in 20 days through taking my bone setting medicinals. The patients natural healing process will last at least 100 days.

TCM observed the tangible part of human body, but it researches or emphasizes the intangible part, which is the brilliant part of TCM.

Taking blood for example. Both TCM and Western Medicine can observe it. In TCM, we considers qi as the commander of blood. Although blood is tangible to us, it is led and driven by qi, which is intangible to us.

I have treated many patients who have lost excessive amount of blood without using hemostatic medicinals. Through the using of *Renshen* (*Radix Ginseng*) which has no function of stopping bleeding but tonifying qi, I have cured some such patients.

In TCM, *Buyang Huanwu Tang* (*Decoction for tonifying Yang and Recuperation*) is used to treat paralyzed patients. In the decoction, adding 120g *Huangqi* (*Radix Astragali seu Hedysari*) to tonify qi. Adding 6g *Dangguiwei* (*tail of Radix Angelicae sinensis*), 4.5g *Chishaoyao* (*Radix Paeoniae Rubra*), 3g *Dilong* (*lumbricus*), 3g *Chuanxiong* (*Rhizooma Ligustici Chuanxiong*), 3g *Taoren* (*Semen Persicae*), and 3g *Honghua* (*Flos Carthami*) to promote blood flow. We can see that the dosage of *Huangqi* (*Radix Astragali seu Hedysari*) is 40 times of other blood flow promoting medicinals, which fully embodies qi as the commander of blood.

The curative effect is remarkable and highly spoken of by the doctors; If we only use medicinals for promoting blood to flow and removing blood stasis without qi tonifying medicinals, positive effects can hardly be achieved. It is the reason why Zhāng Jǐngyuè (张景岳 (Zhāng Zhòngjǐng, 张仲景)) said that 'there's no basis for treatment if a doctor

cannot recognize qi (*Jing Yue's Collected Works* (*Jǐng yuè quán shū,* 景岳
全书)).' There's a saying that all theories of *Huangdi's Internal Classic*
are based on qi-blood theory. *Miraculous·Nine Needles and Twelve
Source Points* (*Líng shū·Jǐu zhēn shí èr yuán,* 灵枢·九针十二原) states
that, 'Inferior doctor cares about the form, superior doctor cares about the
spirit.' That is to say, during the treatment, the inferior doctor only cares
about the tangible form of the patient, the superior doctor cares about the
intangible spirit of the patient. *Huangdi's Internal Classic* also records,
'treating disease should focus on the root.' That 'root' is also intangible.

For example, the tongue tip tumor I've treated is tangible, but the
pathogen of this tumor, heart heat, is intangible. *Daochi San* was used to
solve the problem of intangible 'heart heat', but the tangible tumor also
disappeared then. This therapeutic course belongs to the theory of 'treating disease should focus on the root', and this is the wisdom of TCM.

When treating tumors, modern medicine advocates to remove them
by using surgery and various sorts of medical apparatus and instruments.
Although tumors can be removed, advanced medical science and technology will still bring huge pain and sequelas to the patients. Though it is
advanced at the technical level, it is actually an inferior doctor's work
from the perspective of *Huangdi's Internal Classic.* Because what it
solves is the problem of 'form', not 'spirit'. That's the difference between
TCM and Western Medicine.

Both of them are to solve the problem of form (tumor): one is to
directly remove this 'form', regardless of 'spirit' problem; The other is
to solve the 'form' problem by solving the 'spirit' problem. The purpose is the same but the thoughts are different, resulting in different
consequences.

In summary, we can clearly recognize that studying either TCM or
Western Medicine should include the human body anatomy. However
with the development of science and technology, and the applications of
modern testing instruments, Western Medicine has always been looking
for organic disease along organs, cells and molecules. Western Medicine
confirms diagnosis based on the tangible and visible object, therefore we
might call it the tangible science.

However, under the guidance of 'All internal changes of the body must
have the corresponding manifestations which emerge on the exterior',

TCM has always focused on the human life and disease phenomena of a living person which is intangible. Therefore we might as well call it the intangible science. Because both of their problems are researching and solving the same matter — objective existence of human body, both of them shall belong to human body science.

Both of them research the human body and treat the disease. But why are there two distinct scientific systems? This is determined by the particularity of the human body. All other subjects except the human body, such as astronomy, geography and even physics, chemistry, mathematics, are individual scientific systems. In these fields it will never be the case that the same matter is researched by two distinct scientific systems.

The reason is simple enough: all human beings have their lives, so there are two forms of existence, one is the living person and the other is the dead one. The modern human anatomy studies the structure and morphology of human body, which is called science. However, TCM studies the biological phenomena of a living human body. Shouldn't we call it science too? Both of them study the objective existence of human body, or to say, the truth of the matter. It's only that one observes the structure of the human body that is exact to the cellular, molecular and even genome level, with the help of advanced instruments and test methods. It is still the tangible side of human body no matter how exactly it observes. Therefore, precisely speaking, it shall be called the tangible science. However, TCM observes the 'changeable' biological phenomena of living human body. It is a very mysterious intangible side of human body which cannot be detected by advanced scientific instruments. Therefore, precisely speaking, it shall be called the intangible science. Albert Einstein, the great physicist and thinker who was famous for his 'general theory of relativity' in recent history, had proposed two standards to judge the truth of scientific theory: one is 'Internal completeness', the other is 'External authentication'. However, the classic of TCM, *Huangdi's Internal Classic* had already explained the theories of TCM in all aspects since two thousand years ago. How 'complete' the 'internal' is! Famous doctors and medical schools are enduring from Zhāng Zhòngjǐng (张仲景) to successive dynasties. What kind of 'external authentication' it is! Is there any reason to doubt that TCM has the 'truth of scientific theory'?

The great scientist Sir Isaac Newton had a famous saying: "I do not know what I may appear to the world, but to myself I seem to have been only like a boy playing on the sea-shore, and diverting myself in now and then finding a smoother pebble or a prettier shell than ordinary, whilst the great ocean of truth lay all undiscovered before me."

Although modern science is quite developed, as a part of modern science, modern medicine almost gets to the most detailed point only in the tangible side of human body and disease. It is still utterly ignorant of the intangible side of human body and disease, which is the blind spots in modern science.

However, Chinese people have already formed an independent, complete and systematic theoretical system in this field since two thousand years ago, and it also has the extremely rich and solid clinical foundation. What a miracle in the world this is! Not only Chinese people, but also all mankind will be proud of TCM! TCM is not only the wisdom of Chinese people, but also the wisdom of all mankind.

We can't treat human body science with the viewpoints and methods used for researching other subjects. We can't measure and judge the intangible science of human body with the standard of tangible science of human body either. We can't say only the one observed by eyes (or seen by virtue of instruments and assays) is scientific, and treat the one unable to be seen by eyes (or unable to be seen by virtue of instruments and test) as not scientific. If one only knows the tangible side of human body but doesn't know the intangible side of human body, one just has a one-sided view. Making TCM to be modernized and scientific is equal to making TCM to seek advice from one who can offer none, that is the ignorance of TCM. The ignorance of TCM, after all, is the ignorance of human body science. As the old saying goes, 'People who sail in the sea don't know mountains; people who drive on the land don't know water (by Hé Xiánmíng (何贤明), Ming Dynasty).'

If a doctor of TCM learns western medical knowledge blindly by getting outside of the thought of TCM, it shouldn't be called as 'seeking advice from one who can offer nothing', it should be regarded as 'following advice from one who can offer nothing', leading him astray and nowhere. As a result, one sets foot on the road of no return to what looks like 'science' but actually is very confused westernization of TCM.

Theoretical knowledge is acquired through practice

— Discussing that the intangible science is originated from the practice and talking about the misfortunes of TCM by taking the example of 'contralateral collateral needling method'

In 1980s, I learned acupuncture and moxibustion from Yáng Zhànlín (杨占林), the former superintendent of Shanxi Institute of TCM. Yang had received western medical education and became a Western Medicine doctor before, but he changed to learn acupuncture and moxibustion when he found that acupuncture and moxibustion could cure many diseases that Western Medicine could not.

Yang is good at the contralateral collateral needling. What is contralateral collateral needling? It is a kind of needling method recorded in *Huangdi's Internal Classic*.

As *Plain Questions·Treatise on the Adjustment of Meridians* (*Sù wèn·Tiáo jīng lùn,* 素问·调经论) records, 'If there is pain in body surface, and nine pulse-takings is normal, then contralateral collateral needling method should be used.' *Plain Questions·Treatise on Contralateral Collateral Needling* (*Sù wèn·Miù cì lùn,* 素问·缪刺论) also states that, 'For the patient with collateral disease, his pain is related to the contralateral part of the meridians, therefore the treatment is called contralateral collateral needling.'

In modern words, when treating a patient who has pain in the body surface with a normal pulse manifestation, or has abnormal situation in collateral meridians, instead of needling into his pain point, we should insert the needle into the painless acupoint located at the contralateral part of the pain point.

For example, if the right wrist is contused, the needles should be inserted into Taibai acupoint and Zhongfeng acupoint located at left ankle; if the right ankle joint is contused, the needles should be inserted into Shenmen acupoint located at left wrist.

Yang uses this unique needling method to treat diseases with the localized pain manifested as the cardinal symptom in the limbs, such as general surgical trauma, surgical acute infection, fracture sequela and tenosynovitis, strain, polymyalgia rheumatica, rheumatic arthritis, neuritis. His patients can always get immediate relief after being treated.

This needling method does not use many acupoints and is effective quickly. At the same time, this needling method is safe and easy to learn and it has a wide application. Especially it avoids stimulating the pain site of the patient, thus reducing the pain while inserting the needle.

From whom has Yang learned the method of contralateral collateral needling? He has learned it from Shàng Gǔyú, (尚古愚) who was a doctor from TCM Department of First Affiliated Hospital of Shanxi Medical College, and Shàng Gǔyú, (尚古愚) has learned it from doctor Dù Wéichéng (杜维诚).

Shàng Gǔyú, once said:

"At the beginning of 1951, I learned the acupuncture and moxibustion from my teacher, Dù Wéichéng (杜维诚). Du was good at contralateral collateral needling and could always have amazing curative effects, so this left a deep impression on me.

Thereafter, when I presided over the class of the research institution of acupuncture and moxibustion of Beijing Medical Association, Doctor Yuán Shàngrú (袁尚儒) gave an example of stepping forward with the left leg and moving the right arm simultaneously to explain the relationship between the balance of yin-yang and limbs activities.

Although this was a very common phenomenon in daily life, it gave me great enlightenment. When I was seeking the way to put yin-yang theory of TCM into the clinical practice correctly, my neighbor came to my home to ask for me to cure her scalded left leg.

The woman knitted sweaters for a living at that time. Her right ring finger felt ache and discomfort when she straightened it, for she always seized the knitting woolen yarn by bending right ring finger for a long time. When examined, her scalded part was located at the meridian point of Gallbladder Channel of foot lesser yang. I acupunctured Zuqiaoyin acupoint of her left foot for bloodletting to purge heat; not only her wound relieved pain immediately, but also the disease condition of her right ring finger became better. Her finger became supple gradually.

Through this case, I was familiar with the principle of selecting the acupoints on the same meridian, and the principle of selecting the contralateral acupoints, and at the same time, I realized the curative relationship among the limbs which had the same shape and similar function."

After learning this acupuncture method from Shàng Gǔyú, Yang put it into the clinica use widely. Then he had the outstanding curative effects and countless cured cases.

Taking a simple case example from Yang:

A male patient had suffered from left calf spasm by a gun shot at least 20 years ago. Yang inserted one needle into Zhizheng acupoint located at his right small intestine meridian of hand greater yang, and then kept twirling and rotating the needle for 5 minutes. The patient felt the chill gas passed his left calf right after Yang acupunctured him. After the acupuncture, his spasm had been cured and had never relapsed. A 20-year disease was cured by one needle.

Can the relationship of the selection of contralateral acupoints of human body be detected by the modern scientific instrument? Certainly not. Can it be figured out by autopsy? Certainly not. Because this relationship is intangible. However, it has an objective existence, and it exists in the body of a living person. It is observed by TCM doctors as they are treating patients, which is not fabricated.

Besides, *Huangdi's Internal Classic* records a method called contralateral channel needling, that is to select the acupoints on the right side to treat diseases on the left, and vice versa.

As *Plain Questions·Treatise on the Adjustment of Meridians* records, 'When pain is on the left, and right pulse is abnormal, contralateral channel needling should be used.'

It also records distant needling method, which is also one of nine types of needling, that is to select acupoints of yang meridians on the lower limbs to treat diseases on the upper body.

As *Miraculous·The Therapeutic Principle of Needling Methods* (*Líng shū·Guān zhēn piān*, 灵枢·官针篇) records, 'The distant needling is to select acupoints located at lower limbs, which are the lower sea points of six fu-organs in three yang meridians, to treat diseases on the upper body', 'When the disease is in the upper body, select lower sea points. Lower sea points cure six fu-organs.'

The complicated needling methods of the ancient Chinese reflects the complexity of human body, the inseparable correlation and systematicness of each human organs, which is developed from the yin-yang theory of TCM.

Yin-yang is the unity of opposites originally. No matter the concepts of TCM, like meridian-collateral, qi-blood, zang-fu organs, exterior-interior, or the concepts of human body, such as upper and lower, left and right, front and back, internal and external, physique and spirit, dynamic and static, all these things can be divided into the aspects of yin and yang.

Just as recorded in *Huangdi's Internal Classic*, 'Yin and yang have different names but belong to the same category. Yin and yang meet each other from up and down, they link together from all angles, like a loop that has no port', 'Predominant yang making yin disorder, predominant yin making yang disorder, predominant left making right disorder, and predominant right making left disorder', 'A good acupuncturist will regulate the yang by dispersing the pathogens in the yin and regulate the yin by dispersing the pathogens in the yang. Treating the right will be a good treat to the disease on the left and treating the left will be a good treat to the disease on the right', and so on and so forth.

Although researchers have studied meridian and collateral unremittingly using the modern science detecting instruments for several decades, and have given all kinds of propositions, like nerve, bioelectricity, the regulating function of human fluid, all these have proved the objective existence of meridian and collateral. But no one can totally explain the essence of meridian and collateral.

Why human beings still cannot ascertain the essence of meridian and collateral even though modern technology has been well developed nowadays? The reason is simple: there is no essence of meridian and collateral.

Although modern instruments are advanced, they can only detect the tangible aspect of human body. Meridian and collateral are also called meridian qi. They transport qi and blood, regulate yin and yang, connect zang-organs with fu-organs, associate the external with the internal as well as the upper with the lower, linking the whole body into a network. As the old saying goes, they 'control the death and birth, decide every illness.' These functions are all governed by meridian qi. Qi is intangible.

When doctor Shàng Gǔyú cured the left foot scald of the patient, he also cured disease the condition of the right ring finger unintentionally. Therefore it enabled him to know the principle that selecting one side acupoints on the same meridian can cure the disease located at the other side of the body. In fact, this principle had been recorded clearly in *Huangdi's Internal Classic* 2000 years ago, called contralateral collateral needling.

Hence we know that all the theories of TCM are intangible, but the theories were constructed from the practice. The practice if not related to the anatomy on the dead body, or the observation through a microscope in the laboratory. It is the observations of the living, namely the animate human bodies, and the analyses of the findings shown in the therapeutic processes. With the help of practice, the unique medical theoretical system of TCM finally is formed. This theoretical system could never be fabricated, because it is formed on the solid foundation of practice. It is the truth of intangible science on human body, which has been tested through the practice by the later generations for thousands of years.

Furthermore, the example of doctor Shàng Gǔyú shows that one who wants to truly understand the theories must practice on his own, though the theories of TCM come from the practice. It is because TCM is an intangible science, and no one could truly understand it if they do not put theories into practice. Otherwise, even though one can recite the theories of TCM fluently, it's just superficial learning without practicing. So what's the use of learning it literally?

A friend of mine, majoring in TCM, can recite the whole content of *Treatise on Cold Damage Diseases* so fluently that he knows the exact page of every problem. In one early spring several years ago, a cough patient didn't get better after being treated by my friend for two months. Then he resorted to me, and I cured the patient with 3 doses of the formula.

After reading my prescription, my friend blurted out: "Oh, it's *Xiao Qinglong Tang* (*Minor green-blue dragon decoction*)! Why didn't I think of it?"

I read his prescription and found that he gave a set of medicinals to relieve cough, including *Chuanbeimu* (*bulbus fritillariae cirrhosae*), *Ziwan* (*radix asteris*), *Kuandonghua* (*flos farfarae*), *Baibu* (*radix stemonae*), *Jiegeng* (*radix platycodonis*) and *Gancao* (*Radix Glycyrrhizae*), but he failed in differentiating the right syndrome. No wonder that his prescription didn't work!

In the early 1990s, when I followed Huáng Jiéxī (黄杰熙) as my teacher, a graduate student from a university of TCM in another province came to follow my teacher for studying. However, just a few days later, his supervisor, a well-known professor in TCM circle, called and asked him to return to the university to pursue a PhD degree. The professor said that nothing was more important than the skills of writing papers or making scientific research, and that there was no future for his student to learn medical treatment from a folk doctor.

Therefore, the young student hurried back excitedly.

A few years later, I heard that he not only received a PhD degree, but also managed to get a position as an associate professor in the university. Now, he may have become a full professor, because this student is really smart.

Recently, a renowned professor from a famous university of TCM gave a wonderful lecture in Taiyuan. He talked eloquently about theories of TCM and Western Medicine with fervor and assurance. He said that he had published a great deal of works. At the end of the lecture, he told the audience solemnly: "In this university of TCM, no one is able to win the debate with me!"

After hearing that, one member of the audience stood up and asked, "Which kind of disease are you good at curing?"

The professor replied simply, "I can't cure any disease."

This member of the audience wondered and asked again, "Professor, what's the use of these theories you have said if you can't treat patients?" Instantly, the professor could say nothing at all.

Traditional Chinese Medicine is a medical science coming from practice. The genuine knowledge of the intangible science can only be obtained through practicing.

As the old saying goes, 'theoretical knowledge is acquired through practice.' How can it work just knowing the theory literally?

In retrospect, Fàn Zhòngyān (范仲淹), the famous politician and writer in the Northern Song Dynasty, said that there are 'three misfortunes' in one's life:

- The first one is to receive a government degree in one's youth;
- The second is to secure an official position by taking advantage of the power and position of one's father or elder brother;
- The third is that one has an excellent ability to write, but there is no practical use.

The above three points are deemed as great fortunes of life for common people. However, why did Fan consider them as misfortunes of life?

In the first case, one will become conceited and contemptuous of everything of the world, thinking that nothing is difficult, which will lead to failure. Similar fates are those that make a fortune or make a name in youth.

In the second case, one may act arrogantly and misuse the authority out of one's self-assertion, which will eventually lead to disaster.

I think the third one is more meaningful for people to think deeply.

What does it mean? We can see that in the field of TCM, people with excellent ability to publish can get honor and the title. How lucky he is as for himself! However, when someone is ill, it's hard to find a 'doctor' who can take pulse and prescribe for the patients in our homeland. It is the big misfortune for TCM! It is also the big misfortune for common people!

Traditional Chinese Medicine belongs to Tao-like medical knowledge

— The discussion on the theory of TCM treatment by taking the example of curing a patient with a history of superficial gastritis for 20 years

The patient was a 63-year-old male, who was the professor from Shanxi Provincial Party School. He came to my clinic on May 10, 2005. He claimed that he had suffered pain, fullness and cold sensation in the stomach for 20 years. Although he never ate cold things like cold dishes or fruits even in summer, and he drank hot water all the time, he still felt uncomfortable when he paid less attention.

He was diagnosed with superficial gastritis in a hospital. After that, he had taken metoclopramide, gastropine, domperidone and various anti-inflammatory drugs, but there was no good effect at the end. With the growth of age, the disease condition worsened gradually.

When he came to me, he presented with stomachache which has worsened than before. He also suffered from nausea and bloating. His face was dark yellow with bluish color. His eyebrows became drawn together. His hands were used to push against the epigastrium. He had a light-colored tongue with a white coating. His pulse was deep, thready and slow on both hands. Apparently his symptoms were caused by the syndrome of deficiency-cold of middle energizer. Therefore, I composed *Fuzi Lizhong Wan* (*Aconite Middle Regulating Decoction*) for him.

Here were the ingredients of the formula:

Paofuzi (*Radix Aconiti Lateralis Preparata*) 10g
Ganjiang (*Rhizoma Zingiberis*) 10g
ChaoBaizhu (*Rhizoma Atractylodis Macrocephalae*) 15g
Dangshen (*Radix Codonopsis*) 30g
Sharen (*Fructus Amomi Villosi*) 5g
Zhigancao (*Radix Glycyrrhizae Praeparatae*) 10g

All these drugs should be decocted with water for oral administration, 5 doses in total.

The patient came for the second treatment on May 15. This time, I saw his brows stretched and his face had its luster back. He didn't use his hands to push against his epigastrium. He said that since he took the decoction, he felt that the stomach became warm and comfortable. He also told me that his pain, bloating and nausea had suddenly disappeared. His tongue color started to turn red and the coating was thin and white. His pulse beat 4 beats in a cycle of breath. Since the formula was effective in curing his disease, there was no need to change the formula. Thus I told him to take another 5 doses to strengthen his health.

Seven years later, I met him again in July 2012. He told me with extreme excitement that since he took the decoction that time, he not only never felt stomachache, but also wasn't afraid of cold things when he had meals. What's more, he told me that he dared to eat watermelon in summer now. He invited me to dine at his home at noon. He pointed to the cold dishes on the table and said that he ate two cold dishes, two hot dishes and drank some beer during lunch nowadays, and both his physical strength and spirit exceed his peers.

A 20-year chronic complaint had been resolved; his joy was visible in facial expressions. During the meal, he constantly drank with me, just like the old saying goes, '...Oh, let a man of spirit venture where he pleases. And never tip his golden cup empty toward the moon!'

Superficial gastritis, the name of disease in modern medicine, is a kind of chronic superficial inflammation on gastric mucosa. During the gastroscopy examination, such symptoms can be seen on the gastric mucosa hyperemia, edema, punctate hemorrhage, erosion, or with yellow-ish white exudates, etc. According to the depth of infiltration of the mucous membrane, it can be divided into three stages: mild, moderate and severe.

All in all, with the help of advanced medical instruments, the practitioner can make the meticulous observation on the tangible part of this disease. We believe scientific instruments, because this inflammation objectively exists. In addition, looking at the Chinese character '炎 (inflammation)', it is composed by two Chinese characters '火 (fire)'. Therefore, it is believed that inflammation is related to fire, which means that we have to put out the fire immediately to diminish inflammation! As a result, there must be anti-inflammatory treatments in Western Medicine that can be accepted by everyone.

However, the patient had been taking anti-inflammatory drugs for more than 20 years; this simple inflammation was still not cured. Why? There must be another way to cure it.

Without relying on advanced technological instruments, as an ancient medical science, the image of stomach with superficial gastritis cannot be seen.

Our Traditional Chinese Medicine is indeed not as advanced as modern medicine on the tangible side of observing human body and disease. However, we use another way to observe human body and disease. After the examination, we found that the spleen and stomach of this superficial gastritis patient were deficiency-cold. Deficiency-cold couldn't be detected by any advanced instrument, because it is intangible.

Certainly, we didn't find it by our own naked eyes; we found it by the power of understanding. This power of understanding is derived from the analysis of the pulse and symptoms, which is the result of thinking by 'inspecting exterior to predict interior'.

For treating deficiency-cold syndrome in TCM way, we should use warming interior formula in general. Wasn't this treatment like adding fuel to the fire by prescribing warming interior formula to treat the patient's inflammation? However, after taking the decoction, there was an immediate effect. We did not mean to diminish inflammation but the inflammation was cured. Instead of making the fire stronger, 'adding fuel to the fire' did put out the fire. From the perspective of modern medicine, it is inconceivable.

Someone may ask: "You said that this disease had been cured. But you have no evidence. How would you convince others?"

My answer is this: "The patient's feeling can give enough evidence. He has not felt stomachache or stomach bloating for 7 years. If there are such symptoms as erosion, hyperemia, or edema on his gastric mucosa, can he feel so comfortable? There is no disease in his stomach now, how can we make him get the gastroscopy examination again? Is the examination pleasant to take?"

Someone may also ask, "You are just a TCM doctor. You not only don't understand modern science, but also don't know the chemical components of Chinese medicinals, how can you cure modern diseases? The hot nature of *Paofuzi* (*Radix Aconiti Lateralis Preparata*) and *Ganjiang* (*Rhizoma Zingiberis*) is just recorded in some ancient books, which cannot be proved by modern science. Isn't it metaphysics?"

My answer is as follows: "Modern studies of Chinese medicinals focus on the chemical components. However, it is totally unrelated to the treatment of Chinese medicinals. Thus I don't know about it. Even if I know it, what is the use of knowing it? What the research studies is just about the botanical drugs. People who have not studied the theories of TCM can just classify *Ganjiang* as the botanical drug, not the Chinese medicinal! The use of *Ganjiang* in TCM really doesn't focus on the components. We just focus on the hot nature of *Ganjiang*. Without its hot nature, cold could be dispelled. The hot nature of *Paofuzi* and *Ganjiang* cannot be measured by a thermometer. Only after eating these medicinals can people feel the hot nature of them. Like *Shigao* (*Gypsum Fibrosum*) and *Huanglian* (*Rhizoma Coptidis*), their cold nature also cannot be measured by any thermometer. Only after eating them can people feel the cold nature of them. All these are the feelings of the living people. Four natures of Chinese medicinal (cold, hot, warm, cool), five flavors of Chinese medicinal (pungent, sweet, sour, bitter, salty, and light, in fact there are six flavors), as well as lifting, lowering, floating and sinking of Chinese medicinal are all the feelings of living people, which are the key of TCM to ward off diseases.

No matter how advanced the modern scientific instruments are, they are not the living people, they don't have the function of feeling. Although the instruments can detect the tangible components of some medicinals, they are unable to know the intangible flavors and natures. Therefore TCM and Western Medicine cannot be interconnected with each other."

Someone may ask again, "Modern society is an era of rapid development of science and technology; once the new technology appears, the old technology will be eliminated. Only when there is constant innovation, human lives can be continuously improved. You said that the ancient prescriptions would cure modern diseases, is it contrary to the law of scientific and technological development?"

Here is my answer: "You have got the point. Just like what we often say, 'in the Yangtze River the waves behind drive on those ahead, so each new generation excels the last one.' But TCM is an exception."

TCM is an intangible science, and the intangible science belongs to *Tao-like medical knowledge*. It is the theory of curing disease with the aim of keeping the balance between yin and yang, which is consistent with the 'moderation' thought insisted by Confucianis. Both *Tao-like medical knowledge* and Confucianism are in harmony. Whether an authentic TCM doctor or a modern TCM doctor; whether a young TCM doctor who is at the beginning of learning medicine or an experienced TCM doctor with decades of experience; whether a TCM master or an unknown and ordinary TCM doctor, examining a patient should go through the methods of four examinations (inspection, listening and smelling, inquiry and pulse-taking), and then the patient would be diagnosed and classified into an exact disease syndrome, such as deficiency-yang, deficiency-yin, deficiency-qi, deficiency-blood, cold or heat. These medical terms of the syndromes are the same; the formulas used to treat them are known to all in the TCM circle.

As long as you differentiate the syndrome and then compose the formula correctly, the ancient formula can also cure modern disease. But if you do something wrong, even the modern formula cannot cure modern disease. Taking the formula of treating this superficial gastritis patient as an example, *Renshen* (*Radix Ginseng*) and *Huangqi* (*Radix Astragali*) were used to tonify qi, *Fuzi* (*Radix Aconiti Lateralis Preparata*) and *Ganjiang* (*Rhizoma Zingiberis*) were used to restore yang, *Dahuang* (*Radix et Rhizoma Rhei*) and *Mangxiao* (*Natrii Sulfas*) were purgative, *Huangqin* (*Radix Scutellariae*) and *Huanglian* (*Rhizoma Coptidis*) were used to clear heat, all the Chinese medicinals listed above focused on adjusting the imbalance between yin and yang of human body. When the symptoms were relieved by taking the decoctions, then the patient should stop taking them. As *Internal Classic* records, 'prescribing drastic and toxic medicinals strictly according to the pathogen will do no harm to the pregnant woman and the fetus.' Thus, there would be neither the trouble of harming the body nor the anxiety of medicine resistance.

TCM and Western Medicine coexist in today's world. In order to make us have a clear understanding of TCM, and to get rid of the misunderstanding caused by the different kinds of theories of TCM, we should call TCM as *Tao-like medical knowledge*; comparatively speaking, we should call Western Medicine as *medical skills*.

Certainly, in both ancient and modern times, TCM doctors have always been praised as the master who possesses the brilliant *medical skills* by the patients for the amazing curative effects. People don't care about the differences between *medical knowledge* and *medical skills*. It is just a mixed call.

Actually, there are big differences between *medical knowledge* and *medical skills*, especially in modern society. Only when we call TCM as *Tao-like medical knowledge* can we have an essential understanding of the scientific attributes of TCM.

What is the meaning of Tao? It is the law of nature, and the origin of the whole universe.

Tao is intangible. Just as Lǎozǐ (老子), the founder of Taoism said: "The greatest form has no shape." Does the law of nature has shape? You can only mange to understand it through your thoughts. Therefore Lǎozǐ (老子) said: "The Tao that can be trodden is not the enduring and unchanging Tao. The name that can be named is not the enduring and unchanging name." He cannot make it clear or name it by using the specific shape.

Of course, as for these words of Lǎozǐ (老子), there are different explanations. Although there are disagreements, our understanding is consistent with the point that the Tao is intangible. All the theories of TCM are intangible too.

But the biggest problem of 'intangible' is that the things cannot be expressed clearly and specifically. TCM studies human body. Unclear expressions will not transmit the research information of human body. Thus many naming patterns of terms of TCM are using the method of analogy, such as yin and yang, wood, fire, earth, metal and water of five elements, the monarch organ (heart) and the general organ (liver) of five zang-organs. Even in the book of *Treatise on Cold Damage Diseases* (*Shāng hán lùn*, 伤寒论), the author used the same method of naming terms, such as the names of six meridians: greater yang meridian (taiyang), yang brightness meridian (yangming), lesser yang meridian (shaoyang), greater yin meridian (taiyin), lesser yin meridian (shaoyin), reverting yin meridian (jueyin), and the names of therapeutic methods: taking away firewood from under the cauldron, returning fire to its origin, etc.

Why do we use the method of analogy? The reason is that the intangible thing is the most difficult thing to express clearly. The only way we can make people understand various kinds of theories of TCM is to take the method of analogy. Western Medicine doesn't take this method to name medical terms, for Western Medicine studies the tangible part of human body, which can be seen clearly with the help of instruments and tests. Therefore the tangible part can be named directly. There is no need to understand it.

TCM and Western Medicine are two different medicine systems; the differences between intangible parts and tangible parts are the watershed in these two systems. Only when we know this can we truly understand that although they all study the same object — human body, their respective theoretical systems are definitely different. The combination of them is just like inventing a perpetual motion machine, which sounds reasonable, but in fact it is impossible.

We call TCM as *Tao-like medical knowledge*, so the therapeutic features of *Tao-like medical knowledge* are like what Laozi said: "The law of the Tao is its being what it is."

This so-called *Tao-like medical knowledge* is to recover human body from unnatural state (sick and unhealthy state) to natural state (disease-free and healthy state), namely recover human body from the state of 'inharmony of yin-yang' to the state of 'yin-yang balance'. This is the endpoint of all principles of curing disease of TCM.

Of course, here is the same word 'disease', but the concept in TCM and Western Medicine is very different. The word 'disease' in Western Medicine must be the tangible pathogen (the intangible parts are generally called as syndrome). But the word 'disease' in TCM refers to the symptoms. In other words, TCM tackles disease by removing symptoms. The symptoms emerge under the unnatural state of human body. Only by removing the symptoms can we make human body recover to the natural state. However, there are many false appearances among the symptoms, which are not the direct reflection of the essence. As a result, a TCM doctor must identify the symptoms through a comprehensive analysis of four examinations, which is called as syndrome differentiation and treatment in TCM. The therapeutic goal of TCM is to treat the root of disease, rather than healing head because of headache or healing feet because of pain in feet. A doctor of TCM certainly will never prescribe by the western medical name of disease either.

Western Medicine only focuses on disease itself. The only problem that Western Medicine solves is disease. Western Medicine does not care that whether human body is in natural state or not. This is also the difference between *Tao-like medical knowledge* and *medical skills*. Western Medicine talks about anti-disease, anti-virus, anti-depression, and anti-cancer. The phrase 'anti' is the whole of western medical thinking. In the words of *Sun Tzu on the Art of War*, we can call that as, 'To win a battle, it's good to destroy an entire army.' What about TCM? On the contrary, it never uses the phrase 'anti', instead, it uses the word 'resolve', such as resolving toxin, resolving depression. It can also be considered as the whole of TCM thinking. In the words of *Sun Tzu on the Art of War*, we can call that as, 'To win a battle, it is better to recapture an entire army than to destroy it.'

Therefore Western Medicine is a medical science that fights diseases, and TCM is a medical science that restores balance in the body.

The target of anti is disease. Whether a patient undergoes surgery or takes medicines, he will always be harmed by these approaches. However, the target of balancing is to recover human body to the natural state. What it resolves is disease, and what it protects is human body.

Chinese people have the thoughts of Taoism and the culture of Confucianism. That's the reason why the 'balanced' medical science — TCM — originated from here, and why it cannot be found in any other countries.

The goal of TCM therapy is to deal with the primary cause of disease

— The discussion on scientific attribute of 'treating disease should focus on the root' by taking the example of curing pediatric hydrocephalus

In November 2007, a pharmacopolist named Chen in Wutai County providing Chinese medicinals for me, hurriedly came for me. He said that his two-year-old sick nephew still didn't feel better after hospitalizations in Provincial Children Hospital and Provincial People's Hospital. They had spent more than 10,000 yuan on treating him for less than half a month in Taiyuan.

I followed him to the pediatric ward in a big hospital of Shanxi province. The child was diagnosed with hydrocephalus based on the CT examination.

I took his pulse, and found that his pulse was deep, thready and weak on both hands. His face color was bluish yellow.

The parents introduced that the child had been suffering from nausea and vomiting for a period of time, so they had to come to the provincial capital to seek for treatment.

Through the examinations, I found that the child was suffering from the syndrome of deficiency-cold of spleen-stomach. Therefore, I prescribed him *Fuzi Lizhong Wan* (*Aconite Middle Regulating Pill*). He took less than two boxes, and then he recovered from the disease. What's more, there was no hydrocephalus any more. The course of the treatment cost less than 10 yuan in total.

In 2011, when Chen was in Taiyuan for delivering Chinese medicinals, he told me that the child was in good health for two years and did not fall ill again.

In 2008, I was invited by a boss to Shenzhen to see a patient. The driver who picked me up at the airport asked me for consultation.

I asked him what the matter was?

He said that because of getting a common cold, he had been receiving the treatment in hospital for a month, and had spent over ten thousand yuan; during the treatment, he even had undergone a bone marrow puncture for testing.

Until then, not only his cold hadn't been cured, but also he had waist and leg pain; when he slept at night, he couldn't turn around; once turning around, the pain was unbearable.

I found that his left pulse was floating and tight, and the right Chi pulse was deficient. I told him that the pathogenic wind-cold hadn't been cured; what's more, his kidneys were hurt after having intravenous drip; therefore, the treatment should not only focus on dispersing wind-cold, but on tonifying his kidneys as well. As a result, I prescribed him *Duhuo Jisheng Tang* (*Pubescent Angelica and Taxillus Decoction*).

After taking the prescription that night, he could causally turn around when he slept, and the pain in his waist and leg was greatly reduced.

Then he took two more doses of the prescription. He spent less than 50 yuan in curing his disease.

When someone gets a common cold, it is not a piece of news of spending thousands or even more than ten thousand yuan on treating the patient in a hospital nowadays. The problem is that spending too much money does not guarantee the complete recovery from the disease.

There is an owner of a supermarket near our house. His mother got a common cold. He sent his mother to a hospital, and told the doctor to use the best medicine he can to cure his mother regardless of money. The best medicine certainly is the imported medicine. Since the patient's relative had this requirement, the doctor would use medicine daringly.

Half a month passed, more than one hundred thousand yuan had been spent on treating the disease. Instead of his mother's illness being cured, it became worse and worse. Finally, she was on the verge of death, and was carried out of the hospital by a stretcher. It is really 'standing in, lying out'.

Such examples are too numerous to mention one by one. What's more, we can occasionally find some cases that the patient died after taking intravenous drip therapy for treating common cold. They not only pay high medical bills, but also lose their lives.

The data shows that each year in our country, there is an increase of medical costs of 80 billion yuan caused by the abuse of antibiotics. At the same time, 80,000 patients die because of adverse drug effects, which is really like the old saying goes, 'drug harm is much more terrible than the beast.' Moreover, the drug resistance of bacteria also makes the antibacterial on the verge of losing efficacy.

Some experts have warned, "Our country needs 10 years to develop a new antibiotic medicine at present. However, bacteria can develop antibiotic resistance in only two years. If we don't control this situation, it won't be long before there is no effective antibiotics to cure diseases."

In fact, the insightful and knowledgeable medical scientists in the world have already issued their warnings. They thought that human would return to the dark age of no antibiotics in the near future. Therefore, in 2007, bacteria resistance was listed as one of the serious public health problems that threaten human security in *World Health Report*.

Due to this, western developed countries are very prudent in the use of antibiotics. There is a popular sentence in the medical circle, 'It is easy to buy a gun in the United States, but it is hard to buy the antibiotics there.'

In our country, however, once you come into a hospital, no matter what illness you've suffered, the doctor will tell you to have the intravenous drip treatment first. Some doctors even treat antibiotics as panacea. The frequency and intensity of antibiotic utilization is 20 to 50 times higher than that of European and American countries. It brings great harm and serious consequences to people's health, and also makes the antibiotics lose efficacy quickly.

It is reported that many big pharmaceutical companies are less willing to pay for the research and development of new antibiotics now. The reason is that antibiotics will lose efficacy in a short term. But the cost of new antibiotics research and development is higher. Thus the pharmaceutical companies cannot make profits from the antibiotics investments, which is also another direct cause of high medical bills.

The vicious inflation of medical expenses is not the problem of a country, but the problem of the whole world.

Data shows that the growth rate of American health care costs is four times the growth rate of other commodity-prices. The increased part of personal income is basically used to pay for the increased part of medical care costs.

It is reported that the average allocation of health care portion of a car cost in the United States is even higher than the steel cost of making the car. The country is bearing the burden of public health insurance expenditure which surpasses its tolerance and is growing continuously.

The costs of health care are steadily increasing. In 2006, the health expenditure of the United States was 2.1 trillion dollars, and it was 2.7 trillion dollars in 2007. It increased 600 billion dollars in just one year. It is reported that in the United States, every 1 in 7 dollars earned will be used in medical treatment.

Recently an article called 'The Way to Develop Traditional Chinese Medicine in the United States' (*China News of Traditional Chinese Medicine,* 2012-11-09) which was written by Tián Xiǎomíng (田小明) in NCCAM (National Center for Complementary and Alternative Medicine) points out, '… more and more patients and their relatives strongly ask the government to attach great importance to the research of difficult and complicated diseases, such as cancer and AIDS. They hope the government can seek all possible new treatments, so as to save the lives of their own and their relatives. Secondly, conventional western medical treatments cannot guarantee the curative efficacies in terms of treating some difficult and complicated diseases, or chronic diseases. Due to the fact that the side effects of long-term use of some western medicines are serious, they hope new treatments can be found to complement western medicines. Thirdly, the health care expenditure of the United States is rising year after year. In 2011, it was as high as 17% of total value of national economic output, which had become the heavy burden of expenses.'

Even the United States, the most developed country, is disturbed by high medical bills. The situations of other countries would not be any better.

According to some relevant people, the hospital in our country has entered into a strange cycle for the pursuit of 'high technology, high cost, and high profit'; moreover, there is almost no supervision or check-and-balance system to restrain this strange cycle. Actually, at the back of the 'three highs', there are such problems as low efficiency, bacteria and virus resistance, drug-induced disease, and excessive medical treatment, which lead to a vicious and irreversible cycle.

Relevant statistical information published on *Health News* on May 10, 2009 suggests, 'Cancer patients in our country spend nearly one hundred billion yuan each year; the expenditure of treating stroke patients is nearly 20 billion yuan each year. One and a half years of income of a farmer is just enough for him to be in hospital for one time.'

There is also a report revealing that 7.5 million people died of chronic diseases in our country in 2005, while the death rates of such diseases as bronchitis, lung cancer, breast cancer, cerebrovascular disease, coronary heart disease, and diabetes are on the rise.

It is true that modern medicine is the mainstream medicine, and it has made great contributions to human health and to the prevention and treatment of disease.

But we can't neglect its disadvantages and treat it as the only science, even as the only choice to treat disease. We cannot regard it as the standard of judging whether TCM is scientific or not too. If we do it that way, the damage to individuals, families, nationalities, and countries even to the entire human race around the world is massive and immeasurable. International authority has issued a clear warning in this respect.

Chén Kǎixiān (陈凯先), the academician of Chinese Academy of Sciences and the president of Shanghai University of TCM, introduced, "In November 1996, a WHO international research team, called the Goals of Medicine (GOM), stated briefly and clearly in a report that according to the survey: 'At present, the development of medicine is the formation of unjust medicine which can't be afforded by the whole world', 'Now many countries have reached the edge of affordability'". He called this a global 'medical crisis'. The solution of this 'medical crisis' in fact is not easier than that of 'financial crisis'. This 'medical crisis' becomes more and more serious.

Except for this simple and cheap but effective TCM, are there any other choices to solve this global 'medical crisis'?

Why is it that modern medicine is expensive, but TCM is cheap?

There are various reasons. But here is what I would like to express: Quite a number of diseases detected by modern scientific instruments are only the results of diseases, not the causes; the results are tangible, the causes are intangible; tangible things can be created from intangible things.

Such treatment that only focuses on the result rather than on the cause of a disease cannot solve the problem of the disease fundamentally. The patient under such treatment would suffer a lifelong medication which may lead to drug-induced disease. In addition, the problem of bacteria resistance is increasingly prominent, so the medical costs have to be steadily on the rise and at a high level.

Taking the above pediatric hydrocephalus treatment as an example. There was nothing wrong with the confirmed diagnosis through CT examination, which we couldn't see with our naked eyes. As a result, scientific and technological progress is necessary.

In the view of modern medicine, in treating hydrocephalus, surgery is needed to drain away the fluid in the head, which would cost a lot. Sequelae would occur after the surgery, and the relevant treatment for the sequelae should also be done. What's more, if the hydrops appear again, surgery would be conducted one more time.

But as a TCM doctor, I could not see hydrops. I diagnosed that the child has the syndrome of deficiency-cold of spleen-kidney through the analysis of pulse and symptoms, which was the true cause of the formation of his hydrops. The deficiency-cold is intangible, which cannot be observed by the instrument. I used *Fuzi Lizhong Wan* (*Aconite Middle Regulating Pill*) to warm his spleen-kidney and dispel deficiency-cold, then the yin-water (hydrops) would be resolved. I did not focus on dispelling hydrops, but hydrops disappeared naturally. Not only the cost was little, but also I had solved the hydrocephalus problem fundamentally.

Take another example of a tumor in human body. The tumor is the result. The formation of the tumor is the cause.

To cure the tumor, instead of concentrating on the cause, the doctor may remove the tumor. When the tumor has been surgically removed, new tumor would grow later and even faster. Why? Because of the stimulation of the surgery.

Why do fruit farmers prune fruit trees' branches in spring? It is because by stimulating fruit trees' branches, this will make fruit trees produce more fruits. There are few fruits, even no fruits on the fruit tree without pruning. This is the same theory of the formation of the tumor.

I once saw a boy who was less than 10 years old. To remove his brain tumor, he had to take brain surgery. Unfortunately, each time after the surgery, the tumor would reappear after a short time. Finally, the boy took six brain surgeries which caused severe damage to his brain. His parents were heartbroken.

How many tragedies have happened like this? Western Medicine focuses on cutting tumor, but it can't eliminate the cause of the formation of the tumor. The surgery is successful, but it only solves the surface problem, not the essence.

Although the science is flourishing, people who suffer tumors are not less than before, and the medical costs are much higher than before. Isn't it worth us reflecting?

An article in *Health News* on February 16, 2007 points out, 'there are about 3,700 kinds of diseases known today, but there are very few of these diseases that people have completely cured.'

Common cold may be the mildest disease, but in modern medicine, it could be one of the top ten mystery diseases. The science has been so advanced, but it couldn't find the cause of the mildest disease.

Actually, this problem is very simple in the view of TCM. Taking autumn-winter cold as an example, most people who suffer from it are affected by pathogenic wind-cold. Pathogenic wind-cold would be dispelled and then common cold would be cured through the treatment of TCM by using pungent-warm medicinals which are good at releasing exterior.

It is not saying that Western Medicine doctors do not know this theory. You can recognize that in such cold seasons as autumn and winter, doctors of Western Medicine also remind people to keep warm, so as to avoid catching a cold. But once people catch cold because of wind-cold, antibiotics are used to kill bacteria through the method of intravenous drip. It is not because Western Medicine doctors forget pathogenic wind-cold, but there is no concept of pathogenic wind-cold in their modern medicine system. Pathogenic wind-cold is intangible. Now, hospitals in western countries do not use antibiotics to treat cold patients, they just ask patients to have a good rest and drink plenty of water. Does it cure the cold? No, absolutely not. But it is better than using antibiotics, because the harm of antibiotics is very dangerous!

When the human body suffers pathogenic wind-cold, skin pores are blocked, causing skin to lose the function of metabolism (called as Kaihe (opening and closing) in TCM), and then harmful bacteria and virus would thrive. Pathogenic wind-cold is the cause; harmful bacteria and virus are the result. TCM insists on letting the disease out from where the disease comes. Since pathogenic wind-cold comes into the body from skin, we shall use pungent-warm medicinals to dispel wind-cold from skin. When there is no distraction of wind-cold in skin, then skin will recover to the normal function of metabolism (Kaihe (opening and closing)). Once those bacteria and viruses lose their living environment, they would disappear naturally. The course of this treatment can be called as, 'To win a battle, it is better to recapture an army entirely than to destroy it.'

Western Medicine doctors do not even understand this simple theory of TCM. A great deal of money would be saved from the treatment of common cold and people would suffer much less pain and fewer diseases if Western Medicine doctors understand this kind of theory!

Let's take the driver I cured in Shenzhen as another example. Although he had been suffering from cold for a month, wind-cold was still in his body (left Guan pulse was floating and tight, pain in the body). What's more his kidneys were harmed by the excessive treatment (his waist was too painful to turn around). Thus I prescribed *Duhuo Jisheng Tang* (*Pubescent Angelica and Taxillus Decoction*) to him, which not only tonified his liver and kidneys, but also dispelled wind-cold (cause). As a result, this decoction had an immediate effect. If he still undergoes the former treatment, the consequence would be hard to imagine.

Have you noticed that in the more developed regions of modern medicine, more patients need to take renal dialysis? In terms of the utilization of medicines, Taiwan is 7 times that of the United States. As a result, renal dialysis in Taiwan is also the highest one. Even the best technology is unable to cure disease and save people in its true sense, and it will harm future generations if we only focus on the result of disease, not the cause.

There is a sentence from Sir Isaac Newton, the most famous scientist in modern times, 'Whereas the main Business of natural Philosophy is to argue from Phenomena without feigning Hypotheses, and to deduce Causes from Effects, till we come to the very first Cause (*Opticks*).'

What I want to say is that the causes of disease, such as the external causes: 'wind, cold, summer-heat, dampness, dryness and fire', the internal causes: 'over-joy, rage, anxiety, pensiveness, sorrow, fear, and fright', are the understanding of disease in the view of TCM; they are intangible; they cannot be detected by any modern scientific instruments; they are the primary causes of disease.

No matter how modern medicine develops and how disease spectrum changes, Traditional Chinese Medicine, which depends on the theoretical system of dealing with the primary cause of disease, can cure diseases that cannot be cured by modern medicine. "TCM treats the root of disease, while Western Medicine treats the manifestation of disease", as said by common people. Sir Issac Newton wrote in *Mathematical Principles of Natural Philosophy*, 'We are to admit no more causes of natural things than such as are both true and sufficient to explain their appearances. To this purpose the philosophers say that Nature does nothing in vain, and more is in vain when less will serve; for Nature is pleased with simplicity, and affects not the pomp of superfluous causes.' According to Newton's conception of nature which consists of the principles of simplicity and causality, science is to explore the simple and harmonious natural law hidden behind complicated natural phenomena.

In terms of human body science, what TCM explores is the 'simple and harmonious natural law' of human body, which is the primary cause of disease. The primary cause is also the essential one of the formation of disease. TCM calls it as 'treating disease should focus on the root'. Ancestors of TCM two thousand years ago are pretty consistent with the modern greatest scientist in terms of exploring scientific ideas of natural mystery. *Huangdi's Internal Classic* (*Nèi jīng*, 内经) tells us what the primary cause of disease is and how to differentiate this primary cause! *Treatise on Cold Damage Diseases* (*Shāng hán lùn*, 伤寒论) tells us how to distinguish the primary cause of disease and how to solve it! Truth is always straightforward and simple! The more complicated it is expressed, the more far away it is from the truth.

Since the primary cause of disease is intangible, tangible things (result) can be created from intangible things! TCM is an intangible science and is the science of solving the primary cause. Human being can never get out of the medical crisis if they cannot solve the primary cause of disease. Going back to the traditional way is the only way to go for so-called 'Modern Chinese Medicine'! Over the last one hundred years, the bad habits of westernization of TCM have become immensely popular. Fashionable scientific terms in the TCM circle appear everywhere making people dazzling. This phenomenon was glamorized as the modernization and scientification of TCM. In fact it has walked far away from the primary cause of disease. It can be summarized by a sentence of Newton, 'For Nature is pleased with simplicity, and affects not the pomp of superfluous causes.'

Kidneys are not the therapeutic region for treating nephrolithiasis

— Discussing that the goal of TCM treatment is to deal with the primary cause of disease by taking the example of curing a patient with a history of nephrolithiasis for 30 years

I was once invited to conduct an academic exchange with some Australian TCM groups on September 6, 2005. My first stop was Melbourne. I was invited to hold a lecture at Royal Institute of Technology of Melbourne University on September 10 at 10:00 a.m. But a group of Australians crowded into the room where I lived around 8:00 a.m. that day. The group leader was an over 70-year-old elder with yellow and grey hair. When I was at a loss, a person behind him suddenly appeared. Then we greeted each other with a smile and a hearty handshake. Who was that person? Jason McGavin, the business assistant of Australian Embassy in China before 2004. Our acquaintance can date back to an experience of treating disease.

After leaving the Embassy, he worked in a foreign company in Beijing and became a colleague with my son-in-law. After several contacts, they were familiar with each other. He knew that I am a doctor of TCM for a long time. One day he asked my son-in-law whether I could treat his daughter's illness. My son-in-law immediately agreed. At the beginning of April, 2005, Jason took his seven-year-old daughter — Elisa, to my home. Jason has worked in China for many years. He is married to a Beijing lady — Ms Yang, and had two daughters. Therefore, he could speak Chinese fluently and we didn't have any language barrier.

He said that his daughter had been diagnosed with eczema for almost three months. Her skin was full of red rashes which tickled her so badly, so she scratched her skin all day and left many blood scabs. Ms Yang is a medical doctor (M.D.). She used various kinds of external ointments to treat her daughter, but none of them worked at all. Therefore he came for me. Elisa was a lovely girl of mixed blood. She had slightly curled golden hair and a pair of big eyes. I told her to stick out her tongue and checked it, which was a slightly reddish tongue with a thin and whitish yellow coating. Then I took her pulse, which was soggy, rapid, and floating on both hands. All the symptoms indicated that she suffered the syndrome of dampness-heat accumulating in blood aspect. Moreover, pathogenic wind blocked her exterior at the same time. Under the mutual contention of wind and dampness-heat, the rashes formed. Because of the stickiness and stagnation of dampness, the disease cannot be cured instantly.

I composed three doses of *Siwu Qingzhen Tang* (*Four Ingredients Clearing Rash Decoction*), invented by Zhāng Zǐlín (张子琳), one of the four famous doctors in Shanxi before he died.

Here were the ingredients of the formula:

Danggui Wei (*the tail of Radix Angelicae Sinensis*) 10g
Chishao (*Radix Paeoniae Rubra*) 10g
Chuanxiong (*Rhizoma Chuanxiong*) 6g
Shengdihuang (*Radix Rehmanniae Recens*) 15g
Baixianpi (*Cortex Dictamni*) 10g
Kushen (*Radix Sophorae Flavescentis*) 6g
Difuzi (*Fructus Kochiae*) 10g
Shechuangzi (*Fructus Cnidii*) 6g
Baijili (*Fructus Tribuli*) 10g
Chantui (*Periostracum Cicadae*) 6g
Jingjie (*Herba Schizonepetae*) 6g
Fangfeng (*Radix Saposhnikoviae*) 6g

All these Chinese medicinals should be decocted with water for oral administration.

The first four medicinals of this prescription are the ingredients of *Siwu Tang* (*Four Ingredients Decoction*). The reason of using these four medicinals was following the principle of ancient treatment, 'Treating wind syndrome should focus on blood first. Wind would be relived if blood is invigorated'. Other medicinals with the functions of clearing heat, drying dampness and alleviating itching were all used to remove the toxin in blood aspect. Adding *Jingjie* and *Fangfeng* was to dispel wind in her skin, which could also eliminate dampness. Three days later, Jason telephoned me saying that the formula I prescribed to her daughter was very effective. He told me that after taking two doses, those little red rashes on Elisa's body had all disappeared. His wife said to him happily: "This is a good choice, and we should seek TCM doctors if we are ill in the future!"

He has complimented TCM all around for curing this minor disease. One day, my son-in-law talked about this after work: "Dad, you have made Jason a fan of TCM!"

These words above are a digression. This time, Jason took his whole family to Melbourne. He got up very early and came here from his home-town 50 kilometers away. He hoped that I could treat his father.

This over 70-year-old elder was exactly the father of Jason McGavin. He was very strongly built. He had yellow and grey hair, and a red with little wheaty face. His appearance indicated that he was a laboring person. The fact was that he was the owner of a large farm. He gazed upon me. His eyes were filled with confusion and strangeness. Jason McGavin talked with his father in English for a while and then talked with me in mandarin. I understood the situation quite clearly with the help of this good interpreter who used to be a diplomat.

I knew that his father had suffered from kidney stones for 30 years. His waist was tortured by this disease. It was very painful. The western medical treatment of lithiasis is to cut out the lithiasis related visceral organ in the past. Such as the treatment of nephrolithiasis is to cut out kidney, the treatment of cholelithiasis is to cut out gallbladder. Now since the science and technology has developed, lithiasis can be treated by laser lithotripsy. After the big stone is broken into several small stones by the laser, the small ones will pass out of the body. How advanced this technology is! It indeed reflects that the progress of technology brings good news to human being. However, this is not the end of treatment. Human body is like performing conjuring tricks with the patient. When the old stones are broken and pass out of the body, new stones would appear after a period, which means the lithiasis patient would take laser therapy again. The old man continuously talked. He frowned, shook his head, stretched out his hands, and sighed at times. He said that he had to undergo laser lithotripsy every year, which made him too painful to stand; he suffered a lot, but had no other way.

He did not have to tell me. I actually knew the suffering of this disease. Why? I had this disease once as well. It was in the 1990s that I felt great pain in the waist and went to Taiyuan People's Hospital to do type-B ultrasonic for examination. After the examination, there was a stone found in one of my kidneys. There was a department of laser lithotripsy in the hospital, so I went there at once to take laser lithotripsy, which made me hurt to sweat all over my head. After overcoming the great pain, the stone was finally broken. I felt happy that there was such a technology in modern medicine. Otherwise, how could this stone be dealt with? However, a year later, I felt pain in the same old place, and I knew that it must be the stone secretly reappearing again. Because I was afraid of the violent pain of laser lithotripsy, I prescribed myself medicinals for clearing heat and resolving dampness in liver-gallbladder based on my pulse and symptoms. After taking the medicinals, my waist wasn't painful any more. Later, I powdered those medicinals and made them into capsules for the fear of relapse.

Since I do not want to suffer from this kind of pain anymore, I always take these capsules along with me when I go out for business. I am 70 years old now, and this kind of pain has never appeared again for 20 years, which means the nephrolithiasis has been completely cured. Through this treatment, I've known that the cause of lithiasis is the accumulation of dampness-heat in liver-gallbladder. No matter where it grows, liver, gallbladder, kidney or urethra, all lithiases are caused by this factor.

Through advanced modern instruments, modern medicine can only see the pain caused by tangible stones, but cannot see dampness-heat in TCM. Because it is intangible and can only be realized by the analysis of pulse and symptoms. Therefore, I insist that TCM is an intangible science and it aims at dealing with the primary cause of disease. This theory was realized after countless clinical treatments, not deduced from theories at home.

Now I can still clearly remember that, in the last century, I had an university classmate named Wang. Because of nephrolithiasis, one of his kidneys was removed, and the function of the other side was not good as well. Besides, there was a steel support on his waist, and into his lower abdomen was a catheter inserted, so he had to be careful in the class and could not attend any activities after class. In winter and summer vacations, everyone could go home except him. His home was in southern Shanxi, and he could not go back home to see his parents after such an operation. During vacations, he could only stay in the school alone, and before finishing his sophomore year, he died. Although many years have passed, every time when I think of him, his face and voice would emerge on my mind clearly, which makes me feel so sad. There could be no more sadness than this in a person's life!

Compared with the modern medical technology of laser lithotripsy, I am much happier that I have studied TCM this life. When the patient takes laser lithotripsy, he has to stand violent pain, but after that, new stone will appear again. Though modern medicine is advanced, the cause of lithiasis can't be found. After breaking the stone, I then took medicinals for clearing heat and resolving dampness in liver-gallbladder, which kept me away from the pain of taking laser lithotripsy again. Otherwise I really could have suffered a lot.

Jason's father told me that he had to undergo laser lithotripsy every year, and I could also understand his painful expression, which was like 'people who have the similar illness sympathize with each other'. I took his pulse and found that, among six positions, only his left Guan pulse was surging, slippery, and rapid. He had a red tongue with a thick and yellow coating. He told me that he always had bitterness taste in his mouth. The symptoms above showed that he suffered excess fire in liver-gallbladder coupled with dampness-heat accumulation. As a result, I prescribed 10 doses of the following formula for him:

Chaihu (*Radix Bupleuri*) 15g
Huangqin (*Radix Scutellariae*) 15g
Longdancao (*Radix Gentianae*) 10g

Baizhu (*Rhizoma Atractylodis Macrocephalae*) 15g
Haijinsha (*Spora Lygodii*) 20g
Jinyinhua (*Flos Lonicerae*) 30g
Jinqiancao (*Herba Lysimachiae*) 30g
Qingbanxia (*Rhizoma Pinelliae*) 10g
Honghua (*Flos Carthami*) 10g
Mutong (*Caulis Akebiae*) 5g
Gancao (*Radix Glycyrrhizae*) 5g

All these medicinals should be decocted with water for oral administration; cook the medicinals in three bowls of water until only one cup remains; each dose of the medicinals should be cooked twice and taken twice per day (once in the morning, once in the evening).

In addition, I told him that he could not think that taking ten doses of the formula was enough for the treatment, and he needed to take these medicinals for a long period. However, it was unnecessary to take them as the form of decoction. After I went back, I would powder these medicinals and make them into capsules for him, which would be convenient to take. All of these orders were interpreted by Jason sentence by sentence. I could tell confusion from the old man's eyes.

He was a foreigner and could not understand the theories of TCM treatment. How could he understand that a TCM doctor did not treat kidneys but treat liver and gallbladder? There were no stones in liver and gallbladder! Could Chinese herbal decoction break stones in the kidneys? Didn't it sound far-fetched? It was fortunate that Jason continuously interpreted and explained for him, and said the eczema his granddaughter suffered for a long period was cured by taking my prescription. Although he was still confused, he expressed that he would obey my orders and take the medicinals seriously. Because he could not stand the pain of laser lithotripsy every year!

However, there is an advantage of curing disease by TCM in Australia: you can find Chinese medicinals everywhere, and Australia is not like other countries where only acupuncture is available but, not Chinese medicinals. What is the reason? After getting there, I've found out that Australia is the first western country in the world that recognizes Chinese medicinals as formal medicines, and a country that formulates laws to manage TCM and Chinese medicinals; some states there also have government agencies whose functions are basically similar to that of Chinese Medicine and Herbs Administration; the difference of this agency to Chinese Medicine and Herbs Administration is that it plays the same social role as the agency of Western Medicine, which means that TCM isn't led by Western Medicine; there are legislations for protecting TCM; diagnostic and therapeutic costs in TCM clinics are also included into health insurance; however, what should be paid attention to is that TCM is what it is and Western Medicine is also what it is; doctors of Western Medicine cannot prescribe Chinese medicinals, and those of TCM cannot prescribe western medicines or order medical tests.

A TCM doctor who wants to practice medicine in Australia can only use authentic TCM diagnostic and therapeutic methods. Who dare not to be authentic? If you westernize TCM, then you disobey the local laws! Most of TCM doctors in Australia that I contact with graduated from domestic universities of TCM. They were talents of integrating TCM with Western Medicine in China, and have become authentic TCM doctors after getting to Australia. After turning into authentic TCM doctors, their treatment efficacies have improved. In Australia, they have got rid of the thinking pattern of Western Medicine, and have started to use the theory of syndrome differentiation and treatment in clinical practices. As a result, many doctors of Western Medicine introduce patients to them! Their incomes even exceed those of the Western Medicine doctors; most of them have their own houses and cars, which makes them so excited that none of them is willing to change this authentic TCM job!

Later, the TCM circle in Australia organized a delegation to visit me in Taiyuan. I once asked them: "There are so many universities of TCM that you can visit. Why do you come to this remote place, Shanxi Province, to visit me?" They said: "We are unwilling to visit them because what they talk about are the big theories combining TCM with Western Medicine. What we want is to find a real doctor of authentic TCM and learn real TCM skills of curing disease!" Considering what they said, it sounded really reasonable!

In Australia, TCM doctors are self-employed, which means they do not have 'steel bowls', namely a regular salary and a job until retirement.

Empty talking about the theories of TCM rather than focusing on clinical efficacy is useless! Having the skills of curing disease is the only way to have food to eat, have houses to live, have cars to drive, and have money to spend! Months later, I contacted with related colleges of TCM in Australia once. I found that they also used the textbooks utilized by Chinese universities of TCM, which means over half of the courses are of Western Medicine. When I asked the graduates of their clinical skills, their answers revealed that they could not cure diseases. After all, they were educated by the same pattern of TCM in China, so the results were the same comparing with the students in domestic TCM universities! How can foreigners understand TCM principles of curing disease? What they only know is that there is TCM in China, and the doctors of TCM are cultivated like this, so they follow the same way! How can they understand what TCM really is?

Some people might say, "Why do they formulate regulations of TCM and include expenses of curing disease in individual clinics of TCM into health insurance? After doing these things, they must understand TCM principles of curing disease clearly!" My answer is: "It is definitely not. Those principles are even not understood by many Chinese people, so how can foreigners understand them? If they can understand those principles, departments of TCM in their universities will not follow the example of ours to set courses of Western Medicine!" Some people may also ask, "Since they don't understand the principles of TCM, why do they give green lights to TCM, why can they develop it in such a radical way?" My answer is: "Although they don't understand the principles, they find that TCM not only can cure disease but the disease will never appear again after that. What's more, it costs less money."

This is not a trivial thing at all, because it is related to national economy and people's livelihood! For example, for a common cold with wind-cold syndrome, a doctor of TCM will prescribe pungent-warm medicinals for releasing exterior, which only cost several yuan or over ten yuan. After pathogenic wind-cold being dispelled, the patient would feel refreshed and better. However, if a patient who suffers from this disease seeks treatment in a modern hospital, he may have an injection and intravenous drips contrary antibiotics and receive antiviral treatment. How much will all of these cost? The cost is not a matter if the disease can be cured in this way. But the main problem is that the more harmful bacteria and viruses are killed, the more resistant they become and the bacteria that are beneficial to the body would also be killed. Although they are killed again and again, pathogenic wind-cold still exists. Once wind-cold transfers into the lung, then common cold would turn into chronic cough. The patient will not only cough but has a fever as well, and then he will be treated time after time!

Australia has health insurance for all citizens. If people have Australian nationality, the expenses of curing disease, hospitalization, surgeries and medicines are all paid for by the government. For example, the lithiasis of Jason's father should be treated every year; it is true that he has to stand the pain each year, and the government needs to pay for those expenses, which will recur year after year! Science becomes more and more advanced, but when it comes to curing diseases, the more diseases that science treats, the more diseases will appear, and the higher expenses of curing diseases become. No matter how much thinking those think tanks carry out, this situation can never be prevented! No matter how much money they spend, they still cannot fill the big hole of high medical expenses!

Foreigners especially know that western medicines are biochemical preparations which may have serious side effects because Western Medicine is invented by them! Although TCM is ancient, the medicinals it uses are mostly herbal medicines, which are natural plants grown in soil and don't consist of synthetic chemicals, so TCM has less side effects. If the patients take the right prescription, the disease will be cured thoroughly. Therefore, people go to clinics of TCM. Given all that, how can it not become popular in foreign countries? After formulating related laws, doctors of TCM in Australia can only prescribe Chinese medicinals, or do acupuncture and massage at clinics; nobody is allowed to prescribe western medicines or order any kind of blood tests; otherwise, you disobey the law! In Australia, doctors of TCM must be ancient and authentic, thus the way of westernization is blocked!

In this way, graduates from those universities of TCM, who have learned so much western medical knowledge, cannot integrate TCM with Western Medicine. But, as the old saying goes, 'lost at sunrise and gain at sunset.' Since they forget western medical knowledge and concentrate on studying how TCM cures disease, their thoughts of TCM become authentic and their curative efficacies have improved a lot. In many clinics of TCM, patients have to make appointments one month in advance to see doctors. To our excitement, doctors find that the way of authentic TCM is not a narrow one but a right one to cure disease and save people! The more they learn, the more eager they are to learn. I was only invited to hold a lecture to talk about some experience of disease treatment in the way of authentic TCM, and after the lecture they even happily discussed, "This time, a real doctor of TCM did come!"

In fact, principles of learning knowledge are not complicated, and there is only one sentence, 'the most important thing of learning is concentration.' Because 'if you can't concentrate, you would gain nothing (*Cai E's Collects* (*Cài è jí*, 蔡锷集))', 'People who don't study widely can gain knowledge; people who don't study variously can understand what he is studying (*Zhōng shuō* (中说) by Wáng Tōng (王通) in Sui Dynasty).' In the short time of a human life, if somebody wants to concentrate on doing something, he should not be involved in too many fields. Therefore, 'learning is not important, what important is to abandon other things while learning. Thus abandoning other things is for better learning (*Comment on Poems* (*Shi Jian,* 诗笺) by Hè Yísūn (贺贻孙) in Qing Dynasty)', 'Only when people are willing to abandon something will he achieve something (*Lí lóu xià* (离娄下) by Mèng Zǐ (孟子))'. From ancient time to now, from China to abroad, every successful scholar does obey this basic principle. 'Concentrating on one thing will be perfect, and distraction may lose all (*Comment on Learning* (*Lùn xué wèn,* 论学问) by Cáo Shì Lín (曹世霖) in Qing Dynasty).'

Even uneducated villagers know that 'people who pursue two rabbits at the same time can't get any one of them', let alone the broad and profound TCM which is an intangible science and is easily disturbed by other tangible sciences. Math, physics and chemistry learned in middle and high school have laid the knowledge base for students studying Western Medicine, but what the students have learned are lack of traditional cultural soil. This indicates that westernization is easy but taking Chinese culture as the core is difficult! It is believed that learning both Western Medicine and TCM can adjust to the needs of modern society. Is it scientific? It just treats science as a game! It is to make you endlessly roll around in the strange circle of this scientific lie of learning both Chinese and western knowledge! Only learning TCM seriously and deeply, and setting thought completely different from Western Medicine can solve the disease problems which cannot be solved by Western Medicine, and can adjust to the needs of modern society. Then, why are there so many graduates from universities of TCM changing jobs? If they can adjust to the needs of modern society, will they still change jobs? Has any doctor of TCM changed a job in Australia? There is no one. How much they adjust to the needs of modern society and how comfortable they live now!

These doctors have got rid of the heavy load of thoughts of Western Medicine, and have walked lightly on the way to learn simple, cost-saving, and efficient TCM. The more they've learnt, the better curative efficacies they would have. Once the curative efficacy improves, the income would improve. What's more, they would gain more respects from others. If you ask them about changing jobs, they are unwilling to do so! Ancestors of China left such a treasure of curing disease, let it show its charm in foreign countries. How proud they would be if they could see that now? When we are loudly and continuously discussing about scientification and modernization of TCM, or about whether we should have authentic TCM in modern society, doctors of TCM in Australia have benefited a lot from authentic TCM, just like the poetry goes, 'Yet monkeys are still calling on both banks behind me; to my boat these are ten thousand mountains away.'

Certainly, in terms of the formulation of laws for TCM in Australia, it is the result of deliberate efforts by the people in the circle of TCM in Australia, which has benefited all TCM doctors there. But what I am thinking is that the benefits they have got are little individual ones while Australian government and the local people are actually the best beneficiaries! How much expenses those newly-rising clinics of TCM have saved for their country! They don't understand scientific principles of curing disease in the way of TCM, and I think what they calculate is the great economic account. It is only the State of Victoria that formulates laws for TCM. But, why does Australia's strict immigration policy give green light to the immigrants of TCM doctors and adds marks for them? It is because that they want to attract doctors of TCM to cure diseases for them and save money for them!

This topic has strayed too far, and let's go back to the point of curing nephrolithiasis for Jason's father! Jason is really a dutiful son; he followed me back to China. Based on the formula I composed for his father, I slightly adjusted the dosages and powdered the medicines and made them into capsules which were enough for three months. Jason immediately sent the capsules back and asked his father to carry on taking them. In 2008, Jason ended his work in China and moved to Australia with his family. Before leaving, he specially called me and said that his father never felt pain in his kidneys again since he took the capsules. In 2011, he came to China for business, and he specially expressed thanks to me. He said that his father hadn't taken laser lithotripsy these years and talked about the mystery of TCM; it was marvelous that taking some Chinese medicinals could cure lithiasis. He certainly did not know that the goal of the treatment of TCM is to deal with the primary cause of disease!

TCM is a medical science of meeting changes with constancy

— The discussion on scientific attribute of TCM by taking the example of curing Kawasaki disease

On October 30, 2008, I was invited to treat a three-year-old child named Liu who was hospitalized at the pediatric department of a hospital in Shanxi province. Although the child had been taking intravenous therapy for 6 days, his high fever still couldn't be brought down. He was diagnosed with Kawasaki disease, a recently discovered rare disease. The doctors recommended the child to be transferred to Beijing for further medical treatment.

Although his mother had bought air tickets for the next day flight to Beijing, she asked me to have a try on the child before they left, because I once cured the infertility of her elder sister.

The examination showed that he had a constant cough, a high temperature of 40°C, a few rashes on the body, enlarged lymph nodes, lips that were not only red and swollen, but also dry and cracked; he had a red tongue with a yellowish coating; his pulse was slippery, surging, rapid and a little bit tight on both hands. I was told that the child discharged clear mucus from the nose shortly before he had fever. Thus, I diagnosed the child with the syndrome of wind-cold blocking exterior while heat and phlegm-fluid accumulating in interior. As a result, here was my prescription:

Mahuang (*Herba Ephedrae*) 5g
Guizhi (*Ramulus Cinnamomi*) 6g

Baishao (*Radix Paeoniae Alba*) 6g
Ganjiang (*Rhizoma Zingiberis*) 3g
Xixin (*Herba Asari*) 2g
Shengbanxia (*Rhizoma Pinelliae*) 10g
Wuweizi (*Fructus Schisandrae*) 6g
Xingren (*Semen Armeniacae Amarum*) 10g
Shengshigao (*Gypsum Fibrosum*) 60g
Huashifen (*Pulvistalci*) 10g
Sangbaipi (*Cortex Mori*) 10g
Chaihu (*Radix Bupleuri*) 10g
Gancao (*Radix Glycyrrhizae*) 5g

All the ingredients should be decocted with water, and two doses should be taken in a 4-hour interval.

I composed this formula based on *Xiao Qinglong Tang* (*Minor green-blue dragon decoction*), *Xiao Chaihu Tang* (*Minor Bupleurum Decoction*), and *Maxing Shigan Tang* (*Ephedra, Bitter Apricot, Seed, Gypsum and Licorice Decoction*).

The next day after I prescribed for the child, his parents called me. They told me that after taking my prescription, the child's temperature fell to 36°C. However, they still decided to go to Beijing, because they not only had bought air tickets, but also were afraid of the relapse.

On November 6, I was visited by the parents and their frisky child. They told me that the child did not have any fever in Beijing. After receiving the examination in a hospital, they were told that the child didn't need any kind of therapy, because he was physically sound.

Someone may ask me, "Since you are a '100-percent authentic' TCM doctor, have you ever studied the treatment of Kawasaki disease?"

Frankly speaking, as a doctor of '100-percent authentic' TCM, even if I devote my entire lifetime to study the extensive knowledge of TCM, I merely learn part of it, not to mention the study of Kawasaki disease which belongs to the category of Western Medicine. Before curing the child, I knew nothing about Kawasaki disease.

After checking related information, I've known that Kawasaki disease is named after Dr. Tomisaku Kawasaki, a Japanese doctor who firstly identified the disease, 'Kawasaki disease, an acute febrile disease, is characterized by systemic vasculitis, and has became the leading cause of acquired heart disease of children. Immune mechanism plays a major role in the pathogenesis of Kawasaki disease. The etiology(cause) remains unknown yet. These is also a lack of specificity for diagnosis.'

That is to say, Dr. Tomisaku Kawasaki merely discovered and described the disease. He did not know how to cure this disease, because the cause of disease is yet unknown.

Although I knew nothing about the disease then, I knew the core of TCM treatment was the theory of syndrome differentiation and treatment, and TCM was the medical science of resolving symptoms.

Since Kawasaki disease is mainly characterized by fever, whether the patient suffers from Kawasaki disease or not, as always, I will relieve fever according to the TCM theory. The formula I prescribed for the child was not aiming at resolving Kawasaki disease at all; what my prescription focused on was reducing fever, which is the thought of authentic TCM. If the fever disappears and the patient shows no symptoms of Kawasaki disease, then the disease has been cured.

When I was writing here, I suddenly recalled a story from a book called *Traditional Japanese Kampo Medicine* (*Rì běn hàn fāng yī xué*, 日本汉方医学)(translator's note: Kampo Medicine is the study and further development of Chinese Herbal Medicine in Japan) :

In 1947, MacArthur, the commander-in-chief of U.N. troops stationed in Japan, issued a notice to the Japanese authorities banning the application of massage, acupuncture and moxibustion. The notice aroused a great disturbance in the Kampo Medicine circle which was then known as 'MacArthur whirlwind'.

Then a rescue movement led by the intelligent people swept all over Japan.

Takeshi Itakura, M.D., who had the experience of studying Western Medicine in Europe paid a visit to Brigadier General, Summers, who was in charge of the Ministry of Public Health and welfare of U.N. forces in Japan. He stated the advantages of acupuncture and moxibustion therapy from the academic point of view to Summers. He pointed out that Western Medicine was the medical science of naming different diseases, while Kampo Medicine, whose core thought was syndrome differentiation and treatment, was the medical science of curing disease. These words greatly broadened the horizon of Summers, and he agreed and shared the same feeling with what Takeshi Itakura said. As a result, acupuncture and moxibustion finally had the legal status in Japan.

More than 60 years ago, Takeshi Itakura could hold this correct and penetrating view towards TCM. And Summers, who was not even a medical expert, could accept it and handle this movement in a reasonable manner. I do admire these two people and what they had done.

How could TCM last for thousands of years and be so popular all over the world, if it isn't the medical science of focusing on curing disease?

It is interesting that those who are against TCM also admit its curative efficacies.

Lǐ Kèshào (李克绍), the late professor of Shandong University of TCM, once wrote an article entitled, '*What I Saw and Heard in the Years of Learning and Practicing TCM* (see the first edition of *The Paths of Well-known Traditional Chinese Medicine Doctors*).' In this article, he recalled his experience of learning TCM. Li was a primary school teacher at first when he was young. After experiencing the loss of his uncle who died from the worsened disease condition after taking the wrong prescription for the treatment of a heat syndrome disease prescribed by a quack doctor, he quitted his job and decided to be a doctor.

Without any expert guidance, Li blindly bought the first book, *Diagnostics*, written by Yousai Shimodaira and translated into Chinese by a Zhejiang scholar, Tāng Ěrhé (汤尔和). This is a relatively advanced western medical book at that time. And Tang was opposed to TCM.

There were several sentences he wrote in the preface of the book, 'Of course, I know TCM can cure disease. Sometimes, its curative efficacy is better than that of Western Medicine. However, the only thing that I can see is the result (curative efficacy). No scholar of TCM is able to explain the reason why they treat diseases in this way. If you cannot explain the reason why the disease can be cured, you will convince nobody by using the example of curative efficacy when you argue with people.'

After reading the book, Li realized that even a TCM naysayer had admitted that the curative efficacies of TCM were better than that of Western Medicine. He recognized that they said no to TCM because TCM doctors could cure disease but could not explain, in the perspective of Western Medicine, the reason why TCM could cure disease.

It occurred to him that when a patient was dying, which one was more important, the result (curative efficacy) or 'the reason why'? Because a doctor should regard saving people as the most important thing, he decided to learn TCM without any hesitation.

We should not neglect this 'the reason why' theory, for this is the trump card of all TCM naysayers.

Yú Yúnxiù (余云岫) attributed the reasons of curative efficacies of TCM to the coincidence. According to him, if a scientific truth cannot explain 'the reason why', then this scientific truth should be regarded as pseudoscience, which means TCM doctors are unqualified; if a TCM doctor wants to continue his medical career, he has to renew his medical knowledge, such as modern physiology, anatomy, pathology, pharmacology, microbiology. This seemingly scientific proposition has been widespread and has lasted until present that many scholars nowadays are still following.

Several days ago, I heard from the media that a well-known TCM expert said, "Given the fact that the studies of Modern Medicine have involved genome, so the development of TCM should integrate with Modern Medicine." These incorrect viewpoints can be seen everywhere when I open the magazines of TCM.

Therefore, it's no surprise that many TCM doctors are learning Western Medicine desperately. Because after learning western medical knowledge, a TCM doctor could let the patient understand, in the western medical way, the reason why he suffers from this disease and why the doctor treat him in this way; however, an authentic TCM doctor could not make that happen, what he can do is to save the patient's life with no western medical explanation.

Isn't it the same theory of 'the reason why' as what Tāng ěrhé (汤尔和) proposed?

I don't think that, in this world, there will be any patient who has been critically ill that would choose to take a noneffective treatment of which he can clearly understand 'the reason why' rather than choose to take an effective treatment of which he does not understand 'the reason why'.

Tāng ěrhé (汤尔和) had chosen the former treatment for the patients, but he was not the patient. In order to support his viewpoint he even put the lives of patients at risk; that is to say, he would rather let the patient take the noneffective treatment through which the patient knows 'the reason why' than let the patient be cured by the treatment through which the patient knows nothing. Tāng ěrhé (汤尔和) even said that he would not feel regret about this. Alas! Where is his medical purpose of healing the wounded and rescuing the dying? Where are his medical ethnics?

TCM can cure diseases because of its unique medical theory. TCM doctors know 'the reason why' in its own theory. But Tāng ěrhé (汤尔和) did not know the theory of TCM at all; what's more, he jumped to the conclusion above.

Taking treating Kawasaki disease as an example, I prescribed based on the child's pulse and symptoms. The main therapeutic methods of the formula were: releasing the exterior, resolving the phlegm-fluid retention, clearing the lung heat and relieving cough. High dosage of *Shengshigao* (*Gypsum Fibrosum*) was used to clear heat, and *Huashifen* (*Pulvistalci*) was used to induce heat out of the body through urinating. These two Chinese medicinals were added to accelerate the progress of bringing down the fever so as to deal with the emergency situation. Thus the curative effect could be achieved so quickly.

TCM doctors don't care if a disease is called Kawasaki disease or pneumonia in Western Medicine. If it shows the sign of exterior syndrome, then TCM doctors will relieve the exterior; if it shows the sign of heat (fever), then TCM doctors will clear heat (bring down the fever); if it shows the sign of cold and heat in complexity syndrome, TCM doctors will prescribe both medicinals with cold nature and hot nature according to the syndrome. All in all, TCM doctors will prescribe Chinese medicinals based on syndrome differentiation. No matter what a disease is called in the name of Western Medicine, TCM doctors will be able to calmly adapt the effective treatment to it.

Since the chief manifestation of Kawasaki disease is high fever, if we can bring down the fever, then the minor manifestation like rashes, lymph node enlargement, and others can be cured easily, which means Kawasaki disease will be completely cured. When this child showed no abnormal condition after taking the prescription, it means that he had been cured and was no longer a Kawasaki disease patient.

Knowing nothing about Kawasaki disease but I have cured it. Why? All because of the understanding and application of TCM theory. Not only Kawasaki disease, but also other diseases can also be cured according to the theory of TCM.

Kawasaki disease is the name given by Modern Medicine and it is the latest name up to now. The cause of it still cannot be found until now. However, I have cured this disease according to the formula recorded in *Treatise on Cold Damage Diseases* (*Shāng hán lùn,* 伤寒论) which was written about 1,700 years ago by Zhāng Zhòngjǐng (张仲景). Therefore, TCM is a medical science of meeting changes with constancy.

TCM has a history of thousands of years. The doctrines of yin-yang and wuxing (five elements) handed down by our ancestors thousands of years ago are same as the doctrines on which TCM is based today. The terms that I use today such as yin-yang, exterior and interior, cold and heat, deficiency and excess are the same as what I learned when I was young. Is there any change in the theory of TCM? No. There is no change because TCM belongs to *Tao-like medical knowledge*; the greatest Tao has no shape; the greatest Tao lives forever; the greatest Tao originates from the heaven; if the heaven has no change, then the Tao would change nothing; TCM is a universally adaptive medical science. Although Chinese medicinals are the same as before and formulas are the same as before, medicinals and formulas you prescribed when you were young are somewhat different from what you prescribe when you are an old doctor. From a junior doctor of TCM to a master of TCM, one has to take several decades to accumulate knowledge and experiences.

That is why in China, when a person is ill or when a person wants to see a TCM doctor, he or she always likes to see an elderly one. It is not because this elderly doctor is well acquainted with not only TCM but also Western Medicine; it is not because this elderly doctor can speak English or French; it is also not because this elderly doctor can remember lots of Chinese medicinals and formulas in mind. As far as I know, when talking about the amount and comprehensiveness of knowledge of either TCM or something else, the elderly TCM doctors, such as the masters like Pú Fǔzhōu (蒲辅周) and Yuè Měizhōng (岳美中), are incomparable with the students or the Medical Doctors (M.D.) of universities of TCM. However, the elderly TCM doctors can understand the theory of TCM more thoroughly and deeply. Through their rich experiences and knowledge, they can differentiate the syndrome more accurately and then compose the right formula exactly. As a result, they would have better curative effects. Although they are old, the elderly doctors of TCM do not lag behind the times. On the contrary, they lead the trend of the development of TCM because their rich experiences are not outdated.

TCM belongs to *Tao-like medical knowledge*, which is incessantly renewed in the long history of development. Traditional Chinese Medicine is handed down from generation to generation. Like other disciplines, the development of TCM never stops. But unlike other disciplines, the older generations of TCM will never be replaced by the newer generations, and they will always be the role models for the newer generations to study.

Why do TCM doctors respectfully call Zhāng Zhòngjǐng (张仲景) as the medical sage? The sage is second only to the god, which means eternal existence.

Although he died more than 1,700 years ago, Zhāng Zhòngjǐng (张仲景) still lives in the hearts of Chinese people and his instructions are still followed by today's TCM doctors. Like the old saying goes, 'Although he was dead, he has been missed for thousands of years'. Thus, it is not exaggerating to regard him as the medical sage!

But Zhāng Zhòngjǐng (张仲景) is not the first and the only medical sage. His success was achieved through the accumulation of the knowledge and experiences of the older generations. Before him, we know Shén Nóng (神农) and *Huangdi's Internal Classic* (*Huáng dì nèi jīng*, 黄帝内经) that is also one of the classics of TCM. Countless TCM doctors from various dynasties conduct their treatments according to the theories of this book.

Meeting changes with constancy is the scientific attribute of TCM, and that is the root cause why diseases which cannot be cured by Western Medicine can be completely cured by TCM. TCM is the highest level of intelligence in terms of curing disease.

On the contrary, because Western Medicine is built on the basis of modern science, it is the medical science aiming at the diseases. As a result, we call it as *medical skills*.

Tao-like medical knowledge never changes, but *medical skills* keep changing all the time. From the medical devices to drugs, *medical skills* are continuously developing. As a new medical term or technology comes up, the old one would be replaced. During the eight decades after it was discovered, penicillin has been updated several times. Some newly emerging antibiotics are even replaced by the newer generations within 3 years. According to Zhāng Xiǎotóng (张晓彤), director of Beijing Cuī Yuèlí (崔月犁) Traditional Medicine Research Center, 'Since 1835, more than 7,000 kinds of drugs have been exported into China by western pharmaceutical companies, only about 1,000 kinds of drugs have been used clinically until now while the remaining 6,000 kinds of drugs have been replaced. And this process continues.'

Hippocrates (about 460BC–377BC), the father of Western Medicine, proposed the humoral theory. He suggested that the human's body was made up of blood, phlegm, yellow bile and black bile, different mixture of which leading to different temperaments. But this philosophy has been abandoned for a very long time by Western Medicine. There is no further research on this theory nowadays, let alone the application. People regard him as the father of Western Medicine because he laid the basis for Western Medicine so people want to remember him and pay homage to him. However, it is worthwhile for us to mention one of the heritages of Hippocrates, that is, he insisted that it was the patient who was under the treatment rather than the disease; he held that when treating a patient, the doctor should consider the influence, including the personality, the environmental factors, and the lifestyle, on the disease. His viewpoint resembles the principle of 'Tao is its being what it is'. It is a pity that he did not form a theoretical system based on this seemingly correct approach. People have already abandoned his viewpoint thanks to the rapid development of modern medicine. Resorting to the continuously evolving technology, they unduly advocate the treatment of a disease rather than the treatment of a human. I suddenly recall the sentences from *Sān guó zhì — Wú-biography — Lù kàng* (三国志 • 吴志 • 陆抗传), 'The emperor has spent countless money and mobilized all the troops and ordinary people to fight with the enemy. Although our troops and people are exhausted by this situation, the power of the enemy is not weakened.'

Despite that humans have invented numerous kinds of antibiotics, the bacteria and virus have developed more resistance. The more dosages of antibiotics a doctor prescribes to the patient, the more resistance the bacteria develops inside the body. The current antibiotics seem to be useless to the superbacteria. Even worse, antibiotics inflict great damage to kids. Why is it more difficult to buy antibiotics than a gun in the United States? It is because antibiotics are more likely to be misused.

Next to heart attack, cancer, and stroke, adverse drug reaction is the 4th killer in the United States and about 125,000 people die from it each year. Misuse of antibiotics is likely to be one of the main reasons for the deaths. According to the estimation, China is the No. 1 country where antibiotics are misused. Many children will be harmed by this situation in our country.

Given the fact that Chinese people have been taking Chinese medicinals for thousands of years and we even take smaller dosages today than our ancestors did, why don't Chinese medicinals have drug resistance problem inside the human body? It is because TCM is the medical science based on the principle of 'Tao is its being what it is'. It is because the TCM theory does not advocate anti any bacteria or virus. It is because TCM doctors use Chinese medicinals to balance yin and yang. How can the drug resistance problem come into being?

Drug resistance problem will never emerge in the world of TCM! The theory of TCM will never change! No matter how many symptoms a disease will appear or change, 'observe complexion and take pulse, differentiating yin and yang first' has always been the primary diagnostic and therapeutic principle of TCM. TCM is a medical science of meeting changes with constancy!

TCM is a medical science of simple solutions to complicated problems

— Discussing that TCM contains great wisdom and thought by taking the example of curing disease with *Poge Jiuxin Tang* (*Breaking the Rule and Heart-Saving Decoction*)

When I started learning TCM, I could memorize almost all the facts from the textbooks taught in universities of TCM. But when coming to the clinical practice, I could not guarantee my curative effects at an ideal level. After apprenticing with several elderly experienced TCM doctors, and learning their clinical experiences, I could gradually handle the clinical cases with high proficiency.

I used to avoid using Chinese medicinals to treat severe acute diseases. When I was an apprentice to Lǐ Kě (李可), the well-known elderly experienced TCM doctor, I found that he could always make his patients in severe acute diseased condition get better through the use of high dosage *Fuzi* (*Radix Aconiti Lateralis Praeparata*).

In the past, for its toxicity, I had never dared to prescribe my patients *Fuzi* (*Radix Aconiti Lateralis Praeparata*) for about 10 years. After Li's words and deeds, I've gradually learned how to properly use *Fuzi*. I especially have got deep understanding of the use of *Fuzi* in the formula, *Poge Jiuxin Tang* (*Breaking the Rule and Heart-saving Decoction*), which was invented by my teacher Lǐ Kě (李可). The following is one of the examples.

On October 6, 2000, when I treated patients in a hospital in Linfen, I met a 65-year-old male patient who was hospitalized for rheumatic heart disease (enlarged ventricle) and renal failure. Here were the chief mani-festations: at 6:00 p.m., he suddenly became incapable of speaking and pointed towards his heart giving the sign of extreme pain in this position; the cold areas of his upper limbs were from the fingertips to beyond the elbows, the cold areas of his lower limbs were from the tiptoes to beyond the knees; he had shortness of breath with inability to lie flat, a dry and dull complexion, blue and purple lips and nails, sticky and oily sweating, a smooth tongue with no coating, a floating, feeble, surging, and rapid pulse (the pulse beat about 260 times per minute); his blood pressure (BP) was unable to be measured. Thus, I prescribed *Poge Jiuxin Tang* to him based on these manifestations with no hesitation.

Because of the severe acute diseased condition, the formula was decocted with boiled water by the strong fire. The patient was given the formula right after decocting. At about 8:00 p.m., the patient's condition did not get better. Therefore I added more dosage of *Fuzi* in the second formula, and the patient's diseased condition became relatively stable.

At 11:00 p.m., the patient took the third formula with an even higher dosage of *Fuzi* than the second one. After that, the patient's condition gradually improved. Until 6:00 a.m. of the next morning, the patient had no difficulty in breathing; the blue and purple color on his lips and nails faded away; his limbs became warm; he was able to sit up and talk; his pulse beat slowed down (the pulse beat about 90 times per minute); his blood pressure was 21/9.3kPa (160/70mmHg). He was finally out of the severe acute diseased condition. Then I prescribed him some medicinals for tonifying qi and activating blood. One week later, he was discharged from the hospital.

The reason why I dared to prescribe so many dosages of *Fuzi* to treat the patient was all because of the words and deeds of my respectful teacher Lǐ Kě (李可). *Poge Jiuxin Tang* was frequently used by teacher Li for treating severe acute diseases. He told me that this formula was based on *Sini Tang* (*Cold-Extremities Decoction*) recorded in *Treatise on Cold Damage Diseases* (*Shāng hán lùn*, 伤寒论) and *Laifu Tang* (*Recovering Decoction*) composed by Zhāng Xīchún (张锡纯).

Teacher Li had been devoting his entire life to the study of severe acute diseases. According to his clinical experience, heart failure patients suffer not only yin exhaustion, but also yang collapse. *Sini Tang*

(*Cold-Extremities Decoction*) is good at tonifying yang, but it is not effective enough to nourish yin; *Laifu Tang* (*Recovering Decoction*) is good at nourishing yin, but it is not effective enough to tonify yang. As a result, the integration can realize the mutual complementation of the functions of these two formulas. Particularly, teacher Li broke the normal rule of avoiding overdosing on *Fuzi* and *Shangzhuyu* (*Fructus Corni*) and brought the fundamental change of *Poge Jiuxin Tang. Cishi* (*Magnetitum*) and the powders of *Longgu* (*Os Draconis*) and *Muli* (*Concha Ostreae*) are used to maintain yin and yang. *Shexiang* (*Moschus*) is used for resuscitation and tonification, and only with the use of *Shexiang* could this formula achieve the function of restoring yin and yang to stop collapsing.

The key role of this prescription is *Fuzi*, and only when it is used in a high dosage level can it be effective to the diseased condition. High dosage of *Gancao* (*Radix Glycyrrhizae*) is combined with *Fuzi:* on the one hand, *Gancao* can decrease or moderate the toxicity of *Fuzi;* on the other hand, its sweet flavor and mild nature can keep *Fuzi* and *Ganjiang* stay in the middle energizer longer so these medicinals can warm the body from inside to outside thoroughly, through which the effect of restoring yang will last longer.

Teacher Li composed this formula precisely and comprehensively, so when we treat heart failure patients we may compose this formula for them without worries.

The Album of Lǐ Kě (李可)*'s Experience in Treating Severe Acute Diseases* (*Lǐ kě lǎo zhōng yī jí wēi zhòng zhèng yí nán bìng jīng yàn zhuān jí,* 李可老中医急危重症疑难病经验专辑) published in 2002 has aroused strong feedback and continuous praises in the TCM circle. The formula, *Poge Jiuxin Tang,* recorded in this book has been particularly praised by the readers and has been successfully tested countless times in clinical practices.

How many diseases can this formula actually treat? Only in the book, *Clinical Application Examples,* teacher Li had listed many cases as follows: pulmonary heart disease coupled with heart failure, respiratory failure coupled with cerebral crisis, acute heart failure, rheumatic heart disease coupled with heart failure, brucella acute heart failure, acute myocardial infarction, coronary heart disease coupled with frequent premature ventricular beat, atrial fibrillation and cardiogenic shock, etc.

In conclusion, the patient who has no therapeutic treatment in the view of Western Medicine can be saved by TCM which is regarded as a medical science being specialized at nursing chronic diseases. It shows that TCM not only can cure chronic diseases that Western Medicine cannot cure, but also can cure acute diseases that Western Medicine cannot cure.

People had always been cautious about using *Fuzi* for the fear of its toxicity. But when teacher Li treated patients, he always used high dosages of *Fuzi* and turned it into some kind of panacea.

Although Lǐ Kě (李可) was an elderly experienced TCM doctor, when treating severe diseases he was more like a fearless warrior. *Poge Jiuxin Tang* composed by him will certainly be one of the most famous formulas in our TCM history in terms of treating severe acute diseases.

He not only invented *Poge Jiuxin Tang*, but also had cured many dubious and acute diseases. What is the theoretical basis of his treatment?

As a matter of fact, the basis is very simple. It is the sentence from *Huangdi's Internal Classic* (*Nèi jīng*, 内经), 'With quiet and even yin harmonizing with sturdy and solid yang, man will be energetic and vigorous'. In this sentence, 'Sturdy and solid yang' is the key point. What's more, *Neijing* also records, 'The key in balancing yin and yang is to keep a sturdy and solid yang', 'Yang in the body pertains to the sun in the Heaven. When it loses its normal circulation, long life will be cut shot' to lay stress on the importance of 'Sturdy and solid yang'.

Yin-yang represents the general principle of understanding the human body and treating diseases in TCM. No matter how complicated the diseases are, and no matter how disease spectrum changes, the TCM treatment always remains unchanged, focusing on yin and yang.

When you know how yin and yang works, you know the theories of TCM.

When you get to know how yin and yang works, you know how to treat diseases. Yin and yang represents the general principle of TCM treatment. Only by following this principle can you completely treat diseases.

Therefore, *Huangdi's Internal Classic* (*Nèi jīng*, 内经) says, 'Observe complexion and take pulse, differentiating yin and yang first.' It is the precondition for a TCM doctor before he makes prescriptions, which is like a situation that before a person wants to go to some place, he should firstly be clear about the direction, and only when he selects a right direction can he arrive at the destination. If a doctor runs in the opposite direction, the prescription he makes will be ineffective and even life-threatening. That is the reason why we say TCM is a medical science of simple solutions to complicated problems.

Besides this general principle, there are also eight syndrome differentiation principles in TCM, which include, 'yin, yang, exterior, interior, cold, heat, deficiency, and excess'. Although the symptoms of diseases are always changing, they are closely associated with these eight principles. What a concise and clear thought for diagnosis and treatment.

Adding high dosage *Fuzi* in *Poge Jiuxin Tang* is to expel pathogenic cold. Only if we see some of the symptoms listed as follows can we prescribe this formula for the patients: a profuse cold sweating, cold limbs, a pale and shallow yellow complexion, blue and purple lips and nails, a deep, slow, and weak pulse, no rhythm pulse, sparrow-pecking pulse, roof-leaking pulse or irregular-rapid pulse. The main symptoms that we should pay attention to are: the cold areas of upper limbs cover from the fingertips to beyond the elbows, the cold areas of lower limbs cover from the tiptoes to beyond the knees. In the book of *Plain Questions* (*Sù Wèn*, 素问), ancestors also expressed the relationship between limbs and yang qi, 'Four limbs are the root of yang qi in human body'.

These main symptoms mentioned above indicate a specific moment: in this moment, the patient is on the verge of death; but pathogenic cold does not reach the chest where it is still slightly warm, which means that yang qi is still remaining inside the body though very little. *Fuzi* is extremely hot in nature, and only through the use of this nature can pathogenic cold be expelled and then life can be saved. If prescribing without *Fuzi*, pathogenic cold will reach the chest rapidly and then the whole body will turn cold. And then the heart beat will stop, the patient will be dead. No matter how much *Fuzi* a doctor uses at this time, he still cannot save the dead. Without yang qi, people will be dead and become cold in temperature. How can a doctor turn a cold corpse into a warm and living body?

It is a very simple principle, but it is incomprehensible from the viewpoint of Western Medicine, because Western Medicine focuses on the evidence.

What exactly is yin-yang in the view of TCM? What is really pathogenic cold in the view of TCM? Since these things are undetectable by advanced scientific instruments, they are invisible and intangible. Isn't this metaphysics? In Western Medicine, cardiac stimulants are ineffective for saving a patient whose heart is to stop beating, while in TCM, the use of high dosage *Fuzi*, which is extremely toxic in Chinese medicinals, can save this heart failure patient. This is incomprehensible for Western Medicine. That is the issue concerning the differences between two medical science systems.

From the perspective of Western Medicine, TCM was, is, and will always be incomprehensible, which is like the situation that when we stand on the earth, we see the sun revolving around the earth, and in fact, when you leave the surface of the earth, you will see the earth revolving around the sun. This is the reason why we draw completely different conclusions when we think about an issue from different perspectives.

Teacher Li once said: "If you want to truly understand TCM, you should brainwash yourself first." His words actually mean that people should think about the issues from different perspectives, otherwise, they could never understand TCM.

As a matter of fact, be it Chinese people or foreign people, be it white race, black race, or yellow race, be it TCM or Western Medicine, we all live in the same nature and are originated from the same nature. And the theories of TCM obey this nature.

In summer, the weather becomes hot indicating the excess of yang qi, so people wear vests and shorts.

In winter, the weather becomes cold indicating the excess of yin qi, so people wear cotton-padded jackets or down jackets.

People will dress different clothes due to season changes, and no one can do it against the law of nature, which is called as 'the nature and man unite as one'. However, with supernormal wisdom, only our ancestors applied the principle of 'the nature and man unite as one' to the eternal theme of conquering diseases and delaying aging. Our ancestors invented, or more accurately, they discovered this special medical science system, TCM. This system summarizes the complicated relation between human life and disease as 'yin and yang'. Although *Tao-like Chinese medical knowledge* is complicated, if you could understand the core of TCM, you will be able to handle it. Although there are different diseases with numerous changes, what you should do when treating patients is to creatively study and apply eight-principle syndrome differentiation (yin, yang, exterior, interior, cold, heat, deficiency, and excess). TCM doctors have been following the same diagnostic and therapeutic thinking patterns from ancient times to today. Thus, TCM can meet changes with constancy and TCM is a medical science of simple solutions to complicated problems.

For collecting the knowledge of etiology and pathology of Western Medicine, scholars published many thick books. But when talking about the causes of diseases from the perspective of TCM, there are only two: internal damage and external contraction.

The external contraction includes wind, cold, summer heat, dampness, dryness, and fire.

The internal damage includes over-joy, rage, anxiety, pensiveness, sorrow, fear, fright, yang deficiency, yin deficiency, food damage, and so on.

No matter how frequently the disease spectrum of modern medicine changes, the causes of it in the view of TCM are always the problem of 'internal damage and external contradiction'. Besides internal damage and external contradiction, there is another cause of diseases in TCM called the cause neither internal nor external, that is, traumatism, which is another matter.

The therapeutic methods of TCM can be summarized into only eight methods, that is, sweating method, emetic method, purgation method, harmonizing method, warming method, clearing method, tonifying method, and resolving method.

In all ages, there are large numbers of famous TCM doctors, and they follow different schools. There are approximately millions of Chinese classic herbal formulas and current herbal formulas, but all of the therapeutic methods from these formulas are all closely associated with the eight methods mentioned above. And this is exactly like the old saying goes, 'Eight methods can derive out all therapeutic methods.'

In the book of *Huangdi's Internal Classic* (*Nèi jīng*, 内经), it records, 'the man who can grasp the main point may solve the problem directly; the man who can only grasp the minor point may not solve the problem or solve it laboriously.'

TCM belongs to *Tao-like medical knowledge*, is an intangible science, and is a medical science which has simple solutions to complicated problems. TCM doctors should concentrate on the main point, so they cannot mix western medical theories with those of TCM; if they once mix these theories together, it is difficult for TCM doctors to return to what they were before.

The phrase 'simple solutions to complicated problems' is easy to understand, but it is difficult to put it into practice. There are so many nations and so many countries around the world, and every country has its own herbal medicines. Nicolaus Copernicus, the great Polish astronomer, who proposed the 'Heliocentric Theory' and rejected the 'Geocentric Theory' which had dominated for more than one thousand years in western countries, and who unveiled the mystery of the universe, was once a physician. When he studied at the University of Padua, he was very interested in folk medicine which focused on herbal medicines. Therefore he collected large amounts of folk prescriptions. He always put himself out of the way and never cared about the monetary rewards when he treated patients. He not only didn't charge but also sent medicinals to the poor patients who could not pay for the bills. Copernicus's noble medical ethics is so consistent with the spirit of 'saving people wholeheartedly' that Sūn Sīmiǎo (孙思邈) advocated.

However, although we can find herbal medicines in use around the world, only the Chinese people had summarized the use of herbal medicines into theoretical level, such as four properties and five flavors, ascending, descending, floating, sinking, and channel tropism. Only the ancestors of Chinese nation discovered the intangible relation between human body and disease; based on these discoveries, they formed a complete theoretical system which regards yin-yang as the core; as a result, they initiated TCM which has been widely spread through all the ages and which has been well-known around the world.

On February 20, 2008, Chang Yu, a reporter of *China News of Traditional Chinese Medicine,* published an article based on an exclusive interview with Lǐ Kě (李可). The title was '*Seeing through the Mystery; Treating Diseases among the Masses*'. This 'mystery' represents that giving priority to restore yang at the critical moment. This 'mystery' also indicates the use of high dosage of Chinese medicinals of restoring yang to cure all kinds of severe acute diseases of modern medicine.

Only one therapeutic method, restoring yang, can cure countless severe acute diseases of modern medicine.

Both TCM and modern medicine are treating illness, but why when the illness is cured by a TCM doctor, we say that he has seen through the mystery? 'The mystery, existing in everywhere reconditely, is intangible (*The Mysterious Sutra* (*Tài xuán·Xuán lí,* 太玄·玄离) written by Yáng Xióng (杨雄)).' This 'yang' undetected by any high-technology instrument is also intangible.

Using an instrument, we may see tangible pathogenic factors such as cells, molecules, bacteria, viruses. However, in the view of TCM, complicated diseases can be simplified, which indicates the great wisdom and thought of human beings in terms of conquering disease.

This great wisdom and thought of TCM coincides with the world remarkable scientific thoughts of western scientists.

Sir Isaac Newton once said: "Therefore to the same natural effects we must, as far as possible, assign the same causes (*Newton's Philosophy of Nature Selections from His Writings,* Shanghai People's Publishing House, 1974:3)."

This thought was praised highly by Einstein that the concept of 'logical simplicity' had become one of his most important rules of evaluating scientific theories. He said: "The logically simple does not, of course, have to be physically true, but the physically true is logically simple, that is, it has unity at the foundation (*Collected Works of Albert Einstein,* Volume 1, The Commercial Press, 1976:380)."

He further explained, "Although it is true that it is the goal of science to discover rules which permit the association and foretelling of facts, this is not its only aim. It also seeks to reduce the connections discovered to the smallest possible number of mutually independent conceptual elements. It is in this striving after the rational unification of the manifold that it encounters its greatest successes, even though it is precisely this attempt which causes it to run the greatest risk of falling a prey to illusions. But whoever has undergone the intense experience of successful advances made in this domain is moved by profound reverence for the rationality made manifest in existence (*Collected Works of Albert Einstein*, Volume 3 The Commercial Press, 1979:85)."

Not only did Newton and Einstein give the logical simplicity a lofty scientific status, but also all scientists of all ages consciously or unconsciously follow this important methodology when they construct scientific theories, 'Via the observation and research of lots of natural phenomena, Newton found the similarity and unity in the nature. Based on the similarity and unity, he had been seeking after the common cause behind the phenomena. No matter in the past or at the present, this rule, assigning the same cause to the same natural effect as far as possible, always plays a methodological role in enlightening and helping people to explore the law of the nature. There is a possibility that the special cause can be converted to the general cause through the reasoning from the effect to the cause, that is considering there is a certain relation between the cause and the effect (*Newton's Enlightenment,* Shanxi Science and Technology Publishing House, 1999:90).'

The ancient and intangible TCM shares the same methodology with Newton and Einstein, that is not just a coincidence in the history. TCM represents the real scientific thought and methodology!

Why do so many people love TCM for their entire lives? In Einstein's words, it is because, 'whoever has undergone the intense experience of successful advances made in this domain is moved by profound reverence for the rationality made manifest in existence.'

Nowadays, some diagnostic and therapeutic thoughts of TCM have been completely westernized through some people's push towards the scientization of TCM. These people seem to insanely abandon their tradition. They also defy and trample Einstein's core scientific thought, 'the only and the most critical thing is the logical simplicity of the foundation'.

In 1998, I ran a TCM clinic in West Bingzhou Street, Taiyuan. In order to make me a better doctor, between 2002 and 2003, my teacher Lǐ Kě (李可), who was then 70 years old, came to my clinic for patients from Lingshi County that is 150 km away every week. I have always appreciated that until now.

My clinic was not far from Shanxi Institute of TCM (the current Shanxi Academy of TCM). The directors and professors of the institute frequently came to learn the clinical experience of teacher Li. On the one hand, they were astonished at the use of high-dosage *Fuzi*, on the other hand, they expressed their doubts when they saw that patients were safe and sound and their diseases were cured after taking high-dosage *Fuzi*. A senior member of them sighed, "Although Lǐ Kě (李可) is an extraordinary talent, he did not attend any university of TCM. What a pity."

His words are totally wrong in my opinion. It is fortunate that my teacher Li did not attend any university of TCM. Otherwise, instead of finding out the importance of restoring yang in the treatment of severe acute diseases, or inventing the formula of *Poge Jiuxin Tang*, Lǐ Kě (李可) would just become another normal TCM professor or director in some TCM university.

Appendix: A birthday speech for Lǐ Kě (李可) by Guó Guānghóng (国光红)

Today, we celebrate the 80th birthday of Lǐ Kě (李可).

Mr. Li was born and bred in Lingshi County, Shanxi province while I come from Jinan, Shandong province. The reason why I'm here to celebrate his birthday is to show my great sincerity on both public and private sides. As we all know, a gifted person will surely choose a career not for a common person. What Mr. Li chose to be is an authentic TCM doctor for which a common person cannot be equally competent. Moreover, he always treats those fake doctors and those doctors focusing on making money as the pollution in the TCM circle. In his medical career, he not only doesn't stick to the stereotypes of ancients for prescribing medicinals and formulas, but also has created many new therapeutic methods for saving lives. Through his creative thoughts and innovative applications of *Fuzi (Radix Aconiti Lateralis)*, *Mahuang (Herba Ephedrae)*, and *Xixin (Herba Asari)*, he can always save lives of others in the severe acute situations. No one except Mr. Li can be regarded as the reincarnation of *Bian Que*, and he deserves this honor. Therefore, there is a saying that goes among the masses, "Mr. Li always acts on conscience and is a highly-skilled doctor."

As the old Chinese saying goes, 'It is easy to find a qualified prime minister, but it is not easy to find a qualified doctor.' In peaceful and prosperous times, a country can be governed orderly without any qualified prime minister or general; when a tough time is coming, and when the country needs the qualified prime minister and general, they will emerge at the right moment and will be found easily; however, when the country is in the heyday of peace, it is inevitable that people will fall ill for the unhealthy lifestyles; therefore, people in peaceful and prosperous times will be eager to find qualified doctors, but qualified doctors may not emerge at every generation; that is why finding a qualified doctor is difficult to accomplish.

Thanks to the introduction of Lè Kǎi (乐凯), I could, with my great honor, make acquaintance with Lǐ Kě (李可). Lè Kǎi (乐凯) is one of the favorite pupils of Li, and he is a TCM doctor well-known in Shandong province. He also founded Lǐ Kě (李可)'s Academic Thought Inheritance Base on December 22, 2008, the Chinese winter solstice festival of that year. I remember Lè Kǎi (乐凯) once asked me whether I would like to join him and spread Lǐ Kě (李可)'s thought. When I heard his words, I agreed instantly without any hesitation. Without the passion and the experience of researching Chinese classical culture, I dare not take over this glorious task of heavy responsibility.

I seldom attend birthday celebrations. Today, accompanied by my wife, I come to the birthday celebration because we want to pay our respect to Mr. Li. In Mount Meng, we had exchanged words with each other for about half a month, but it was too short for me to fully understand his great and profound thought. Therefore, on the public side, I come here this time to show my respect and admiration. On the private side, I want to take this opportunity to motivate and spur on myself. Now, I wish Mr. Li to be happy as immense as the east sea and live a long and happy life! He is the fortune of TCM, and the fortune of Chinese classical culture! His existence and his thought are the fortune for the common people, and the fortune for us who have the responsibilities to inherit and spread his thought.

Guó Guānghóng (国光红)
Jinghuahuidian TCM Research Institute,
Shandong Jinan Lǐ Kě (李可)'s Academic Thought Inheritance Base

Notes by the writer: December 15, 2009, was the 80th birthday of my beloved teacher, Lǐ Kě (李可). On that day, Lǐ Dàníng (李大宁), the vice director of State Administration of Traditional Chinese Medicine of the People's Republic of China, Zhōu Rán (周然), the vice president of CCCP of Shanxi province, Wén Yuān (文渊), the director of State Administration of Traditional Chinese Medicine of Shanxi province, were coming here for Lǐ Kě (李可)'s birthday celebration. I, as the first disciple of Lǐ Kě (李可), accompanied by more than 50 disciples all over the country, came here for the ceremony of worshiping our mentor. During the ceremony, I led the fellows to recite the pledge for expressing our ambitions of being a TCM doctor, 'inheriting the teachings from our mentor, revitalizing Traditional Chinese Medicine, treating diseases and saving lives, we will insist on obeying these rules till we die.'

Guó Guānghóng (国光红), a former professor of Qilu Normal University, a scholar specializing in the research of the ancient Chinese hieroglyphics, the ancient phonology, and the explanations of ancient classics, traveled hundreds of kilometers in the cold winter accompanied by his wife to attend the birthday celebration and delivered this speech. Although Mr. Guo does not belong to the field of TCM, he has always cared and contributed to us a lot. While attending the birthday celebration, Mr. Guo took this opportunity to call us to further develop Traditional Chinese Medicine. We have been greatly impressed by what he has done. Therefore, I attach the speech he delivered at the birthday celebration.

TCM is a medical science of handling difficulties with great ease

— The discussion on the advantage of scientific attribute of TCM by taking the example of curing advanced prostate cancer with bone metastases

The patient was a 67-year-old male named Fang, who was a retired officer from the Department of Public Security of Shanxi Province. During the time he was living in Changzhou, Jiangsu Province in May, 2012, Mr. Fang went to the First People's Hospital of Changzhou (out-patient No. 8874163) because of the difficulty in urination and the pain in legs. Tumor markers showed that TPSA (total prostate-specific antigen) was higher than 100.000μg/ml (the reference range of TPSA is lower than 4.000μg/ml), FPSA (free prostate-specific antigen) was 8.720μg/ml (the reference range of FPSA is lower than 1.000μg/ml). These two are the core indexes used by modern hospitals to diagnose prostate cancer. Therefore, Fang was diagnosed with advanced-stage prostate cancer.

As the patient could only use his medical insurance in Taiyuan, he went back there preparing for the operation as well as dealing with formalities related to medical insurance of critical illness. On May 25, he was hospitalized in the Urology Department of the First Affiliated Hospital of Shanxi Medical University (admission No. 618740).

On May 26, the tumor markers showed that TPSA was 76.8μg/ml, FPSA was 8μg/ml. What's more, the bone scan showed that hot spots were found in the left side of the sacrum joint and right side of the pubic bone.

Given these examinations, he was diagnosed as advanced prostate cancer coupled with bone metastases.

It was useless to have the operation, so the hospital just suggested the patient taking a kind of medicine imported from Germany. This medicine, however, was out of stock for the moment, so Fang had to wait for more than one month.

At that time, the patient could neither have the operation nor take the medicine, so waiting was the only method. He did not believe in TCM then, while his wife Ms Sun (a teacher in a middle school of Taiyuan) held the opposite opinion, persuading him to seek for treatment from me. On June 3, the patient, without other choices, came to my clinic for treatment.

When he came to my clinic, I noticed a urine collection bag with bloody urine inside hanging on his leg.

He staggered toward me with great difficulty, just like a prisoner with heavy shackles.

His main complaints were as follows: his crotch and waist were painful, his groins and private part were also distending painful, blood clots which were as large as rice grains could be seen in the bloody urine catheterized via the urinary catheter, blood also could be found in his excrement.

The examination revealed that he had an extremely exhausted and swelling face, a dry and dull complexion, an enlarged dull purple tongue with a thick yellow coating, slippery and rapid pulses, which were also deficient at Cun and Guan positions under heavy pressure.

These symptoms were caused by qi deficiency after a long-term illness, and the accumulation of dampness-heat and stasis-toxin in lower energizer. The treatment should primarily concentrate on tonifying qi with high dosages of medicinals, and secondarily focus on clearing heat and eliminating dampness, activating blood and removing toxin. As a result, I composed the formula as follows:

Huangqi (Radix Astragali seu Hedysari) 60g
Yedangshen (Radix Codonopsis) 30g
Baimaogen (Rhizoma Imperatae) 100g
Cangzhu (Rhizoma Atractylodis) 15g
Huangbai (Cortex Phellodendri) 10g
Cheqianzi (Semen Plantaginis) 30g

Yedanshen (Radix Salviae Miltiorrhizae) 30g
Chishaoyao (Radix Paeoniae Rubra) 15g
Dangguiwei (tail of Radix Angelicae sinensis) 15g
Zhizi (Fructus Gardeniae) 10g
Dengxincao (Medulla Junci) 6g
Zhuye (Herba Lophatheri) 10g
Chuanniuxi (Radix Cyathulae) 15g
Baizhu (Rhizoma Atractylodis Macrocephalae) 10g
Fuling (Poria) 30g
Zhuling (Polyporus) 30g
Baihuasheshecao (Herba Hedyotis) 60g
Gancaoshao (Radix Glycyrrhizae) 30g

All these medicinals should be decocted with water for oral administration. Three doses should be taken.

On June 6, 2012, he came to my clinic for the second visit. Rice-sized blood clots could still be seen in the urine collection bag, but there was clear yellow urine instead of fresh bloody urine in it.

He told me that he got relief from those symptoms and felt much better both physically and mentally after taking the formula. He also emphasized that the first dose helped him become more confident in my treatment because there was no more blood in urine immediately. Afterwards, he only sometimes felt exhausted and painful in waist and legs.

Since the prescription had positive effect, I just followed the original formula with slight changes of some dosages and adding some new ingredients for strengthening bones and muscles. Besides, the prescription also increased the proportion of medicinals for removing toxin and eliminating dampness. Here were the ingredients of the formula:

Huangqi (Radix Astragali seu Hedysari) 60g
Yiyiren (Semen Coicis) 30g
Dangguiwei (tail of Radix Angelicae sinensis) 15g
Chishaoyao (Radix Paeoniae Rubra) 15g
Chuanduan (Rasix Dipsaci) 30g
Duzhong (Cortex Eucommiae) 15g
Yedangshen (Radix Codonopsis) 30g

Qumai (Herba Dianthi) 20g
Zhuling (Polyporus) 30g
Zexie (Rhizoma Alismatis) 20g
Gancaoshao (Radix Glycyrrhizae) 20g
Baihuasheshecao (Herba Hedyotis) 120g
Banzhilian (Herba Scutellariae Barbatae) 60g

The last two medicinals should be decocted with water first for half an hour and then the other medicinals should be decocted in it. Three doses should be taken.

On June 10, 2012, he came to my clinic for the third visit. He said he felt a steady improvement of his health after taking the formula, during which time he once removed the catheter and still maintained unob-structed urine flow, but the difficulty of urination appeared again two days later; he then inserted the catheter and got clear urine without small blood clots. Therefore, I composed the third formula for him with added medicinals for elevating:

Huangqi (Radix Astragali seu Hedysari) 60g
Yedangshen (Radix Codonopsis) 30g
Chenpi (Pericarpium Citri Tangerinae) 10g
Gancaoshao (Radix Glycyrrhizae) 15g
Huangbai (Cortex Phellodendri) 10g
Zhimu (Rhizoma Anemarrhenae) 20g
Rougui (Cortex Cinnamomi) 10g
Huashifen (Pulvistalci) 10g
Zexie (Rhizoma Alismatis) 20g
Fuling (Poria) 30g
Shengma (Rhizoma Cimicifugae) 10g
Chuanniuxi (Radix Cyathulae) 30g
Yedanshen (Radix Salviae Miltiorrhizae) 30g
Baihuasheshecao (Herba Hedyotis) 120g
Banzhilian (Herba Scutellariae Barbatae) 60g

All these ingredients should be decocted with water for oral administration. Six doses should be taken.

The fourth time he came to my clinic was on June 17, 2012, and there was no urine collection bag on his leg. The patient said he maintained unobstructed urine flow as healthy people without the catheter, and he even took a bus this time for more than one hour from Hexi District of Taiyuan to my clinic located on the east hillside. I could tell he was much better from the glow on his face. Yet he said he had no pain in waist and legs but felt exhausted and got a dry mouth. I found that he still had a dull purple tongue; the pulses, which beat 7 times in a cycle of breath, were still weak at Cun and Guan positions under heavy pressure. Therefore, I continued composing the third formula with the original therapeutic thought for tonifying and elevating qi, clearing heat and eliminating dampness, activating blood and resolving stasis:

Huangqi (Radix Astragali seu Hedysari) 60g
Machixian (Herba Portulacae) 40g
Chuanniuxi (Radix Cyathulae) 30g
Mutong (Caulis Akebiae) 6g
Banzhilian (Herba Scutellariae Barbatae) 60g
Huashifen (Pulvistalci) 30g
Dongkuiguo (Fructus Malvae) 30g
Shengdihuang (Radix Rehmanniae Recens) 30g
Shengma (Rhizoma Cimicifugae) 6g
Chaihu (Radix Bupleuri) 6g
Zexie (Rhizoma Alismatis) 30g
Fuling (Poria) 30g
Yedanshen (Radix Salviae Miltiorrhizae) 30g
Xianlingpi (Herba Epimedii) 10g

All these medicinals should be decocted with water for oral administration. Six doses should be taken.

On June 24, 2012, he came to my clinic for the fifth time. He said he continued to maintain unobstructed urine flow and felt increasingly better. He now had bloody excrement, the prolapsing sensation of the anus, skin numbness, turning red suddenly on his face, excessive sweating (all over the body). His tongue was red and slightly dull. His tongue coating at the root of tongue was yellow. The pulses were still weak at Cun and Guan positions, and were huge and slippery at Chi positions. I changed the formula based on the previous one and increased the proportion of medicinals for clearing heat and removing toxin, tonifying and elevating qi:

Huangqi (Radix Astragali seu Hedysari) 60g
Chenpi (Pericarpium Citri Tangerinae) 10g
Gancao (Radix Glycyrrhizae) 10g
Machixian (Herba Portulacae) 60g
Cheqianzi (Semen Plantaginis) 30g
Huashifen (Pulvistalci) 30g
Chuanniuxi (Radix Cyathulae) 30g
Mutong (Caulis Akebiae) 6g
Shengma (Rhizoma Cimicifugae) 10g
Chaihu (Radix Bupleuri) 10g
Yedanshen (Radix Salviae Miltiorrhizae) 30g
Dongkuiguo (Fructus Malvae) 20g
Zhimu (Rhizoma Anemarrhenae) 15g
Huangbai (Cortex Phellodendri) 15g
Fuling (Poria) 30g
Zexie (Rhizoma Alismatis) 20g
Diyu (Radix Sanguisorbae) 30g
Huaijiao (Fructus Sophorae) 20g
Banzhilian (Herba Scutellariae Barbatae) 60g
Baihuasheshecao (Herba Hedyotis) 120g

All these medicinals should be decocted with water for oral administration. Six doses should be taken.

On July 1, 2012, at the sixth time he came to my clinic there was no blood in excrement and he felt much better than ever both physically and mentally. His pulses, which beat 5 times in a cycle of breath, were weak at Cun and Guan positions and were huge and slippery at Chi positions. His tongue was still dull red, the coating at the root of tongue was yellow. On June 28, the patient took a PSA examination reporting that TPSA was 7.144μg/ml, FPSA was 0.716μg/ml, which indicated that the values of tumor markers significantly decreased. He was delighted and encouraged with lots of confidence. Since the excrement did not contain blood, so I did not use *Huaijiao* (*Fructus Sophorae*) this time, and slightly reduced the dosages of other medicinals.

Huangqi (*Radix Astragali seu Hedysari*) *60g*
Chenpi (*Pericarpium Citri Tangerinae*) *10g*
Gancao (*Radix Glycyrrhizae*) *10g*
Machixian (*Herba Portulacae*) *60g*
Cheqianzi (*Semen Plantaginis*) *30g*
Huashifen (*Pulvistalci*) *20g*
Chuanniuxi (*Radix Cyathulae*) *30g*
Shengma (*Rhizoma Cimicifugae*) *6g*
Chaihu (*Radix Bupleuri*) *10g*
Yedanshen (*Radix Salviae Miltiorrhizae*) *30g*
Dongkuiguo (*Fructus Malvae*) *20g*
Zhimu (*Rhizoma Anemarrhenae*) *15g*
Huangbai (*Cortex Phellodendri*) *10g*
Diyu (*Radix Sanguisorbae*) *15g*
Baihuasheshecao (*Herba Hedyotis*) *90g*
Banzhilian (*Herba Scutellariae Barbatae*) *30g*

All these medicinals should be decocted with water for oral administration. Six doses should be taken.

On July 8, 2012, the seventh visit. He told me that he did not feel heavy and exhausted in his right leg, but felt so in his left leg. Sometimes, his face turned red and he begun to sweat all of a sudden. His tongue was red. His pulses beat 7 times in a cycle of breath, and were still weak at Cun and Guan positions. I still composed him the former formula with a little change for adding some astringent medicinals:

Huangqi (*Radix Astragali seu Hedysari*) *60g*
Dangshen (*Radix Codonopsis*) *60g*
Chenpi (*Pericarpium Citri Tangerinae*) *10g*
Gancao (*Radix Glycyrrhizae*) *10g*
Shanyurou (*Fructus Corni*) *30g*

Shenglonggu (Os Draconis) 30g
Shengmuli (Concha Ostreae) 30g
Huashifen (Pulvistalci) 20g
Mahuanggen (Radix Ephedrae) 10g
Chuanniuxi (Radix Cyathulae) 30g
Dongkuiguo (Fructus Malvae) 20g
Diyu (Radix Sanguisorbae) 30g
Shengma (Rhizoma Cimicifugae) 10g
Chaihu (Radix Bupleuri) 10g
Yedanshen (Radix Salviae Miltiorrhizae) 30g
Xianlingpi (Herba Epimedii) 10g
Mutong (Caulis Akebiae) 10g
Baihuasheshecao (Herba Hedyotis) 60g
Banzhilian (Herba Scutellariae Barbatae) 60g

All these medicinals should be decocted with water for oral administration. Six doses should be taken.

On July 15, 2012, he came to my clinic for the eighth time. He said that though he was hospitalized in the First Hospital of Shanxi Medical University, the medical insurance of critical illness actually should be handled in the Shanxi Provincial Cancer Hospital, so he went there to handle related formalities on July 11. He also took a PSA examination in the hospital, reporting the following: TPSA: 0.8µg/ml, FPSA: 0.01µg/ml. The two indicators fell into the normal value range (TPSA: 0.000~4.000µg/ml, FPSA: 0.000~1.000µg/ml). According to western medical criteria, when two indicators are both lower than 0.2µg/ml, no follow-up treatment is needed, that is to say, the patient should not be diagnosed as having the prostate cancer any more.

He called the director of urology department of the First Hospital of Shanxi Medical University who was responsible for his treatment to tell him about the result, but the director did not believe it, regarding it as a mistake in the examination result.

The expert of Shanxi Provincial Cancer Hospital insisted that the result was correct, saying that the hospital is specialized in the diagnosis and treatment of cancer and operates that examination every day.

Moreover, the patient himself also considered that the examination result given by Shanxi Provincial Cancer Hospital was correct, because he felt as good as a healthy person both physically and mentally.

Up till then, the patient had come to my clinic for eight times and taken formulas of more than 30 doses. He was completely cured both on the perspective of modern medicine and according to the modern scientific instrument testing.

However, I still persuaded the patient that he suffered such a severe disease that he should constantly be very careful and take the formula continuously for enhancement.

I asked him whether he had some discomfort. He told me that sometimes his face turned red and he begun to sweat all of a sudden as before. He said that although his legs were not painful, his left leg was still heavy. His pulses beat 7 times in a cycle of breath, his right pulse at all three positions was normal, and his left pulse was still weak at Cun and Guan positions. I followed the previous formula and slightly added some medicinals for stopping sweating:

Huangqi (Radix Astragali seu Hedysari) 60g
Yedangshen (Radix Codonopsis) 60g
Chenpi (Pericarpium Citri Tangerinae) 10g
Gancao (Radix Glycyrrhizae) 10g
Shanyurou (Fructus Corni) 30g
Shenglonggu (Os Draconis) 30g
Shengmuli (Concha Ostreae) 30g
Huashifen (Pulvistalci) 30g
Mahuanggen (Radix Ephedrae) 10g
Chuanniuxi (Radix Cyathulae) 30g
Dongkuiguo (Fructus Malvae) 20g
Diyu (Radix Sanguisorbae) 30g
Shengma (Rhizoma Cimicifugae) 6g
Chaihu (Radix Bupleuri) 10g
Yedanshen (Radix Salviae Miltiorrhizae) 30g
Xianlingpi (Herba Epimedii) 10g
Mutong (Caulis Akebiae) 10g

Baihuasheshecao (Herba Hedyotis) 60g
Banzhilian (Herba Scutellariae Barbatae) 60g

All these medicinals should be decocted with water for oral administration. Six doses should be taken.

On July 15, 2012, the ninth visit. He told me that he had no profuse perspiration problem any more, and the heavy and exhausted sensations of his left leg had alleviated. Therefore, based on the former prescription, I took out *Shanyurou (Fructus Corni)*, *Shenglonggu (Os Draconis)*, *Shengmuli (Concha Ostreae)*, and *Mahuanggen (Radix Ephedrae)*, which were for stopping sweating, and added 15g of *Shihu (Herba Dendrobii)*, 10g of *Dangguiwei (Radix Angelicae Sinensis (Tail))*, 30g of *Cheqianzi (Semen Plantaginis)*, and also changed the dosage of *Banzhilian (Herba Scutellariae Barbatae)* to 30g. This time, I asked him to take 10 doses of the formula.

I left for Weihai, Shandong Province from Taiyuan the next day. Mr Fang called me from Taiyuan, saying that he took the PSA examination a second time in the First Hospital of Shanxi Medical University after taking those medicinals, and the result was as follows: TPSA: 0.114μg/ml, FPSA: 0.0023μg/ml, which indicated that he was much better than before. Not until this time did the doctor in that hospital completely believe the test result from the cancer hospital. And the latest result turned out to be even better than the former one.

I asked whether he still felt ill or not, and the patient told me that everything was fine except for the exhausted and heavy sensations still in his left calf.

I composed another formula for him on the phone for further treatment as consolidation.

Huangqi (Radix Astragali seu Hedysari) 60g
Yedangshen (Radix Codonopsis) 60g
Shengma (Rhizoma Cimicifugae) 10g
Chaihu (Radix Bupleuri) 10g
Jiegeng (Radix Platycodi) 10g

Baizhu (Rhizoma Atractylodis Macrocephalae) 15g
Chenpi (Pericarpium Citri Tangerinae) 10g
Shihu (Herba Dendrobii) 15g
Chuanniuxi (Radix Cyathulae) 30g
Fangji (Radix Stephaniae Tetrandrae) 10g
Yedanshen (Radix Salviae Miltiorrhizae) 30g
Dongkuiguo (Fructus Malvae) 20g
Huashifen (Pulvistalci) 20g
Chishaoyao (Radix Paeoniae Rubra) 10g
Gancao (Radix Glycyrrhizae) 10g
Baihuasheshecao (Herba Hedyotis) 30g
Banzhilian (Herba Scutellariae Barbatae) 30g

All these medicinals should be decocted with water for oral administration. Ten doses should be taken.

My treatment, by then, for that patient with prostate cancer and bone metastases had been basically completed.

All of the above are original records for curing this disease. I just made a copy of them based on the fact, especially the test results of TPSA and FPSA that I totally had no idea of.

Some of you may wonder if I am an expert who specializes in treating cancer.

Of course not, I am just an ordinary doctor of TCM. What I know about cancer is that it is one of the most difficult medical problems in the world.

Someone then probably doubts that why I was able to cure such a severe cancer since I am not an expert in that area.

If I have to answer this question, I can, without any hesitation, say that I cure this disease based on my primary knowledge about syndrome differentiation and treatment of TCM. It is the knowledge of syndrome differentiation and treatment that enables me to handle difficult problems with great ease. That is why, in the view of common people, TCM is regarded as the medical science which is 'simple, convenient, inexpensive, and effective'.

Only TCM, the intangible science, can be regarded as a medical science that handles difficult problems with great ease.

What does 'handling difficult problems with great ease' actually mean? Taking this case as an example, we doctors of TCM have neither scientific knowledge of treating cancer nor any modern instruments. However, simply with feeling the pulse, composing the formula and the thinking pattern of syndrome differentiation and treatment, such a fatally severe disease was gradually cured by us. This is definitely 'handling difficult problems with great ease'.

Someone may therefore consider whether modern medicine as a comparison should be called 'handling simple problems with complex methods' or not?

In terms of this, in my opinion, some understandings about modern medicine shall also be explained.

For example, in the above case, considering the severity of prostate cancer, modern hospitals probably perform an operation of excision, followed by radiotherapy and chemotherapy, with plenty of imported medicines. Even the radical operation is not able to completely cure the disease. Most of the cancer patients have to continuously suffer from the spread of cancer cells.

A wave of patients suffering from treatments live in poverty because of their diseases but eventually lose their lives. What's more, it is increasingly difficult and expensive for patients to treat their diseases. The core problem is still the therapeutic effect.

Spending lots of money is not equal to curing diseases.

I accidentally read a report '*the Morbidity Rate of Prostate Cancer in China Rises Rapidly*' by Wáng Xiǎodōng (王晓冬) from *Zhongguo Yiyao Bao* (a Chinese newspaper about pharmaceuticals) published on 21 April, 2009. The report cited the words of Yè Dìngwěi (叶定伟), a professor of Fudan University Shanghai Cancer Center that, '[…] in Shanghai, for example, the morbidity rate of prostate cancer has ranked first among all cancers of the urogenital system. According to the statistics of cancer in Shanghai in 2004, the morbidity rate of prostate cancer ranked fifth among male cancers in Shanghai, while it accounted for the largest part (40%) in cancers of the urogenital system with its onset age decreasing gradually as other cancers.'

The treatment of cancer is a recognized medical problem. The efforts that modern medicine has spared to study it are countless.

During the fourth Plenary Session of the Tenth National People's Congress, Wáng Yǒngyán (王永炎) (a member of the Standing Committee of the National People's Congress, academician of Chinese Academy of Engineering, honorary president of China Academy of Chinese Medical Sciences, vice president of China Association of Chinese Medicine, and professor) said through an interview that according to a report on the studies of cancer in the last 30 years published in the third issue of *Fortune* in 2004, the studies cost $20 billion, over 1.5 million papers were published, and thousands of lead compounds were selected, but only little effect was achieved. People who did that research admitted that no substantial progress was made and therefore considered that they should change their ideas to learn from eastern culture about the harmony between man and nature as well as personalized diagnosis and treatment experience.

As the birthplace of Western Medicine, the West, including America, the country with the most developed science and technology as well as economy, has faced a large economic cost on the study of cancer, let alone numerous lives that were sacrificed for this, before a conclusion was drawn 'that the road is blocked ahead'.

Not until faced with this ruthless fact did they start to rethink, and they summarized TCM as the medical science which is harmonious with nature and possesses the experience of personalized diagnosis and treatment.

This is foreigners' understanding of TCM, which in us common people's words, in a more straightforward way, is 'simple, convenient, inexpensive, and effective'.

Why can TCM handle difficult problems with great ease? The reason is that TCM is a scientific medicine emphasizing on the entirety. As long as the balance between yin and yang in one's body is well-adjusted through syndrome differentiation and treatment, cells and molecules would metabolize in a normal way automatically like 'domino effect'.

If, however, people only concentrate on studying cancer cells with high-tech methods, it is ineffective even though thousands of lead compounds are selected.

In terms of the treatment of cancer, modern medicine, though applying high technology, is on the wrong track, which has got deeply trapped into 'complex philosophy'. If modern medicine is regarded as handling easy problems with complex method, the 'complex method' is indeed complex, which is equal to 'expensive medical bills and difficult access to quality medical services'. This is what WHO once said that modern medicine has been 'on the brink of affordance', which in economics is 'health care crisis'.

With the highly development pace of science in the 21st century, it is western countries that should send people to China to 'eliminate their illiteracy' of TCM, an intangible science, instead of us sending people with doctorate of TCM to western countries to study modern medicine. After all, they lack knowledge of TCM.

It is disappointing that the westernization of TCM has dominated the TCM circle in China, the birthplace of TCM.

I neither know how much research funding those experts who propagandize the modernization and scientification of TCM have received, nor how many of them have read some of 1.5 million papers on the study of cancer by America. I notice, however, as long as they find one or several 'lead compounds', they would be praised and advocated as being outstanding and successful. It seems that only in this way can the ancient TCM find its development direction and get rid of traditional methods to make innovations.

As for patients' feelings and lives, they have already ignored.

We should not criticize Western Medicine doctors who have no idea about TCM, because what was learnt does not contain intangible science, i.e. no blame attached to innocents.

On the contrary, a TCM doctor fails to study TCM intensively but pays much attention on learning Western Medicine. Could it happen that with such little knowledge of Western Medicine you can cure the disease that the true Western Medicine doctors are not able to? If a patient comes and requests you to feel his pulse and compose a formula, are you going to ask them for many examinations and tests, or will you prescribe some irrelevant Chinese medicinals and some western medicines and call it 'the combination of TCM and Western Medicine'? If you do so, you will not only betray your vow of 'life-saving', but also delay the treatment of the disease. Such act cannot be treated as ignorant, but as intentional and guilty!

Provided you are a senior TCM doctor, if you do not teach the students the scientific attribute of TCM, but propagandize the failure of adapting to the society due to unawareness of Western Medicine, much western medical knowledge will misguide the students who were supposed to master the real skills of TCM and such students will become the 'gravediggers of TCM'. This is misleading the youth and having negative effect on the development of TCM, which is very guilty.

Here, I want to say more about the patient Mr Fang.

Mr Fang and I were classmates of the School of Foreign Languages of Shanxi University at the same period. During the 'Cultural Revolution', he was the leader of the faction which opposed Liú Méi (刘梅), the principal, while I was the 'initiator' of the faction that supported the principal. At that time, we were 'enemies'. However, after I was recalled to Taiyuan in 1984, we became next-door neighbors. What a fate.

Nonetheless, time flies, we became close friends instead of enemies, and he visited the principal even more frequently than I did.

Having retired, he went back to his hometown, Changzhou, Jiangsu Province, and we had lost contact for over 10 years since then.

This time he suddenly suffered from prostate cancer and was hospitalized in the First Hospital of Shanxi Medical University. Since the cancer reached an advanced stage, no operation would be effective. Having heard of this bad news, many classmates visited him, a long-lost friend, but they were not as happy as in the old times, only with bitter smiles and asking him to take care.

When they left the ward, they sighed, saying, "this will be the last time we see Fang."

Coincidently, I just returned to Taiyuan at that time, and after being informed of his condition, I visited him immediately, having the same feeling as other classmates.

For many times, I called my wife in Beijing and told her my sorrow after I visited him. Seeing that a happy family was going to be hopeless instantly, my wife felt very sad too.

It was unexpected that Mr Fang's son was admitted to the same hospital at the same time. A few years ago, due to splenomegaly, he had his spleen excised in this hospital. However, the spleen is not an independent organ in the body, it is a part of the digestive system similar as liver.

Therefore, after his spleen was excised, the liver had to bear heavier loads. Several years later, he suffered from the cirrhosis of liver and ascites, so he had to have his liver treated. However, the cirrhosis of liver failed to be completely cured, and even became more and more serious.

Thus, the hospital told them that the liver must be transplanted, which was the only hope. At that time, both Mr Fang and his son received treatment in the hospital and prepared for the liver transplantation. What a hapless family.

Mrs Fang was one of my schoolmates in the School of Chemistry of Shanxi University. She was a very outgoing person. Although she had retired, she danced and sang in Yingze Garden (Taiyuan) with the aged every day, even more energetic than the young.

When Mrs Fang met me, she was very grieved and murmured, "What a miserable life I have."

Surprisingly, Mr Fang came to me and asked me to compose formulas, carrying a bloody urine collection bag. I knew he came to me as a last resort, because he hadn't believed in TCM.

However, after receiving the treatment for the first time, he was confident in TCM due to positive effects, so that he always took Chinese medicinals to prevent the relapse after he was clinically cured. At this time, he not only believed in TCM, but was also 'addicted to' taking TCM decoctions.

He did accept my suggestions, and started to eat more vegetables, but sometimes still could not help eating some meat and fish. Afterwards, his son would come to me and asked me to 'teach his father a lesson'. Now his diet is 'monitored' by all his family members. It is more difficult to 'keep a diet' than to 'do some exercise'. At present, Fang's son does not intend to transplant his liver, but sticks to taking TCM decoctions I prescribe. He is only 30 years old with a sallow and dark face and no energy. Fortunately, he feels better and better now after taking those medicinals.

TCM, as an intangible science, is invisible to people. Only therapeutic effects are most trustworthy. Therefore, TCM masters always emphasize therapeutic effects. TCM has been inherited for thousands of years due to its therapeutic effects. It is the therapeutic effects instead of theories that TCM depends on to gain trust of and to conquer the world.

TCM is an intangible science, while Western Medicine is a tangible one

— The discussion on the differences between the theories of TCM and Western Medicine by taking the example of curing complete deep venous thrombosis (DVT) of both lower extremities

The patient was a 27-year-old female named Guo, working as a teacher in North University of China. She lived at Wuyi Road, Xinghualing District, Taiyuan, Shanxi Province.

I was invited to attend to the patient at her home on June 1, 2009. Upon arrival, I got the information that she was just discharged from the hematology department of the Second Hospital Affiliated to Shanxi Medical University. Patient Identification Number was 436702.

Primary discharge diagnosis: Complete deep venous thrombosis (DVT) of both lower extremities.

Secondary discharge diagnosis: Inferior vena cava (IVC) filter placement; Connective tissue disease (CTD); Sjogren's syndrome.

The patient was hospitalized at Linfen Municipal People's Hospital before being transferred to the Second Hospital Affiliated to Shanxi Medical University. She received the same diagnostic result in and out of the hospital.

The diagnosis was confirmed on May 12, 2009 after being hospitalized.

Here is her medical record: four months ago, the patient suffered postpartum hemorrhoea after cesarean delivery, and received treatment at

Linfen Municipal People's Hospital. After doctors prescribed coagulant medicines, the hemorrhoea was immediately prevented. One month later, however, the patient was unable to walk because of oedema and pain of both lower extremities. Therefore, she continued her medical treatment at that hospital and was diagnosed as deep venous thrombosis (DVT) of both lower extremities.

Two months later, she was transferred to the hematology department of the Second Hospital Affiliated to Shanxi Medical University, where she was hospitalized for 22 days.

What Western Medicine doctors had prescribed for her were as follows: low-molecular-weight heparin calcium, sodium chloride, urokinase, cefmetazole, buflomedil hydrochloride and sodium chloride, levofloxacin, warfarin, dexamethasone, series of antirheumatic and anticoagulant drugs and so on.

The patient told me that due to her legs, she was 'palsied' for about 3 months. Western Medicine doctors once told her that there was no effective therapy anymore, so she had to spend the rest of her life in bed.

Her mother's hair turned grey because of the worry. Her mother told me that if her daughter in such a young age had to be paralyzed for the rest of her life without any effective treatment, she herself did not have the courage to live anymore.

I was informed that the reason she could not move the legs was that her lower extremities and joints were too painful, swelling and heavy to lift up. What's worse, every time she tried to stand up, the lower extremities would become cyanotic and she was drenched in sweat due to the pain. However, the patient would feel better if she elevated the lower extremities when sleeping.

The pulse diagnosis showed that her pulses were deep, slippery and rapid, and the pulses at her Cun and Guan positions were weak under heavy pressure.

Deep pulse indicates the depression and sinking of qi.

Slippery and rapid pulse indicates dampness-heat.

Weak pulse under heavy pressure at Cun and Guan positions indicates the deficiency of both qi and blood.

Heavy sensation of the legs indicates the problem of dampness-heat is severe.

The sensation of swelling pain indicates the stagnation of qi and the stasis of blood, as the old saying goes, 'When there is pain, there is no free-flow.'

Based on comprehensive analysis of the pulse and the symptoms, she was diagnosed with the syndromes of qi deficiency resulting in sinking, qi stagnation and blood stasis, and dampness-heat obstructing qi movement.

The principle of treatment should primarily focus on tonifying and elevating qi, and secondarily focus on clearing heat and draining dampness, activating blood and resolving stasis.

Here were the ingredients of the formula:

Huangqi (Radix Astragali seu Hedysari) 60g
Dangshen (Radix Codonopsis) 30g
Baizhu (Rhizoma Atractylodis Macrocephalae) 10g
Chenpi (Pericarpium Citri Tangerinae) 6g
Shengma (Rhizoma Cimicifugae) 10g
Chaihu (Radix Bupleuri) 15g
Dangguishen (Radix Angelicae sinensis) 20g
Cangzhu (Rhizoma Atractylodis) 15g
Huangbai (Cortex Phellodendri) 12g
Chuanniuxi (Radix Cyathulae) 15g
Yiyiren (Semen Coicis) 30g
Shihu (Herba Dendrobii) 10g
Fuling (Poria) 15g
Xiangfu (Rhizoma Cyperi) 15g
Chishaoyao (Radix Paeoniae Rubra) 15g
Mudanpi (Cortex Moutan Radicis) 15g
Mugua (Fructus Chaenomelis) 15g
Fangfeng (Radix Saposhnikoviae) 10g
Taoren (Semen Persicae) 10g
Guizhi (Ramulus Cinnamomi) 6g
Gancao (Radix Glycyrrhizae) 6g

All these ingredients should be decocted with water for oral administration.

The patient couldn't stand the swelling pain anymore in the legs at first. She decided to go to the hospital for intravenous therapy (with vaso-dilators and anticoagulants, so hospital always treated her in this way every time she felt painful. But it only worked for a short while).

Surprisingly, in the midnight after she took my medicinals, the pain was gone, so she did not need to go to hospital. She was so excited that without concerning about time she shouted repeatedly, "magical doctor!" The next day she was even able to walk slowly.

On June 8, the second visit. After taking 6 doses of the formula in a row, she told me that all the symptoms were improved apparently, which means that the formula I composed for her was effective. Therefore, I slightly altered the formula this time. I changed *Dangguishen* (*Radix Angelicae sinensis*) for *Dangguiwei* (*Radix Angelicae sinensis(tail)*) and added 10g of *Honghua* (*Flos Carthami*) to enhance the efficiency of acti-vating blood and resolving stasis. Adding 15g of *Qingpi* (*Pericarpium Citri Reticulatae Viride*) to enhance the efficiency of regulating qi, because the movement of blood is based on the movement of qi. Adding 15g of *Zexie* (*Rhizoma Alismatis*) to enhance the efficiency of promoting urination (water) and removing dampness (water). According to the TCM theory, blood and water originated from the same substance, if water can-not move, then blood will not move. Ten doses of the formula should be taken this time.

On June 20, I visited the patient for the third time. She could walk as normal but the lower extremities still appeared cyanotic and felt numb when she squatted. All indicators of the coagulation test were back to normal.

The examination showed that he had a red tongue with a slightly yel-low coating; her pulses were slightly deep beating 4 times in a cycle of breath, her pulses at Cun and Guan positions were slightly weak under pressure. Thus I slightly changed the former formula and the ingredients of the newer one were as follows:

Huangqi (*Radix Astragali seu Hedysari*) *60g*
Dangshen (*Radix Codonopsis*) *30g*
Baizhu (*Rhizoma Atractylodis Macrocephalae*) *10g*
Jiegeng (*Radix Platycodi*) *10g*
Chaihu (*Radix Bupleuri*) *10g*

Shengma (Rhizoma Cimicifugae) 10g
Zhimu (Rhizoma Anemarrhenae) 20g
Shihu (Herba Dendrobii) 15g
Yedanshen (Radix Salviae Miltiorrhizae) 30g
Mudanpi (Cortex Moutan Radicis) 20g
Chuanniuxi (Radix Cyathulae) 10g
Dangguiwei (Radix Angelicae sinensis(tail)) 15g
Chishaoyao (Radix Paeoniae Rubra) 15g
Taoren (Semen Persicae) 10g
Chuanxiong (Rhizoma Chuanxiong) 10g
Guizhi (Ramulus Cinnamomi) 10g
Qingpi (Pericarpium Citri Reticulatae Viride) 10g
Zexie (Rhizoma Alismatis) 10g
Honghua (Flos Carthami) 10g

Ten doses of the formula should be taken this time.

Meanwhile, I composed him another formula for fumigating and washing:

Haitongpi (Cortex Erythrinae) 15g
Weilingxian (Radix Clematidis) 15g
Xixiancao (Herba Siegesbeckiae) 15g
Honghua (Flos Carthami) 30g
Chuanxiong (Rhizoma Chuanxiong) 30g
Sanleng (Rhizoma Sparganii) 30g
Ezhu (Rhizoma Curcumae) 30g
Taoren (Semen Persicae) 30g
Chuanshanjia (Squama Manis, pangolin scales) 20g

The medicinals should be decocted with water for 15–20 minutes; the decoction should first be used to fumigate then to wash the lower extremities every morning and evening; 3 doses of the formula should be used to fumigate and wash.

Ten days later, the patient came to me, saying that everything, including the lower extremities, has been back to normal. On May 11, 2012, when I was writing this article, the patient visited me a second time and told me that she had no longer received any treatment from the hospital since taking my prescription.

I asked, "Has the filter been taken out?"

She answered: "Not yet".

"Why not", I wondered.

She said: "The doctors told me that this filter was a hi-tech device which was hard to be taken out. Otherwise, it would cost too much. Therefore, I have to keep it in my body."

All of the above is the whole process of curing deep venous thrombosis (DVT) of both lower extremities. This case should have been ended there; however I would like to take more time to share my experience with readers.

Firstly, to be honest, the first time I visited this patient, I took no glimpse at her medical record. All I did was composing the formula according to her pulse manifestation.

I was an authentic practitioner of TCM, so I ignored numerous medical records and various test reports provided by the patient. Even if I did read them, I could not understand a word of that. Moreover, even today, I still don't know how to use a computer or access the Internet, not to mention learning and understanding those test reports. I have devoted myself to ancient TCM books so much that I have become more and more ignorant of those modern stuff.

It was when I prepared for this article that I accidentally found these medical records left by the patient. I briefly read them and copied some vital reports in my article.

Why could I crack the hard nut without the support of any test reports?

It was because of the differences of medical science between TCM and Western Medicine instead of my own ability. Western Medicine, with its high technology, always focuses on the tangible aspect of man's body and illness while simple TCM dwells on the intangible aspect.

All in all, TCM is an intangible science, while Western Medicine is a tangible science. This is the boundary between TCM and Western Medicine.

Western Medicine, focusing on tangible aspects, deals with illness itself rather than finding the cause of the illness.

It is because the cause is intangible, hardly to be found through advanced scientific instruments. On the contrary, TCM dwells on intangible aspect, focusing on the cause of the illness. According to western philosophy, everything is born in a tangible way. Thus, Western Medicine spares more and more efforts to observe 'everything'. Through their observations, illness names, test statistics, and even the biochemical drugs have been updated several times. All for anti-diseases.

However, according to our philosophy, all tangible things come from intangible ones. Tangibility is the result while intangibility is the reason. That is why TCM emphasizes that 'superior doctor cares about the spirit', for the spirit is the primary reason. If the primary reason of intangibility (the cause of disease) could be solved, then the problem of tangibility (disease) would recover itself without being treated with.

Taking this case as an example, the cesarean operation caused uterus hemorrhage. To stop bleeding, doctors used coagulant, and it worked immediately.

As for uterus hemorrhage (metrorrhagia and metrostaxis in TCM), it was cured. However, thrombi were formed, blocking the vessels of lower extremities, which resulted in swelling pain. Western Medicine therefore diagnosed this as deep venous thrombosis (DVT) of both lower extremities.

In order to cure thrombi, doctors of Western Medicine used anticoagulant (thrombolytics) specifically, attempting to dissolve the thrombi, but it did not work as expected. Due to the fact that the thrombi remained inside the intravenous vessels of the lower extremities, though not very fatal, the patient was unable to walk. However, if any thrombus breaks off and migrates to the lung through the blood vessels, it will result in the pulmonary embolism, that is life-threatening.

To avoid the thrombus moving up with blood towards the lung, doctors implanted an umbrella-shaped filter in the vein at the root of the leg.

Being blocked by this filter, the thrombus could never move up. Therefore, there would be no life threatening danger.

What an advanced technology this is to implant a filter in such a narrow vein. However, it is even more difficult to take it out. As a result, she had no choice but to keep it in her body for the rest of her life.

This should be the last step for her treatment. No matter how complex it was, doctors saved her life though she had to lie in bed for the remaining lifetime due to the existing deep vein thrombus. Nevertheless, the more the thrombus aggregated, the more painful the patient's legs were. To release the pain, she had to receive infusion treatment of vasodilators and anticoagulants, which would help to widen the blood vessels and to alleviate pain temporarily.

Although the blood vessels are widened, they would still shrink to normal size. That is to say, every time when she feels swelling pain, she has to receive infusion treatment. Consequently, she would rely on treatment for the rest of her life. Such a treatment not only would bring her a miserable life, but also would have negative effect on her health.

Doctors in all modern hospitals follow the same way for treatment of lower extremity deep venous thrombosis. Since they all diagnose and treat blood diseases and thrombus depending on high-tech medical devices, I hold the view that Western Medicine is a tangible science.

Facing this tangible science, I, as a TCM doctor, regard myself as an illiterate, especially for blood diseases. But I do admit that Western Medicine is scientific, just like other people in this world do, for it is based on the modern science. I just think it would be more precise to define it as a tangible science.

On the contrary, what if the patient had asked for treatment from a TCM doctor? I am afraid that would be a very different situation.

According to the TCM theory, postpartum causes the deficiency syndrome and hemorrhage damages qi. When talking about the TCM principle of treating hemorrhage, doctors must use high dosages of medicinals for tonifying qi, such as *Huangqi* (*Radix Astragali*) and *Renshen* (*Radix Ginseng*). Because in the view of TCM, 'qi is the commander of blood', which means that if qi is sufficiently tonified, then the bleeding would be stopped due to the command of qi. If so, how could the thrombus appear?

Huangqi (*Radix Astragali*) and *Renshen* (*Radix Ginseng*) do not have the function of coagulating blood; even the use of hemostatic medicinals like *Zonglvtan* (*Pétiolus Trachycarpi Carbonisatus*) and *Xueyutan* (*Crinis Carbonisatus*), as far as I know, never results in forming the thrombus; especially, *Sanqi* (*Radix et Rhizoma Notoginseng*), as the hemostatic medicinal, has the advantage of stopping bleeding without stasis; since the function of these medicinals is only to stop bleeding but not to coagulate blood, how could they lead to thrombus?

Once the deep vein thrombus of lower limbs has been formed, Western Medicine doctors will use anticoagulants and begin to implant filters in case it affects the upper body. However, TCM doctors still emphasize on tonifying qi, not only ignoring the risk that the thrombus may move up to the lung, but also adding medicinals like *Chaihu* (*Radix Bupleuri*), *Shengma* (*Radix Bupleuri*), and *Jiegeng* (*Radix Platycodi*), etc. These medicinals are used to improve some qi-tonifying medicinals' function for elevating qi like *Huangqi* (*Radix Astragali*) and *Renshen* (*Radix Ginseng*), and then to promote the blood flowing upwards.

In Western Medicine doctors' perspective, this is definitely contrary to scientific theory. In their opinion, they implant the filter to avoid the thrombus moving upward, but the TCM doctors yet make it go upward. They may wonder whether the TCM doctors consider the risk of the thrombus moving upward to lungs and may also doubt our knowledge of general science.

Actually, they have worried too much. TCM has its own theory and method.

Let's think about the process of forming the thrombus, the blood stagnating downwards instead of moving upwards, then the thrombus appears. How could the thrombus appear if the blood flows normally?

Through elevating qi by large dosages of medicinals, the blood would move upwards, then the blood circulation would be normal. When the blood circulation is normal, the blood would not stagnate downward, which means, there would be no thrombus and the illness would be cured. Therefore, the patient can act as normal people, except that the high-tech filter is still kept in her body which needs to be concerned.

It is after the patient is able to walk as a normal person that we may regard it as completely cured. After all, normal people do not have thrombus.

Nonetheless, the TCM theory has mentioned many things about toni-fying qi and elevating qi and so on, which are too intangible to be explained specifically to others.

In comparison with Western Medicine, which only controls and alle-viates the disease instead of curing it, TCM can completely cure the disease but it is not considered as the real science. This is unreasonable. Therefore, I would rather call TCM an intangible science.

However, one academician of the Chinese Academy of Sciences who opposes TCM argued that, the theory of TCM had lagged behind, and the concepts of TCM such as, deficiency and excess, qi and blood, tonify and reduce, yin and yang, five elements, and so on, were incorrect and unsci-entific; what's worse, he even said far more irrelevantly that, "Marxism has already progressed with the times, but TCM refuses to do so."

This academician is much 'greater' than Isaac Newton. Newton, even as one of the greatest scientists, still told himself time after time, "the great ocean of truth lay all undiscovered before me", but this academician dares to judge what he does not know improperly.

Confucius once said: "When you know a thing, hold that you know it, and when you do not know a thing, allow that you do not know it — this is knowledge." If the academician had a bit of scientific spirit or a little knowledge of this famous saying, he would not make such a fool of himself.

In addition, I would like to question those experts of integrated Chinese and Western Medicine who often criticize that it would be so ridiculous for present TCM doctors to not understand the indicators of modern medical tests.

In terms of this, could you kindly tell me what Chinese medicinals should be prescribed to return the abnormal indicators back to normal?

Moreover, I would like to question experts of modern TCM education who keep on saying that to adapt to modern society, one must master modern medical knowledge. In terms of this, could I definitely cure a patient with a severe disease after I spare all my efforts to master the modern medical knowledge of blood disease, to understand all test reports, and to reach a high level attained by a hematologist? Western Medicine is tangible, while TCM is intangible. They are totally different.

Whether it is tangible is the line that separates Western Medicine and TCM, which leads to complete differences in the diagnosis, treatment and even the medical ideas for patients' physiology, pathology and diseases. They cannot be mixed up, otherwise it would cause confusion of understandings, thoughts and orientations, which would result in a situation of 'losing yourselves after listening too much' that makes people feel puzzled and has very negative effects.

It is just because TCM is an intangible science that the dispute about TCM has been increasingly heated from modern times after Western Medicine was introduced to China. If the theoretical system of TCM can be tested by instruments and examinations, there will not be any skeptical arguments of TCM.

People only know the truth that 'seeing is believing', but ignore the truth that 'seeing is not always believing'.

People only think that 'seeing is believing' is objective, but does not think 'seeing is not always believing' is also objective. Moreover, there are more illusions among what you see through your own eyes.

Those who are against TCM and who support westernizing TCM are not so much as ignorant of TCM as of the human life science. They all deny the scientific attribute of TCM in essence, the former directly denying it while the latter indirectly doing it. The common point they share is that they all set people's sufferings aside, and the latter one brings even more serious harm, because it leads the whole development process of TCM astray in the excuse of science, thus satisfying those people who are against TCM.

Manfred Porkert, the world-renowned sinologist, the TCM educationist and tenured professor of Ludwig Maximilian University of Munich, held the view that TCM so far is the most integral, most coherent and most accessible representative manifestation of Chinese Medicine, so he used abundant and existing materials to illustrate that Chinese Medicine provides the most useful patterns for all life sciences to establish the univocal characteristic of expression.

The U.S. Food and Drug Administration (FDA) (FDA guidelines) claimed in its document in 2001 (FDA Guidance) that Chinese medicine, like western mainstream medicine, has 'complete systems of theory and practice that have evolved independently from or parallel to allopathic (conventional) medicine' rather than a simple complementary medical product of mainstream medicine.

As far as I am concerned, it should be the most impartial comment from the west or even from the whole humankind.

I do not know whether those native-born Chinese who advocate scientification among the Chinese Medicine circle will feel ashamed of themselves when hearing this.

Although I have cured this patient with DVT of lower extremities, I have no idea of the blood disease of modern medicine. I do not know when there exists such a disease name in modern medicine; but for the patient I treated, I do know the disease that she suffered from is a consequence of mistreatment by modern medicine or modern science.

What makes me think of this? This disease appeared after postpartum hemorrhage (PPH). TCM calls it metrorrhagia and metrostaxis; sudden and profuse uterine bleeding is called metrorrhagia; gradual uterine bleeding with moderate amount of blood is called metrostaxis. In a word, stop bleeding as soon as possible is the common medical principle both TCM and Western Medicine share. However, despite their same purpose, their specific treatment is dramatically different.

This patient's bleeding was due to the qi deficiency being unable to control blood. In the view of TCM, qi is the commander of blood and more bleeding will definitely have a bad effect on qi, for blood is the mother (source) of qi, and disorder of mother-organ would affect child-organ. Thus the more the patient bleeds, the less qi the patient has. At this moment, more *Huangqi* (*Radix Astragali*) and *Renshen* (*Radix Ginseng*) were needed to tonify qi. When qi is sufficient, it will command the blood, which means the bleeding will be stopped and the blood will normally circulate in the vessels. Also, *Zonglvtan* (*Petiolus Trachycarpi Carbonisatus*), *Xueyutan* (*Crinis Carbonisatus*), and other hemostatic medicinals could be added to help qi-tonifying medicinals stop bleeding faster. This is the course of curing this case, nothing more. Though tangible bleeding could be observed, people should treat the intangible qi which causes the bleeding, and then the bleeding would be stopped. That is so called syndrome differentiation and treatment.

Hemostasis in TCM is just to stop bleeding without stasis; it is different from the therapeutic method of blood coagulation in Western Medicine. Blood coagulation is to coagulate the blood into static blood, which refers to the thrombus in blood vessels inspected by modern medicine.

During my career life, I have cured numerous patients with different diseases, but never witnessed a patient suffering from the thrombosis caused by hemostasis in TCM.

In terms of Western Medicine doctors, they know nothing about the intangible science, so they can only see the tangible side of the disease. Actually, it is impossible for them to change their thinking patterns, because there is not any statement of syndrome differentiation in Western Medicine world. Western Medicine doctors will not waste their time on considering the reason of hemorrhage, they will never consider the invisible stuff like deficiency and excess; instead, they will use coagulants regardless of the reason. As long as they use it, the bleeding will be controlled.

Coagulant works immediately. Once used, it will show its positive effect, and uterine hemorrhage is treated then. Though cured, blood coagulation and hemostasis in TCM are quite different. Hemostasis just means stop bleeding, yet blood coagulation means coagulating the blood. Once the blood is coagulated, there must be blood clots, named static blood in terms of TCM and thrombus in Western Medicine. This blood clot is very tiny, so Western Medicine doctors can only see it via the instrument, but TCM doctors have already been aware of its existence. Because they understand that pain comes from the stagnation, and the stagnation comes from the static blood.

Then why does this thrombus stay in the lower limbs rather than the upper limbs? It is caused by qi deficiency. Qi is the driving force for blood circulation. Qi deficiency syndrome is first manifested as qi being lack of driving force for the blood, which is responsible for promoting the blood to move upwards. Once it fails, the blood will stay below and not move to the upper limbs, so the incidence of upper extremity deep vein thrombosis is far less than the lower one.

But why does it stay in the deep vein of lower limbs? Because the arterial blood flows quickly, and the fast-flowed blood will not be coagulated, there is no thrombus naturally.

Nevertheless, the venous blood does not flow as quick as the arterial blood does. The stagnant blood is the easiest one to be coagulated; the deeper the vein is, the narrower the blood vessel is; the slower it flows in the narrower vessels, the easier it is going to be coagulated. At that time, the thrombus will be formed and then DVT will appear. All deep veins were blocked by thrombi, so adding a word 'complete' in this case. It means that the disease was severe. Therefore, after her postpartum haemorrhage being cured, the patient suffered DVT of both lower limbs, which is an incurable disease in Western Medicine. Since the thrombi had formed, it was useless to use anticoagulants when the blood had already been coagulated, and then the doctor had no other choice but only to use vasodilator to ease the swelling pain temporarily.

In order to prevent thrombi from moving upwards and save her life, the doctor had to place a sophisticated filter in the vein at the end of her legs. There would be no further treatment in the view of Western Medicine, and then there would be a word 'recovery' written on the patient's hospital discharge report. However, even though the patient had been cured according to scientific evidence, the patient had to go to the hospital to get vasodilator when she couldn't bear the pain and this would be a lifetime treatment.

In contrast to Western Medicine who fears that it will threaten life when the thrombus moves upwards, TCM holds that the patient should not only be greatly tonifying qi, but also be prescribed qi-elevating medicinal like *Chaihu* (*Radix Bupleuri*) and *Shengma* (*Rhizoma Cimicifugae*) and other medicinals for clearing heat and draining dampness, activating blood and resolving stasis to promote the blood moving upwards.

Don't TCM doctors fear that it would cause pulmonary embolism? Of course, I am afraid, and I am even terrified. However, after greatly tonifying and promoting qi, the stagnant blood would be commanded by intangible qi, and thrombi would disappear when the blood of lower limbs could flow upwards. Therefore, the patient would walk as a normal person after taking this formula. This time, we can exactly say that she has been cured.

Turning an ill person (disorder of qi and blood circulation) into a healthy one (normal qi and blood circulation) who does not suffer DVT of lower extremities, is the scientific basis of TCM and also the reason why I, as an ordinary TCM doctor, who knows nothing of modern blood disease, can cure this modern incurable disease.

Afterwards, I've heard several more similar cases of DVT of lower extremities which cannot be cured by modern medicine.

I, with great sympathy, was informed that such kind of diseases has been on an increasing trend. Through the treatment and analysis of this disease, I consider we all should understand that this new disease appears after the invention of the powerful coagulant by modern medicine! However, who can work out the number of diseases caused by abuse of antibiotics, hormones, operations and even vitamins?

It is valuable of curing a coronary artery disease patient without the heart stent implantation

— Discussing that TCM cures the patient who is ill, while Western Medicine cures the disease of the patient by taking the example of curing coronary artery disease

On January 29, 2003, Mr Chen, deputy director of the local police station in one district of Taiyuan, Shanxi Province, rushed to my clinic, saying that his father was too ill to come here by himself so that he invited me to treat his father at home.

Upon arriving at his home, I just saw his father lie in bed like a walking skeleton with a pale face. Eyes slightly closed and breathing low, he was so weak that he could hardly speak clearly. He moaned to me about his illness.

This patient, Mr. Chen, was 69 years old and was born in Zhengding County, Hebei Province. He engaged in farming in the village throughout his life.

Several years ago, he had already realized he had a feeling of tightness and pain in his chest sometimes, but he did not care it too much in the early time. Afterwards, that kind of feeling had been annually aggravated and he scarcely did any job gradually. More than ten days ago, the pain in his chest, just like getting an electric shock, was so terrible and extended to his back, and he could not bear it anymore, so he asked his second son working in Shijiazhuang, Hebei Province to arrange for him to have a cardiography in the First Hospital of Hebei Medical University.

The medical test showed that the coronary artery in his heart was quite narrow, and the percentage of obstructions was nearly 70% and 80% respectively in two areas. What is worse, the blood vessel had already shrunk to some extent with severely insufficient blood supply, so two stents had to be implanted into his body.

The chief doctor however said that there might be a certain risk to implant stents because the blocked area just lied in the coronary arterial intersection. In addition, one stent cost RMB 80,000 at that time. The patient was a farmer all his life, so he was unable to pay for the high operation cost and finally had to only receive the conservative treatment.

What can be seen as the conservative treatment? Of course, they had no other choices but to find a TCM doctor. That is why the deputy director thought of me and specially took his father to Taiyuan from his hometown.

After telling the whole event, the deputy director continued to say that besides the feeling of tightness and pain in the chest, his father felt general weakness and could not move. Once he moved, he would excessively sweat, feel dizzy, flustered and short of breath, as well as constantly choke and cough, having to lean on the wall to walk his way when going to the toilet.

Then, he showed me his father's hands and said: "Look, his hands tremble so much that he could not wash his own face but has to be washed by me every day."

"My father also has another stubborn problem for 30 years: he has lower abdomen pain and diarrhea at five in the morning every day", he said.

I felt his pulse very carefully. He had an extremely deep, slow, thready, and weak pulse on both hands. His pulse sometimes beat slow with occasional and irregular intermittence, sometimes beat slow with regular and longer intermittence. His tongue was dark-purple with a white coating. His pulse and tongue manifestations showed that he suffered yang deficiency and the deficiency-cold of spleen-kidney. That's the reason of the stasis and obstruction of his heart-vessel, and the stasis and obstruction lead to his pain. It is quite similar to the case recorded in the

Synopsis of the Golden Chamber (*Jīn kuì yào luè*, 金匮要略), 'chest impediment, can be manifested as heart pain and short of breath.'

According to his pulse and symptoms, the treatment should primarily focus on tonifying qi and warming yang, regulating qi and dissipating mass, activating blood and dredging collateral, and secondarily focus on nourishing yin and blood, astringing lunge and recovering vessel.

Here were the ingredients of the formula:

Huangqi (*Radix Astragali*) *30g*
Dangshen (*Radix Codonopsis*) *20g*
Fuzi (*Radix Aconiti Lateralis Praeparata*) *15g*
Gualou (*Fructus Trichosanthis*) *30g*
Xiebai (*Bulbus Allii Macrostemi*) *20g*
Guizhi (*Bulbus Allii Macrostemi*) *10g*
Chuanxiong (*Bulbus Allii Macrostemi*) *15g*
Yedanshen (*Radix Salviae Miltiorrhizae*) *20g*
Honghua (*Flos Carthami*) *10g*
Jiangxiang (*Lignum Dalbergiae Odoriferae*) *10g*
Xiangfu (*Rhizoma Cyperi Preparata*) *10g*
Fuling (*Poria*) *10g*
Xianlingpi (*Herba Epimedii*) *10g*
Maidong (*Radix Ophiopogonis*) *10g*
Wuweizi (*Fructus Schisandrae*) *10g*
Shuizhi (*Hirudo*) *10g*
Dilong (*Lumbricus*) *10g*
Gancao Zhi (*Radix Glycyrrhizae Preparata*) *10g*
Wugong (*Scolopendra*) *5g*
Shengjiang (*Rhizoma Zingiberis Recens*) *3 slices*
Dazao (*Fructus Jujubae*) *30g*

All these medicinals should be decocted with water for oral administration. One dose for one day.

Ten days later, the father, accompanied by his son, came to my clinic. He told me that the pain in his chest was greatly relieved after taking the medicinals and he was much more comfortable. His pulse was a bit stronger and much better than before, though sometimes it still beat slow with occasional and irregular intermittence, and sometimes it beat slow with regular and longer intermittence. The formula was not changed after that, except for increasing the dosage of *Dangshen* (*Radix Codonopsis*) to 30 grams. I told him that he should continue taking this formula till his illness was completely cured.

Thereafter, the patient went home to Zhengding County of Hebei Province, and continued to take the formula. During that period, he called me for 7 times to tell me about the condition after taking these medicinals. I did not change the prescription except taking out *Fuzi* (*Radix Aconiti Lateralis Praeparata*), and adding *Buguzhi* (*Fructus Psoraleae*), *Roudoukou* (*Semen Myristicae*), and *Wuzhuyu* (*Fructus Evodiae*) for warming and tonifying spleen-kidney, astringing intestines and stopping diarrhea.

On August 20, 2005, Mr. Chen took a special trip to my clinic together with his son from hometown. It was only two years and eight months, but he turned into such a different person that I could hardly recognize him.

I could only see his florid face, healthy body and his passion and power to talk.

He was very glad to say that he was even stronger than when in his youth so that he could do any kind of farm work. He not only went to the fair a few kilometers away from home but also helped the villagers to build the house. He was just like a healthy person to do daily work. Feeling his pulse, I found it was gentle in sensation, powerful in rebounding. Besides, he said that he would keep a record on the notebook after taking the formula and he had taken 340 doses of the formula.

He also told me that what surprised him most was not only that his coronary heart disease had been cured but also that the 30 years' stubborn disease of aching and cold stomach and dawn diarrhea had also been cured; in the past, he would easily catch a cold, but things had changed in these two years; in the past, he dared not eat any cold food, but now he could eat watermelon in summer.

The deputy director remembered that in his childhood, his father always let him step on his stomach because of the pain, which indicates how painful the patient suffered from this stubborn disease. He also said that the shank and feet of his father used to be very cold, but now it was better.

On August 6, 2012, Mr. Chen came to my clinic from Zhengding county to thank me with his family of five, saying that he was quite healthy and that I gave him the second life.

I asked him, "Haven't you done cardiography again to see whether there's any change?"

He told me that his children also persuaded him to do so. However, he had no discomfort and could energetically do the farm work in recent ten years; he said he was healthy and had no reason to do the cardiography. He needed not to experience that kind of pain; besides, it would take thousands of yuan to do the examination. He was delightful effusively and explained that he had been so strong since he took the medicinals for nearly ten years.

Taking another case as an example. On August 25, 2007, when I was at home in Beijing, I suddenly heard that the 67-year-old co-mother-in-law, Ms. Zheng, was seriously ill. Since I lived on the second floor in a building with no elevator, her children told me that she was so weak that she could not get upstairs and the patient would wait for me in her younger daughter's home on the fifth floor with an elevator. Therefore, my wife and I went there in a hurry.

Ms. Zheng used to be hospitalized in Chengde People's Hospital in Hebei Province due to angina, where she was diagnosed with old myocardial infarction. Since there was no positive effect by transfusing the blood-activating and stasis-eliminating medicines, the doctor suggested that she go to Beijing for heart stent implantation surgery.

On August 20, she arrived at the 304 Hospital of the PLA in Beijing to do colorized Ultrasound and was diagnosed as severe myocardial infarction that needed heart stent implantation. But the doctor there advised her to go to Qingdao Hospital or Beijing Anzhen Hospital to receive the surgery because those two hospitals were more authoritative in dealing with stent surgery.

As is known to all that it is the children that worry the most when the parents get sick. My son-in-law was the youngest son of the patient. His eldest sister just rushed in Beijing after hearing the situation. He with his two elder sisters talked about their mother's condition together to decide which hospital they should go to. They however after a long discussion, made an unexpected decision that they would ask me for TCM treatment of their mother instead of the surgery.

In what circumstances did they come to such a consensus?

In my opinion, they made that decision due to the following two reasons: firstly, since we became relatives by marriage, all their family members came to me for prescriptions when they were sick and fortunately they were all cured so that they did believe in my medical skills; secondly, my son-in-law witnessed how I cured the patient Mr. Chen, so he clearly knew that heart stent could relieve the pain for a short while, but Chinese medicinals were the effective solution to cure that disease. Relying on the above two reasons, they made such a decision.

It's not household affairs, but a matter of life and death. Therefore, even if we were the closest relatives, it was hard for her to give up those various modern standard hospitals in the capital city but to come to me for TCM treatment. Apparently, this was not just a simple treatment but she had to entrust her life to me.

In that situation, how could I not treat her seriously? Treating this illness was somehow similar to fire-fighting.

She told me that her angina attacked every ten minutes and that kind of pain lasted 1-2 minutes each time, which could be relieved by taking nitroglycerin. The pain was not fixed and was migratory, located everywhere around the heart area. Her hands were swollen and numb, chest felt oppressed. She felt so exhausted that she could hardly climb the stairs and was out of breath. During the night, she could not lie flat on her back and had frequent urination. Her average blood pressure was also high at night (160/70mmHg on average). Her pulse was deep, wiry, thready, and a bit rapid on both hands. Her tongue was slightly red with a thin white coating. According to what were manifested above, her symptoms belonged to the syndromes of chest-yang deficiency, stasis and obstruction of heart-vessel. These syndromes were caused by the deficiency and stagnation of qi.

The treatment should focus on tonifying and benefiting qi-blood, soothing liver and relieving depression, activating blood and resolving stasis, activating yang and dissipating mass.

The ingredients of the formula were as follows:

Huangqi (Radix Astragali) 60g
Dangshen (Radix Codonopsis) 60g

Gualou (Fructus Trichosanthis) 30g
Danshen (Radix Salviae Miltiorrhizae) 30g
Xianlingpi (Herba Epimedii) 15g
Xiebai (Bulbus Allii Macrostemi) 15g
Zhishi (Fructus Aurantii Immaturus) 10g
Guizhi (Ramulus Cinnamomi) 10g
Shengdihuang (Radix Rehmanniae) 30g
Zisugeng (Caulis Perillae) 10g
Bayuezha (Fructus Akebiae) 15g
Yujin (Radix Curcumae) 15g
Gancao Zhi (Radix Glycyrrhizae Preparata) 10g

All these medicinals should be decocted with water for oral administration, and 20 doses should be taken.

On October 12, 2007, she came to my clinic for the second visit. She told me that after taking the first dose of the formula, she passed gas frequently and felt that the frequency of angina attacks had greatly reduced, nearly once every 3–4 hours; after taking 15 doses, her attacks had completely gone and she had no feeling of swellness and numbness on her hands; what's more, she could lie flat on her back and had overcome the frequent urination at night; however, she still couldn't fall asleep until midnight; even when she had fallen asleep after midnight, her sleep time could not last more than 4 hours; though her exhausted feeling was much better than before, she was still out of breath and had aching and weakness sensation in her loin and knees when she climbed stairs; other uncomfortable feelings were dizziness, shedding tears, wandering mind, amnesia, and tinnitus; she also had chest oppression and palpitation sometimes. Her pulse was deep, thready, weak, and a bit wiry on both hands. Her tongue was not red, the coating was thin and white. All the manifestations showed that her qi-blood and yin-yang were still deficient, and her heart-spirit was harassed by up-floating yang.

This time, the treatment should primarily focus on tonifying qi-blood, activating yang and dissipating mass, activating blood and resolving stasis, subduing yang and returning fire to its origin, and secondarily focus on regulating qi movement, nourishing yin and moistening lung, relaxing bowels and removing stagnation.

Here were the ingredients of the formula:

Huangqi (Radix Astragali) 50g
Dangshen (Radix Codonopsis) 60g
Danggui (Radix Angelicae Sinensis) 20g
Cishi (Magnetitum) 60g
Danshen (Radix Salviae Miltiorrhizae) 30g
Xianlingpi (Herba Epimedii) 10g
Gualou (Fructus Trichosanthis) 30g
Xiebai (Bulbus Allii Macrostemi) 10g
Zhishi (Fructus Aurantii Immaturus) 10g
Wulingzhi 15g
Maidong (Radix Ophiopogonis) 15g
Wuweizi (Fructus Schisandrae) 10g
Baizhu (Rhizoma Atractylodis) 10g
Chaihu (Radix Bupleuri) 10g
Shengma (Rhizoma Cimicifugae) 10g
Yujin (Radix Curcumae) 10g
Fuzi (Radix Aconiti Lateralis Praeparata) 6g
Xiangfu (Rhizoma Cyperi Preparata) 10g
Dahuang (Radix et Rhizoma Rhei) 6g
Gancao Zhi (Radix Glycyrrhizae Preparata) 10g

All these medicinals should be decocted with water for oral administration, and 30 doses should be taken.

The third visit was on June 2, 2008, the patient said that she had a regular bowel movement after one dose of the formula and enjoyed a sound sleep at night, falling asleep at ten in the evening and waking up at six the next morning. The other symptoms were also eliminated after 5 doses. In addition, since she could not find me for the moment, she decided to continue the first two prescriptions which she thought highly of and took 83 doses in total.

She also excitedly told me that her blood pressure remained stable at 120/80 mmHg without dizziness or giddiness. Besides, her eyes were not always filled with tears and she had no hardness of hearing and tinnitus. Without shortness of breath anymore, she could climb to the fourth floor carrying a bag of 20 kg of flour on her shoulder. In addition, she would dance an hour and a half every evening without any feeling of exhaustion. She also attended the elderly performance team organized by the local community in Weihai and it was easy for her even to change 14 costumes during the show one night sometimes. She had no experience of angina attacks any more since taking the medicinals. She looked healthy. Therefore, I wondered why she came to me again.

She said that she had a fatty liver with the indicator of the blood fat higher than standard one for more than 3 mmol/L. Moreover, her fasting blood-glucose maintained at 7 to 8 mmol/L that was also higher than the standard level. Therefore, she asked me for another treatment.

According to her pulse and symptoms, I composed the formula for her which emphasized on regulating three energizers (upper, middle, and lower), and harmonizing the natures of medicinals.

On October 2, 2008, Ms. Zheng came to the clinic again because of the bitter taste and dry tongue recently, saying that her fasting blood-glucose level returned to the standard level after taking 20 doses of the formula prescribed last time.

Based on her pulse and symptoms, my treatment focused on nourishing yin and moistening dryness, harmonizing lesser yang. After taking the formula, she felt better.

Whenever the old have any discomfort, they should take Chinese medicinals to improve their physical conditions.

Since Ms. Zheng came for treatment five years ago till now, we made phone calls to each other several times and she has not relapsed so far. She once told me that she was busy doing the housework and taking care of her husband every day and also participating in the Guang Chang Wu (Chinese public square dance) together with other old people, as well as other entertainment performances.

On August 25, 2012, I called her again when I was writing this article and she said she was very healthy; she even had not shown any cardiac diseases when taking the regular medical check-ups in recent years.

The coronary heart disease, also being called atherosclerosis of coronary artery or ischemic heart disease, was named by modern medicine. It is regarded as 'the top-one killer' of human health due to its high mortality and morbidity rates.

Facing this 'top-one killer', with the progress of technology, the modern medicine created heart stent and bypass to clear the blocked cardiovascular areas immediately with an effective result in a very short time, which has received lots of applauses. Therefore, the fast spread of the stent surgery since its invention has made it everywhere on this earth.

Nevertheless, can this invention indicate that we human beings have already conquered this 'top-one killer' of human health? I do not think so.

A male friend of mine, Mr. Li, 67 years old, was implanted with a stent three years ago due to coronary heart disease and the chest pain disappeared at once after its implantation. However, he felt comfortable for just one month, and then he got chest congestion and heart pain, so he went to the hospital for a second time and was told that the other cardiovascular area was blocked, which required another stent implantation. He had no other choice but to receive that operation though he was very angry. Back and forth, he was implanted with ten stents within only three years. Finally, he died because of a heart attack, which was so depressing.

Why a patient with coronary heart disease who has already been implanted with stents or has had a heart bypass operation will relapse in only a month or two or up to a year or two? In the words of modern medicine experts, the main reason is that although the clinical symptoms of stenocardia caused by coronary heart disease can be improved and eliminated after stents or bypass surgery, the pathology of atherosclerosis and blood viscosity has not been changed. Therefore, when there are negative factors, the disease will reappear, which means a considerable number of patients will suffer stenocardia again and again. That's why modern medicine experts appeal that patients with coronary heart disease should take good care of themselves and should continue receiving treatments especially after stent-implantations or heart bypass operations, because the stent here can prevent this certain area from being obstructed but cannot prevent other areas from being blocked.

Briefly speaking, what Western Medicine treats is only the disease people suffer from. Western Medicine regards disease as the unhealthy part of the whole body. But human being is an organic whole body, not just a combination of parts. Specific to coronary heart disease, high-tech methods treat the obstructed cardiovascular area, which can be seen by cardiography or ultrasound scans and other advanced imaging technologies. However, Western Medicine doctors have no idea of the whole body. It is not caused by others, but simply by the limits of this medical system.

However, the idea of TCM is completely different from that of Western Medicine in treating diseases. Taking the above two cases as an example, I did not know which specific cardiovascular area was blocked, but what I concentrated on was treating the human body as a whole.

Heart, as the specific uncomfortable part of these patients, is not isolated from the whole body; it shares a close relationship with other organs, such as the liver, the spleen, the lung, the kidney, and even to qi, blood, yin and yang of the whole body; they are indispensable and constraining, so we should not only treat the heart regardless of the whole body.

When treating these two patients, the reason I added large dosages of medicinals for tonifying qi was that only through the command of qi can blood circulate to the heart, the brain, and the whole body; why I added medicinals for regulating qi was that only resolving the stagnation of qi can the blood stasis be resolved; adding medicinals for activating blood and dredging collaterals was to promote the therapeutic effect of tonifying and regulating qi and to relieve the pain caused by the stagnation of blood.

However, the reason of adding *Roudoukou* (*Semen Myristicae*), *Buguzhi* (*Fructus Psoraleae*), and *Wuzhuyu* (*Fructus Evodiae*) in the first case of Mr. Chen was to stop his diarrhea before dawn caused by the deficiency-cold of kidney. In the view of China's five elements and TCM, the kidney which controls the metabolism of water of the body is similar to water in properties; the heart, which governs blood of the body, is similar to fire in properties. Therefore, the deficiency-cold of kidney can lead to the discordance of water and fire. In other words, the deficiency-cold of kidney can cause the functional disturbance of heart governing blood, then the blood will stagnate in the vessels. The reason why adding yang-tonifying medicinals in these two cases was that the impairment of yin caused by the chronic illness will affect yang; adding yin-nourishing medicinals was based on the theory that, 'solitary yang failing to grow, solitary yin failing to increase.'

All in all, the choices of the medicinals, the formulas, and the dosages were all strictly based on the pulse and symptoms.

I could not say how brilliant my combination of medicinals (sovereign, minister, assistant, and guide) was, but what I could guarantee is that the general direction of my therapeutic thought was definitely right — keeping yin and yang in equilibrium. The theory of curing diseases also follows this thought. As a result, when a person's yin and yang are in equilibrium, how can he have stenocardia? These two stenocardia patients I discuss above both have taken more than 100 doses of the formulas. Quantity is important in leading to changes in quality.

Patient Chen and Zheng both suffered from severe heart attack not in a sudden situation but it developed gradually to the extent of implanting stents at last. Though it worked immediately after one dose of the formula, a long-term treatment should still be taken to make heart return to the 'normal state'. It is just like in time of war, people have to consolidate 'base areas' after securing them; otherwise, they will lose what they have just obtained. 'Seizing' takes a short period of time while 'consolidating' needs a longer one. Although this has no relation with TCM, they share the same principle. Otherwise, how can Mr. Chen, who has already been treated by TCM for more than ten years, energetically do a lot of farm work or how can Ms. Zheng still be physical agile five years later?

TCM regards symptoms as 'disease'

— The discussion on the differences between the concepts of disease in TCM and in Western Medicine by taking the example of curing a patient with a history of abdominal pain for 15 years

In 1984, I was transferred from Traditional Chinese Medicine Department of Shanxi Linfen People's Textile Factory Workers Hospital to Medicine & Hygiene Editing Sector of Shanxi People's Publishing House (renamed as Shanxi Science and Technology Press in 1985) as an editor. At that time, I met Mr. Zhao who was born in Nanyangdian Village, Guo County (now Yuanping County), Shanxi Province in 1928, 15 years older than me.

Mr. Zhao has a rough life. He suffered from the miserable era of Sino-Japanese War during his youth, experiencing the unexpected family calamity; he left the hometown at the age of 15 and had a terrible and homeless life, tasting the hardships in the world.

However, he, though without adequate food and clothing in an unhealthy life, has a very smart brain and an extraordinary retentive memory. In particular, he only studied English for several years at Taiyuan Young Men's Christian Association (YMCA) from 1974, but he could skillfully tell the English and Latin names of different medicines, which was even admired by graduates from English major.

Modern nutriology advocates that different food contains different vitamins and microelements, and that scientific eating habit can provide balanced nutrition for the human body. This scientific truth is really convincing.

However, there was not enough nutrition for Mr. Zhao during his adolescence. He always suffered from starvation and only ate bran for some years. In that situation, he still kept a smart mind and healthy body. He is 85 years old now and has a clear mind that helps him be familiar with TCM, *the Classic of Changes* (*Yì jīng*, 易经) and Western Medicine.

Mr. Zhao is not the only one that has built up a well-developed brain under the circumstance of lacking enough nutrition.

For example, Huining County was a nationally designated poor county in Gansu Province with 580 thousand people. However, there were 200 people receiving doctorate degrees, more than 1000 masters degree holders and 10000 bachelors degree holders from this poorest county from 1977 to 2005. Dating back to the Ming and Qing dynasties, there were over 20 Scholars and 113 provincial graduates, which made this place the nationally renowned township of scholars and doctors.

In particular, one modern nutritionist even claimed that one person should eat 40 kinds of vegetables daily to absorb enough vitamins needed by the human body.

Fàn Zhòngyān (范仲淹), the famous politician and literature figure in the Northern Song Dynasty, lived in a very poor situation in his youth that porridge was the only food he had every day, but his brain was quite well-developed. Not only did he have outstanding political achievements, but also had widespread poetries and poses, one of which was *Fan Wenzheng Collection* (*Fàn Wénzhèng gōng jí*, 范文正公集) that contained numerous wisdom words to enlighten and inspiring later generations.

How can the modern nutriology explain all these situations?

This slightly strays from the point. To return to the subject, I will introduce Mr. Zhao, the person inspired me most, to readers. He used to learn TCM from Zhāng Zǐlín (张子琳) (1894–1983), one of the most famous doctors in Shanxi Province at that time, and was Mr. Zhang's best student.

Mr. Zhao not only gave the clinical notes recorded during his follow-up clinic with Zhāng Zǐlín (张子琳) to me for my study, but also taught me Mr. Zhang's medical experience at his spare time.

Despite the fact that I have never met Zhāng Zǐlín (张子琳), thanks to Mr. Zhao, I can also be called the disciple of Mr. Zhang. Therefore, I always respected Mr. Zhao as my teacher and often visited him. Every time when talking about TCM, we would be so dedicated that we even forgot the time.

On September 29, 2008, I visited him at his home and he unintentionally said that his wife Ms. Wang (82 years old) had suffered the lower abdominal pain with nausea and vomiting for 15 years. There were no obvious abnormal findings except the gallstones after several B-ultrasonic examinations. As we all know, the gallstones may cause intense pain, but the pain position is in the upper-right side of the abdomen not the lower abdomen. Every examination reported that she was physically sound, but she still felt pain in her lower abdomen. This abdominal pain came and went not regularly; sometimes it occurred every 10 days, sometimes it occurred every 3–4 days; the interval time of next abdominal pain was no longer than half a month; the duration of pain sometimes took one hour, sometimes took a whole day; the abdominal pain could be accompanied by nausea and vomiting sometimes. She had taken a lot of western and Chinese medicines like Belladonna tablets, Vitamin B1, and Inflammation-Resolving Gall-Bladder-Excreting Tablet, etc., but none of them could take any effect.

The doctor also felt that this was strange, wondering why Ms. Wang's lower abdomen was in pain for so many years without any lesion or exact disease.

Mr. Zhao asked me to see her. I found that she had a red tongue with no coating, her pulse was wiry and huge on both hands. Her symptoms could be classified as the syndrome of liver depression and qi stagnation in TCM. In the view of China's five elements, liver is similar to wood in properties, and spleen is similar to earth in properties. According to the restriction among five elements, wood is able to restrict earth, especially when the liver (wood) is in the abnormal condition. Therefore, her lower abdominal pain, nausea, and vomit were caused by wood restricting earth due to liver depression, which resulted in the functional disturbance of ascending lucidity and descending turbidity of the spleen-stomach. Here were the ingredients of the formula:

Danggui (Radix Angelicae Sinensis) 20g
Baishao (Radix Paeoniae Alba) 20g
Baizhu (Rhizoma Atractylodis) 15g

Fuling (*Poria*) 20g
Chaihu (*Radix Bupleuri*) 15g
Xiangfu (*Rhizoma Cyperi*) 15g
Qingpi (*Pericarpium Citri Reticulatae Viride*) 20g
Yuanhu (*Rhizoma Corydalis*) 30g
Chuanlianzi (*Fructus Toosendan*) 15g
Qingbanxia (*Rhizoma Pinellase*) 15g
Chenpi (*Pericarpium Citri Reticulatae*) 10g
Gancao (*Radix Glycyrrhizae*) 10g
Bohe (*Herba Menthae*) 6g
Shengjiang (*Rhizoma Zingiberis Recens*) 3 slices

This formula was composed based on three classic formulas, *Xiaoyao San* (*Peripatetic Powder*), *Jinlingzi San* (*Toosendan Fruit Powder*), and *Erchen Tang* (*Decoction of Two Old Ingredients*). The treatment should focus on smoothing liver and regulating qi, harmonizing stomach and descending adverse qi, clearing and discharging liver-fire.

Mr. Zhao mentioned that his wife had always been in a deficiency condition and suggested me adding some qi-tonifying medicinals.

I said that the lower abdominal pain was caused by liver depression and qi stagnation, and qi-tonifying medicinal might exacerbate the stagnation of qi. That is the reason why our seniors said that 'all pain should not be treated by tonic'.

Mr. Zhao asked that whether the dosages of *Yuanhu* (*Rhizoma Corydalis*), *Qingpi* (*Pericarpium Citri Reticulatae Viride*) and *Baishao* (*Radix Paeoniae Alba*) in this formula were excessive, and would they consume qi?

I said that your wife's abdominal pain was a kind of chronic and serious illness, so only large dosages of medicinals for elimination could take it out; after the pain was cured, she could take tonic.

After taking four doses of the formula, her lower abdominal pain and vomit was relieved, but she felt tired and exhausted. Thus, Mr. Zhao let her wife keep taking *Xiyangshen* (*Radix Panacis Quinquefolii*) for two to three days, and then she recovered gradually.

This case can be regarded as the treatment which primarily focuses on elimination and secondarily focuses on tonification.

This lower abdominal pain never happened till Ms. Wang passed away two years later. While talking about it, Mr. Zhao still felt amazing that such a few doses of formula prescribed by me could cure that chronic disease. He even recorded this case in his book, and addressed me as 'Mr. Guo' respectively, but actually he should call me as 'Guo'. This is the clear evidence to show Mr. Zhao's modest personality.

The reason why I quote this case is mainly to illustrate that the same word of 'disease' has completely different meanings although it is used both in TCM and Western Medicine.

In Western Medicine, the disease must be diagnosed by using advanced instruments or laboratory detection to test tangible pathogenic 'factor', such as ulcer, inflammation, bacteria or virus infections. The disease names are very accurate, precise and appropriate, to fully embody the scientific attribute of Western Medicine.

If no pathogenic 'factor' can be found via the examinations, the disease is often called as the syndrome with certain probabilities, or called as sub-health, and so on.

Moreover, the disease may be named after a person who finds a group of symptoms, such as Kawasaki Disease. However, the authoritative study of modern medicine shows that scientific testing method in modern times is not a panacea, which still leaves 40% of diseases without known cause. In terms of this, Western Medicine has no appropriate 'remedy' medicines and TCM will play a role.

In contrast with Western Medicine, TCM names the diseases according to the body discomfort status including a variety of symptoms (such as headache, emesis and dizziness).

The reason why our ancestors created TCM is to solve the problems related to body discomfort. Therefore, in my opinion, TCM is the solution to medical symptoms, i.e. as long as there are symptoms, TCM will regard it as a 'disease'.

For example, Ms. Wang's lower abdominal pain is called as 'pain in lower abdomen' in TCM, which is quite unclear to some extent.

The disease names by TCM are not unclear on purpose, but because it is an intangible science.

The pathogenic 'factors' of this 'pain in lower abdomen' included liver depression and qi stagnation, functional disturbance of ascending lucidity and descending turbidity, which were so intangible that could not be detected by the modern scientific instruments.

In fact, even those diseases that have pathogenic 'factor' in modern medicine can be cured via relieving the symptoms in TCM.

After the physical discomforts (symptoms) disappear and yin-yang balance is restored, the human body returns to a healthy state of a healthy person. Will such a person have any pathogenic 'factor' as stated in Western Medicine?

The thinking of the development of integrating TCM and Western Medicine has been misled

— The discussion on the mistakes of the development of TCM in the past one hundred years by taking the example of curing aplastic anemia

Mr. Han, 56 years old, the director of a national bureau, was found to have hematologic disorder during the physical examination. On August 6, 2009, he went to Peking University People's Hospital for treatment. The test report showed that his blood platelets (PLT) were only $2.1 \times 10^9/L$ and he was diagnosed with 'aplastic anemia'.

At that time, the relevant specialist told him that he needed to inject 'cyclosporine' and the number of the blood platelets (PLT) would immediately increase then. The effect could maintain for a month, so he had to receive the injection once a month.

Mr. Han asked: "How long does the course of treatment last?"

"For a year", the doctor answered.

"Then what will happen after one year?" Han inquired.

"Renal failure, probably", the doctor replied.

Han continued to ask: "Would I die then?"

The doctor's answer was yes.

Han said: "I will refuse to take cyclosporine if this treatment could be effective for only one year."

"That may lead to death at any time", the doctor said.

Mr. Han frankly told his families his condition. All his family members were astonished, some of whom were Western Medicine doctors and even the director of a hospital. They got together trying to find out a method but failed.

Then Mrs. Han said firmly: "Since we could not figure out a good idea, I decided to ask Senior Guo for treatment."

All others were stunned, but could not come up with any better opinions.

Senior Guo mentioned by Mrs. Han was just me. She and my wife were both the intellectual youths sent down from Beijing to Xing County, Shanxi Province in 1968. In 1980s, Mr. and Mrs. Han worked in Shanxi provincial government first before being transferred back to Beijing. She then became the director of Beijing Municipal Commission for Economic Restructuring in a district. Because of her own experience, she quite believed in TCM.

During the time she was sent down to the countryside, she was in a coma due to serious illness once. Villagers thought she was dying, so they moved her to a cave dwelling particularly for the dead. At that time, there was a dying old man lying on a wooden board in the cave. The villagers probably found the old man and Mrs. Han still had the breath though their eyes were closed, so they awakened the old man and gave him a needle, showing him that Mrs. Han was still alive. Actually, this old man was a TCM doctor. He struggled to acupuncture Mrs. Han and then immediately died. Mrs. Han however survived.

Every time when Mrs. Han mentioned this, she always said with great emotion: "My life was saved by that dying TCM doctor!"

Mrs. Han was in poor health, so she always took Chinese medicinals prescribed by me if she was ill.

In 1994, her 78-year-old father-in-law suffering from cerebral thrombosis was hospitalized in the senior-official ward of the First Hospital of Shanxi Medical University. However, he was still in right hemiplegia and unable to move after the injection and transfusion for one month.

Mrs. Han invited me to treat him. By using three doses of *Buyang Huanwu Tang* (*Yang-Tonifying Five-Returning Decoction*), in which the dosage of *Huangqi* (*Radix Astragali*) was 150g, the patient could move, and then acted as an ordinary people after taking an extra ten doses of such decoction.

The daughter-in-law of Mrs. Han had failed to conceive for a long time after getting married. In 1998, through my treatment, she was pregnant in less than three months, and finally gave birth to a cute infant. The family was very pleased.

Through the practical experience for many years, she extraordinarily trusted TCM. Therefore, when her husband was suffering from aplastic anemia, she invited me to give the treatment without any hesitation.

On September 1, 2009, Mr. Han, accompanied by Mrs. Han came to my clinic for treatment.

Mr. Han said that he had been suffering from gastric ulcer for more than 20 years, with the symptoms of recurrent stomachache, severe pain after eating, diarrhea for 2–3 times a day, poor appetite, and distending pain in both sides of hypochondria. I found that he had a bluish yellow and dull complexion, a fatigued and weak body, a red tongue with a yellow and greasy coating, and a salty mouth. His left Guan pulse was deep, thready, and wiry, while the right Guan pulse was wiry and feeble.

All the symptoms manifested above showed that he suffered from spleen-kidney deficiency, coupled with wood (liver) restricted earth (spleen), which resulted in the failure of qi transformation, and the internal forming of dampness turbidity.

The treatment should focus on tonifying qi-blood, invigorating spleen-stomach, soothing liver qi, and removing dampness turbidity. Here were the ingredients of the formula:

Huangqi (Radix Astragali) 30g
Yedangshen (Radix Codonopsis) 20g
Chenpi (Pericarpium Citri Reticulatae) 10g
Banxia (Rhizoma Pinellase) 10g
Fuling (Poria) 15g
Chaihu (Radix Bupleuri) 10g
Chuanlianzi (Fructus Toosendan) 10g
Yuanhu (Rhizoma Corydalis) 15g
Zhishi (Fructus Aurantii Immaturus) 10g
Zhuru (Caulis Bambusae In Taeniam) 6g

Buguzhi (Fructus Psoraleae) 15g
Xiangfu (Rhizoma Cyperi) 10g
Gancao (Radix Glycyrrhizae) 10g

All these medicinals should be decocted with water for oral administration. Twenty doses should be taken.

The second visit was on October 11, 2009. He told me that his stomach pain was greatly reduced, appetite had increased, but he still had diarrhea. This time, the treatment focused on soothing liver and tonifying spleen, uplifting the middle qi, and astringing intestines. Here were the ingredients of the formula:

Huangqi (Radix Astragali) 30g
Yedangshen (Radix Codonopsis) 30g
Fangfeng (Radix Saposhnikoviae) 10g
Buguzhi (Fructus Psoraleae) 20g
Shengma (Rhizoma Cimicifugae) 10g
Shenqu (Massa Medicata Fermentata) 6g
Cangzhu (Rhizoma Atractylodis) 10g
Baizhu (Rhizoma Atractylodis Macrocephalae) 10g
Chaihu (Radix Bupleuri) 10g
Fuling (Poria) 15g
Baishao (Radix Paeoniae Alba) 15g
Kezi (Fructus Chebulae) 10g
Chenpi (Pericarpium Citri Reticulatae) 10g
Gancao (Radix Glycyrrhizae) 10g

All these medicinals should be decocted with water for oral administration. Ten doses should be taken.

The third visit was on October 24, 2009. His abdominal pain and diarrhea were relieved. His appetite had improved, though he still had a full sensation in his stomach occasionally. Through the examination, I found that he had a slight red tongue without a greasy coating; his right Guan pulse was deep, slippery, and huge, right Chi was weak, left Guan was wiry and thready. According to his pulse and symptoms, I continued using the same therapeutic method for tonifying the middle and replenishing qi. What's more, the therapeutic methods also included warming and tonifying spleen-kidney, clearing heat and draining dampness. Here were the ingredients of the formula this time:

Huangqi (Radix Astragali) 30g
Yedangshen (Radix Codonopsis) 30g
Cangzhu (Rhizoma Atractylodis) 15g
Baizhu (Rhizoma Atractylodis Macrocephalae) 15g
Chenpi (Pericarpium Citri Reticulatae) 6g
Shengma (Rhizoma Cimicifugae) 6g
Chaihu (Radix Bupleuri) 10g
Danggui (Radix Angelicae Sinensis) 20g
Fuling (Poria) 15g
Chuanpo (Cortex Maganoliae) 10g
Sharen (Fructus Amomi) 5g
Xianhecao (Herba Agrimoniae) 30g
Buguzhi (Fructus Psoraleae) 30g
Pugongying (Herba Taraxaci) 20g
Gancao (Radix Glycyrrhizae) 10g

All these medicinals should be decocted with water for oral administration. Twenty doses should be taken.

The fourth visit was on December 6, 2009. All symptoms continued improving except having a diarrhea at 4:00–5:00 every morning and having a slightly full sensation in stomach sometimes. I found that his pulse at right Guan position was a little slippery and huge; at right Chi position was still weak; at left Guan position was a little bit wiry. Therefore, I composed the formula this time basically based on the former formula except for adding some medicinals for warming kidney and spleen. Here were the ingredients of the formula:

Huangqi (Radix Astragali) 30g
Yedangshen (Radix Codonopsis) 30g

Baizhu (Rhizoma Atractylodis Macrocephalae) 15g
Fuling (Poria) 15g
Chenpi (Pericarpium Citri Reticulatae) 10g
Xianhecao (Herba Agrimoniae) 30g
Pugongying (Herba Taraxaci) 20g
Danshen (Radix Salviae Miltiorrhizae) 20g
Fangfeng (Radix Saposhnikoviae) 15g
Baishao (Radix Paeoniae Alba) 15g
Buguzhi (Fructus Psoraleae) 30g
Roudoukou (Semen Myristicae) 5g
Wuweizi (Fructus Schisandrae) 6g
Wuzhuyu (Fructus Evodiae) 6g
Chuanlianzi (Fructus Toosendan) 10g
Wuyao (Radix Linderae) 10g
Gancao (Radix Glycyrrhizae) 10g

All these medicinals should be decocted with water for oral administration. Twenty doses should be taken.

The Fifth visit was on January 26, 2010. All symptoms he manifested before were completely relieved, and both his mental and physical conditions were back to normal. I asked him to take extra 15 doses of the formula for strengthening his health.

On April 2, 2010, Mr. Han came from Beijing to Taiyuan specially for my prescription, and showed me the lab report given by the Hematology department of Shanxi Coal Hospital which manifested that his blood platelets (PLT) had risen to 8.5×10^9/L. He then took me to meet with the director of the hematology department.

The director said that though the number of blood platelets (PLT) of Mr. Han in this examination was still not standard, his aplastic anemia could be identified as being cured in theory. The director also expressed his surprise at the magical effect of TCM, asking, "Which Chinese medicinal did you use to let the number of platelets increase?"

I said: "The concepts of treatment in TCM and Western Medicine treatment are quite different. No matter what disease it is called in Western Medicine, the TCM doctors only know to adjust the balance of yin-yang in one's body according to the patient's pulse and symptoms, making him recover from the discomfort state to the normal state as a healthy person. A healthy body of course has the standard number of platelets."

She nodded her head with a confused expression, and said: "Miracle!"

Traditional Chinese Medicine and Western Medicine are two distinct medicine systems. I know nothing about blood diseases, while she is an expert of blood diseases in Western Medicine without the knowledge of Traditional Chinese Medicine. Therefore, there are definitely difficulties between us talking about this disease.

Later, Mr. Han took out seven hematology test reports of Peking University People's Hospital. During the period of taking medicinals, he went to take the examination once every other month, and the number of blood platelets rose rapidly. Therefore, he had the confidence to take the medicinals again and again. In accordance with the former therapeutic methods, I made other prescriptions for him based on his pulse and symptoms in Beijing. There were more than one hundred doses taken by him during this period.

On December 6, 2010, Mrs. Han called me from Beijing saying that her husband had been healthy as usual and been busy at work all day and sometimes on business trips, and that recent test records showed that the number of platelets (PLT) had risen to $12.0 \times 10^9/L$.

In June 2012, I heard that the number of platelets (PLT) of Mr. Han had remained at $13.0 \times 10^9/L$.

In fact, at the beginning of the treatment of this disease, I had not read any test report. Every time when I treated Mr. Han, I always followed traditional four diagnostic methods which respectively are: the inspection, auscultation and olfaction, inquiry as well as pulse-taking and palpation. After the disease had been cured, in order to record the whole disease process, I had to ask the patient (not patient anymore) to take the report copies to me for comparison and just read the rising process of the number of blood platelets (PLT). However, even today, I still know nothing about platelets or which kind of Chinese medicinal could increase blood platelets.

Someone may think that I hold the extreme views about these two medical sciences, saying that Western Medicine is the modern medicine, and the doctor like me not learning that will be eliminated by the society.

They even use *Records of Traditional Chinese and Western Medicine in Combination* (*Yī xué zhōng zhōng cān xī lù*, 医学衷中参西录) written by Zhāng Xīchún (张锡纯) to support their ideas.

In my opinion, however, their views are too one-sided. I adapt to the modern society by curing diseases via the ancient Chinese medical skills, and I only have one magic: totally obeying the authentic TCM skills without any integration with Western Medicine. If I combine TCM with Western Medicine, I will fail to follow the path of Traditional Chinese Medicine and lose the skill of helping me adapt to this society.

There are so many students graduated from Chinese medical universities with master's degrees and doctorate degrees having learnt TCM combined with Western Medicine concepts. Nonetheless, most of them change their career paths because they lack skills to treat diseases.

Few patients now have the opportunity to find an authentic TCM doctor who is good at feeling the pulse and making prescriptions. In fact, patients do not care whether their doctors can understand their test reports or not, they do care about the curative effect.

As for *Records of Traditional Chinese and Western Medicine in Combination* (*Yī xué zhōng zhōng cān xī lù*, 医学衷中参西录) mentioned above, it is very well-known among TCM doctors with significant influence.

In my mind, Zhāng Xīchún (张锡纯) was also a great master doctor admired by me, so his book is also essential to me to read from time to time, with great benefits for my clinical applications.

Frankly speaking, however, I only read the Chinese medicine part in this book and ignore the Western medicine part. Why? On the one hand, there is little information related to Western medicine in this masterpiece; on the other hand, the content related to Western medicine is far-fetched, which the academia has reached a consensus of. Therefore, it is useless for me to study it.

Someone may wonder that since *Asipilin Jia Shigao Tang* (*Aspirin and Gypsum Decoction*), praised generation after generation, has been treated as the model of integrating TCM and Western Medicine, why you still negate its value?

The reason of negating the value and effect of integrating TCM and Western Medicine in this book is that there is nothing useful in the combination of TCM and Western Medicine in the book.

What we all have known is that *Asipilin Jia Shigao Tang* (*Aspirin and Gypsum Decoction*) does receive countless applause and has been regarded as the backbone of integrating TCM and Western Medicine, but what we do not really know is that whether there really exists a patient who has been cured by taking this decoction nowadays.

Countless cases of high fever have been cured in my clinical career for decades, but none of them has ever been cured by using this decoction. Why? Because it is useless.

In the book of *Records of Traditional Chinese and Western Medicine in Combination* (*Yī xué zhōng zhōng cān xī lù*, 医学衷中参西录), it records that *Asipilin Jia Shigao Tang* (*Aspirin and Gypsum Decoction*) is used to 'treat the former syndromes'. What are the former syndromes? It means the syndromes of warm disease which are treated by '*Liangjie Tang* (*Cool Relieving Decoction*)' and '*Hanjie Tang* (*Cold Relieving Decoction*)'. The ingredients of the former one are *Bohe* (*Herba Menthae*), *Chanyi* (*periostracum cicada*), *Shigao* (*Gypsum Fibrosum*), and *Gancao* (*Radix Glycyrrhizae*); the ingredients of the latter one are *Shigao* (*Gypsum Fibrosum*), *Zhimu* (*Rhizoma Anemarrhenae*), *Lianqiao* (*Fructus Forsythiae*), and *Chanyi* (*periostracum cicada*). Because the ingredients of these two decoctions are not the same, the applications are different and the syndrome differentiation is needed. However, the book records that *Asipilin Jia Shigao Tang* (*Aspirin and Gypsum Decoction*) can treat the former syndromes, which means it not only treats what *Liangjie Tang* (*Cool Relieving Decoction*) treats but also treats what *Hanjie Tang* (*Cold Relieving Decoction*) treats. In a word, syndrome differentiation and treatment can be neglected when using this decoction. How ridiculous it is!

In this book, the symptoms treated by *Hanjie Tang* (*Cold Relieving Decoction*) are similar to the symptoms treated by *Baihu Tang* (*White Tiger Decoction*) recorded in *Treatise on Cold Damage Diseases* (*Shāng hán lùn*, 伤寒论), which can be manifested as, 'high fever all over the body, an unpleasant sensation of heat in epigastric area, feeling thirsty, a tongue with a yellowish white coating, a surging and slippery pulse'. As a result, *Shigao* (*Gypsum Fibrosum*) with pungent-sweet flavor and slight cold nature, attributed to the lung and stomach meridians, is used to clear heat in this decoction.

In the view of TCM, the excessive heat leads to the deficiency of water. Given the fact that the curative effect of clearing heat by only using *Shigao* (*Gypsum Fibrosum*) is not enough, so *Zhimu* (*Rhizoma Anemarrhenae*) with bitter flavor and cold nature, attributed to the lung, stomach, and kidney meridians, is added in this decoction for clearing heat and nourishing water. The application of these two medicinals in the theory of TCM is called as 'treating heat with cold'.

According to the symptoms recorded in the book, 'headache, constricted feeling all over the body', we know that warm pathogen attacks the greater yang exterior. Thus, as the key medicinal for treating warm disease, bitter-pungent flavor *Lianqiao* (*Fructus Forsythiae*), which is attributed to the heart meridian, is used to clear heat and expel wind-heat; *Chanyi* (*periostracum cicada*) with sweet flavor and cold nature, attributed to the lung and liver meridians, is used to promote the effect of expelling wind-heat. Through explaining the combination of these four medicinals in this decoction, we can clearly draw the conclusion that syndrome differentiation plays an important role.

However, the symptoms *Liangjie Tang* (*Cool Relieving Decoction*) treats are less severe than the symptoms *Hanjie Tang* (*Cold Relieving Decoction*) treats, which can be manifested as 'a sensation of heat (not high fever) in both interior and exterior, a surging and floating pulse'. Thus, only using *Shigao* (*Gypsum Fibrosum*) is enough to clear heat.

Gancao (*Radix Glycyrrhizae*), with sweet flavor and mild nature, attributed to twelve meridians, is used to tonify spleen and replenish qi; what's more, through its mild nature, *Gancao* (*Radix Glycyrrhizae*) can make the efficacy of *Shigao* (*Gypsum Fibrosum*) penetrate to yang brightness meridian and muscles from the stomach and then the pathogenic heat will be expelled from the pores gradually.

'A surging and floating pulse' indicates the wind-warm pathogen attacks the exterior. As a result, *Bohe* (*Herba Menthae*) and *Chanyi* (*periostracum cicada*), *as well as Heye* (*lotus leaf*), which are pungent in flavor and cool in nature, attributed to the lung and liver meridians, are used to disperse wind and expel heat, as well as clear summer heat and excrete dampness. Considering that the degree of heat the latter decoction treats is less severe than that the former one treats, we call the latter decoction as *Liangjie Tang* (*Cool Relieving Decoction*).

All in all, the applications of these two decoctions should base on the differentiation of pulse and symptoms, and should also evaluate the degree of the disease. Furthermore, treating diseases should completely obey the therapeutic principle of correcting the excessive or deficient condition by making good use of different properties of medicinals.

However, there are only two drugs in *Asipilin Jia Shigao Tang* (*Aspirin and Gypsum Decoction*), which are aspirin and *Shigao* (*Gypsum Fibrosum*). In addition, aspirin, as an analgesic-antipyretic drug in the field of Western Medicine, is composed by chemicals, which means it doesn't have property (four natures, five flavors, and meridian tropism) like Chinese medicinals. When the indication of aspirin appears, it would be prescribed to the patient by Western Medicine doctors without differentiating the patient's disease syndrome. The patient who has taken it would sweat a lot under its pharmacodynamic action. Therefore, it seems neither fish nor fowl to us authentic TCM doctors when *Shigao* (*Gypsum Fibrosum*) is accompanied with aspirin to treat diseases.

Aspirin is only a temporary solution to heat (fever) and pain, but not a medicine for 'eliminating pathogen'.

If a healthy person takes this decoction occasionally, this person may have no serious problem in a short time. If a physically weak person takes it, this person will become weaker, and the resistance to disease also decreases. For this reason, what's the benefit of taking it?

Let's check the medical case of *Asipilin Jia Shigao Tang* (*Aspirin and Gypsum Decoction*) in this book, 'A child suddenly had high fever in the late summer[...]. *Asipilin Jia Shigao Tang* (*Aspirin and Gypsum Decoction*) was prescribed to this child...the fever passed and the clear consciousness was back right after taking it [...] however, the fever came back again in the next afternoon.' From the sentence, 'the fever came back again in the next afternoon', we can draw the conclusion easily that aspirin is only a temporary solution to heat (fever) from the sentence. Thus, when talking about the efficacy of bringing down the fever permanently, aspirin is far less effective than those Chinese medicinals which are prescribed based on syndrome differentiation.

Subsequently, this medical case also records, '*Banxia Qing* (*Rhizoma Pinellase*) and *Niubangzi* (*Fructus Arctii*) were added in the decoction for the child had a cough with profuse phlegm. The child's symptoms had been cured completely after taking it.'

Niubangzi (*Fructus Arctii*), which is pungent and bitter in flavor and cold in nature, attributed to the lung and stomach meridians, is used to disperse wind and expel heat. As one of the key medicinals for treating warm disease, *Niubangzi* (*Fructus Arctii*) has always been added in some famous formulas for treating fever caused by warm disease like *Yinqiao San* (*Lonicera and Forsythia Powder*) and *Qingdu Liangge San* (*Diaphragm Cooling Powder*). *Banxia Qing* (*Rhizoma Pinellase*), which is pungent in flavor and warm in nature, attributed to the spleen and stomach meridians, not only can dry dampness and eliminate phlegm, but can clear heat and remove toxin as well. Just like what *Shennong's Classic of Materia Medica* (*Shén nóng běn cǎo jīng*, 神农本草经) records, 'the major function is to treat the symptom of aversion to cold with fever caused by cold damage diseases [...] to treat swollen and painful throat...to stop sweating.' *Miscellaneous Records of Famous Physicians* (*Míng yī bié lù*, 名医别录) also holds the same opinion, 'dissipating the mass and relieving the full sensation in the thoracic and epigastric area caused by phlegm and heat.' Although the therapeutic method of treating fever caused by warm disease is releasing exterior with pungent-cool, *Banxia* (*Rhizoma Pinellase*), which has a warm nature, should be used when the patient has a cough with profuse phlegm. This is the prescription of Chinese medicinals based on syndrome differentiation. As a result, the reason of curing this child's disease is all because of the use of *Shigao* (*Gypsum Fibrosum*), *Banxia Qing* (*Rhizoma Pinellase*) and *Niubangzi* (*Fructus Arctii*). Without these three medicinals, this child's fever would come back even when the sweat was emitted and the fever subsided at the moment. This medical case reveals the failure of *Asipilin Jia Shigao Tang* (*Aspirin and Gypsum Decoction*), which is difficult for common people to realize it.

What's more, for its pungent flavor, *Shengshigao* (*Gypsum Fibrosum*) can induce sweating. The medicinal with pungent flavor has an action of dispersing the pathogen. That is to say, *Shigao* (*Gypsum Fibrosum*) can disperse pathogenic heat from the pores. Considering the fact that its efficacy of dispersing heat is relatively mild, so *Mahuang* (*Radix Cannabis*) and *Guizhi* (*Ramulus Cinnamomi*), which are pungent in flavor and warm in nature, would be needed to promote the efficacy of inducing sweating and releasing the exterior when facing the syndrome of wind-cold fettering the exterior.

When facing the syndrome of warm pathogen attacking the exterior, with the purpose of promoting the efficacy of inducing sweating and releasing the exterior, *Shigao* (*Gypsum Fibrosum*) must be accompanied with *Lianqiao* (*Fructus Forsythiae*), *Niubangzi* (*Fructus Arctii*), and *Bohe* (*Herba Menthae*), etc., which are pungent in flavor and cold in nature.

In his book, Zhāng Xīchún (张锡纯) declared, '*Shigao* (*Gypsum Fibrosum*) has a slightly cold nature, not the extreme cold one.' He also illustrated that *Zhupi Dawan* (*The pill of Caulis Bambusae In Taeniam*), which contained *Shigao* (*Gypsum Fibrosum*), recorded in *Synopsis of the Golden Chamber* (*Jīn kuì yào luè*, 金匮要略) could treat the symptoms occurring in lactation period like the deficiency of middle qi, dysphoria, and vomit.

However, what *Science of Chinese Materia Medica* records is that *Shigao* (*Gypsum Fibrosum*) is extremely cold in nature. Which one is right? The answer is the former one. Why? Because in the book of *Shennong's Classic of Materia Medica* (*Shén nóng běn cǎo jīng*, 神农本草经), *Shigao* (*Gypsum Fibrosum*) is classified as a medicinal with slightly cold nature.

In Zhang's book, there is an attached medical case below the article talking about *Shigao*. It records the case of a 7-year-old child suffering from a high fever due to the wind-cold pathogen attacking the exterior; through the course of treatment, he only took *Shigao* (*Gypsum Fibrosum*), and the dosage of it was gradually increased at fixed time intervals; totally 6 liang (approximately 300g) of *Shigao* (*Gypsum Fibrosum*) had been taken in 24 hours, and then the fever started to subside, and the appetite increased; what's more, his stomach was not harmed by *Shigao* (*Gypsum Fibrosum*). In my medical career of treating patients with fever after catching a cold, no matter how old or young the patient was, the dosage of *Shigao* (*Gypsum Fibrosum*) I prescribed was never below 60 grams. After the treatment, not only had their fever been cured, but also none of them ever complained about the uncomfortable feeling in stomach after taking the decoction.

Proven by the clinical practice above, the slightly cold nature of *Shigao* (*Gypsum Fibrosum*) is right. Furthermore, in the book of *Science of Chinese Materia Medica*, the safety dosage of it for oral use is 9–60 grams. Is it rational to treat a patient with 60g of an extremely cold natured medicinal?

In the book of *Treatise on Cold Damage Diseases* (*Shāng hán lùn*, 伤寒论), the clinical application of *Baihu Tang* (*White Tiger Decoction*) includes high fever, excessive thirst, profuse perspiration, and a full forceful pulse. In the view of TCM, treating heat syndrome should use cold natured drugs, which means when facing high fever (the syndrome of excess heat), extremely cold natured drugs should be used. This is a constant and immutable truth for treating diseases. If the nature of *Shigao* (*Gypsum Fibrosum*) is slightly cold, how could it cure high fever? Moreover, Zhāng Zhòngjǐng (张仲景) classified *Shigao* (*Gypsum Fibrosum*) as the extremely cold natured medicinal in this decoction. What's the reason that this drug sometimes can be slightly cold in nature and sometimes can be extremely cold in nature?

My answer is that its dosage decides its nature.

In the book, the dosage of *Shigao* (*Gypsum Fibrosum*) in *Baihu Tang* (*White Tiger Decoction*) is 1 jin, approximately 500 grams today; 500 grams of *Shigao* (*Gypsum Fibrosum*) should be taken in three times each day, which means 170 grams of it should be taken each time. Although the nature of *Shigao* (*Gypsum Fibrosum*) is slightly cold, large dosage of it can achieve the curative effect of extremely cold natured medicinals. What's more, 6 liang (approximately 300 grams today) of *Zhimu* (*Rhizoma Anemarrhenae*), which is bitter and sweet in flavor and cold in nature, is added in this decoction to promote the efficacy of *Shigao* (*Gypsum Fibrosum*) for clearing heat and nourishing water. Therefore, high fever can be cured by using this decoction. That's why large dosage of *Shigao* (*Gypsum Fibrosum*) is regarded as the panacea for treating fever.

In one of his medical cases, Zhāng Xīchún (张锡纯) also let his patient take *Shigao* (*Gypsum Fibrosum*) for more than ten times in two nights in a row, and more than 1 jin of it had been prescribed for the treatment. In ancient times, the dosage of it for oral use could reach 14 jin (*Bǐ huā yī jìng,* 笔花医镜), or even tens of jin (*The medical records of Wu Jutong* (*Wú Jútōng yī àn,* 吴鞠通医案)). That's the reason why treating fever should use large dosage of *Shigao* (*Gypsum Fibrosum*).

We all know that treating heat with cold, but there are so many cold natured drugs, and Zhāng Zhòngjǐng (张仲景) only selected *Shigao* (*Gypsum Fibrosum*) as the primary drug for clearing heat in *Baihu Tang* (*White Tiger Decoction*). Why? Because it is sweet in flavor. Generally speaking, most Chinese medicinals for clearing heat will harm spleen and stomach, for the reason that they are bitter in flavor and cold in nature. According to the TCM theory, sweet flavor is associated with the spleen, which means *Shigao* (*Gypsum Fibrosum*) would not harm the spleen and stomach. However, when the dosage of it is large, its slightly cold nature would turn to an extremely cold nature, and its sweet flavor would become less effective. In my clinical career, I've seen several records that people who had taken large dosages of *Shigao* (*Gypsum Fibrosum*) presented with distending and full sensation in stomach.

Taking this into consideration, Zhāng Zhòngjǐng (张仲景) added *Gancao Zhi* (*Radix Glycyrrhizae Preparata*) to promte the efficacy of sweet flavor; he also added *Jingmi* (*Semen Oryzae Sativae*) for protecting the stomach. The method for decocting is also important, 'the medicinals should be decocted with water till *Jingmi* (*Semen Oryzae Sativae*) is well done and take the decoction several times after removal of the residue.' After being well-cooked, the soup of *Jingmi* (*Semen Oryzae Sativae*) is viscous and sticky. Thus, it will stay in the stomach longer and make the efficacy of decoction penetrate to the muscle from the stomach. Subsequently, people would sweat gradually, and then the symptoms would be cured.

The exquisite and delicate formulas created by Zhāng Zhòngjǐng (张仲景) are beyond words.

In the ancient times, *Baihu Tang* (*White Tiger Decoction*) was regarded as the 'miracle cure' for treating fever, and it deserves this honor. For every action (high fever) there is a reaction (cold or cool natured medicinals). Since Chinese medicinals can balance yin and yang harmlessly, there is no need to add aspirin in the decoction.

Aspirin is both the premier drug to reduce fever and relieve pain in Western Medicine and the most widely used drug to prevent heart disease and stroke in the world. It has become a common phenomenon among the old to take aspirin for they believe they benefit from this without any harm. What a terrible mistake!

It is reported that angina pills including aspirin can induce or aggravate angina pectoris (*China News of Traditional Chinese Medicine*, June 23, 1998).

According to Dutch researchers, aspirin use may increase the risk of cerebral micro-bleeds (*Archives of Neurology*, Online First).

In accordance with a latest study by American scientists, 'the potential harm — such as increased risk of stroke, intestinal bleeding and kidney failure — of taking more than 300 milligrams a day of aspirin or nonsteroidal anti-inflammatory drugs (NSAIDs) outweighs the potential benefits in terms of preventing colorectal cancer (*Health News*, April 4, 2007).'

The experts of the 302 Hospital of the PLA also pointed out that at least 200 or more drugs can cause liver and kidney damage, and aspirin, the antipyretic-analgesic drug, ranked at the top. (*China News of Traditional Chinese Medicine*, August 1st, 2005). It is also frequently reported that taking antipyretic-analgesic drugs can cause skin rashes and even be life-threatening.

In particular, doctors must be cautious in prescribing for children.

It is reported that the medical field has found that children taking aspirin may suffer from severe disease — Reye Syndrome. Initially, it shows the symptom as 'viral infection', mainly including respiratory infections, intestinal infections and chicken pox; a few days later, the symptoms develop into persistent vomiting, convulsions and coma and so on, with the mortality rate of more than 30%. In some countries, this used to be one of ten diseases causing the death of children.

As early as the 1980s, the medical field found the relation between aspirin and the Reye Syndrome, and then a number of countries prohibited aspirin use for children under 12 years old.

In the US, 555 cases of Reye Syndrome occurred in 1980, but only 2 cases were reported in 1997 after the issue of prohibition.

In the UK, 81 cases of Reye Syndrome occurred in 1983, and the number decreased to 17 in 1986 after the issue of prohibition.

In 1999, the *New England Journal of Medicine* published a report entitled '*Disappearance of Reye Syndrome — a Public Health Victory*', to celebrate the achievements.

Nevertheless, there were 10 patients over 12 years old among those 17 cases of Reye Syndrome in the United States after the issue of prohibition. Thus, the age limit was changed from 12 to 16.

In China's pharmaceutical market, there are a variety of antipyretics containing aspirin without any cautions for children (see *Aspirin Taking for Children with Caution* written by Xiǎo Yǔ (小雨) for more).

Some reports show that pregnant women with improper medication in the first trimester are prone to fetal malformations, which are mainly affected by aspirin and phenacetin that probably cause the fetal skeletal, neurological and renal abnormalities (*Health Digest News*, April 28, 1992).

In China, a deformed infant is born every 30 seconds. This statistic has exceeded the global average which should arouse the alert to aspirin.

There are other reports expressing that octogenarians often suffer from cerebrovascular amyloidosis with the rate of occurrence as high as 60% and easy bleeding, and the worst danger for taking aspirin is the aspirin-induced bleeding, 'For the old prone to amyloidosis, aspirin can increase the risk of cerebral hemorrhage'.

In addition, patients suffering from ulcer (taking aspirin can cause bleeding or perforation), coagulation disorders (e.g. severe liver damage, hypoprothrombinemia, vitamin K deficiency), preparing for surgery (to avoid clotting disorders in surgery), having asthma (allergic reactions in some asthma patients after taking aspirin, such as urticaria, laryngeal edema, asthma attacks), and after drinking (to avoid gastric mucosal damage causing the bleeding) should not take aspirin (see *Less Aspirin for Octogenarians*, written by Wáng Jìlì (王继立)).

As stated in other reports, the scientists of a school of medicine in Boston, the US, conducted medical experiments on 88,000 persons and the result indicated that people regularly taking aspirin due to headache, flu and other reasons had more chance of suffering from cancer with a risk possibility 86% higher than those not taking aspirin, and this is the most vital factor leading to pancreatic cancer (*China News of Traditional Chinese Medicine*, November 7th, 2003, Zhāng Yíngwén (张莹文)).

Similar reports are frequently published in newspapers.

With further research, the side effects of aspirin are increasingly prominent.

On that account, American experts recently modified the aspirin guideline, and published it on the *Annals of Internal Medicine* on March 17, 2009. The journal illustrated that the low-dose aspirin (75–81mg daily) should be taken to prevent the heart disease and stroke, and suggested that men below 45 years old and women below 55 years old should not take aspirin due to the lower risk of heart disease (*Life Times*, March 24, 2009).

Does this mean low-dose aspirin will be much safer for human health? Not really.

In recent years, research has found that taking low-dose aspirin to prevent cardiovascular and cerebrovascular diseases is not suitable for everyone. The persons with allergic reactions can have dyspnea, wheezing, and severe cases can be fatal, which is specially called 'aspirin asthma'.

Aspirin is not suitable for these people: people who are prone to bleeding such as bleeding gums or skin; people who are suffering from gastric or duodenal ulcers, hepatic cirrhosis, esophageal varices; people who have had surgeries recently, especially the surgery of eyes, internal organs, or brain.

Generally, people aged over 70 suffering from liver function reduction and clotting mechanism insufficiency are prone to bleeding due to long-term use of low-dose aspirin. Besides, people with the blood pressure higher than 170/110 mmHg and suffering from severe arteriosclerosis should not take aspirin in the long term so as not to induce cerebral hemorrhage (see *Low-Dose Aspirin is not for everyone* written by Yì Shànyǒng (易善勇) for more).

British doctors and scientists found that healthy people taking aspirin daily do not significantly reduce the risk of heart disease. Instead, their risk of bleeding doubles that of ordinary people (*Health News*, April 3rd, 2009).

According to the report of United Press International on August 30, 2009, the researchers announced this finding at the meeting of European Society of Cardiology held in Barcelona, Spain. They believed that the general public at this stage are not advised to take aspirin to prevent heart disease. Aspirin may be effective on the prevention of cardiovascular disease, but it can also cause internal bleeding which if severe enough could result in death (*China News of Traditional Chinese Medicine*, September 3rd, 2009).

Through these general analyses, we can draw the conclusion that *Asipilin Jia Shigao Tang* (*Aspirin and Gypsum Decoction*) is the combination of TCM and Western Medicine, which is nondescript, ineffectual and harmful.

Someone may say that the side effects of aspirin are mostly found in the recent two or three decades. Zhāng Xīchún (张锡纯) did not know these at his era. They also wonder whether I hear of the saying that, 'a packet of aspirin is the solution to the fever.'

My answer is that people holding this view are not familiar with the knowledge of medical science. 'A packet of aspirin is the solution to the fever', came from the therapeutic method (antipyretic analgesics) for treating common cold and fever in Western Medicine. The doctors of Western Medicine do not learn about TCM, so it is reasonable for them to follow this method.

But for a doctor of TCM, to treat fever by prescribing aspirin is an unforgivable mistake.

There are many formulas for treating fever in TCM, but they all target to resolve the cause of disease, and they are harmless to the human body. When the cause is resolved, the fever will be cured. When facing the fever due to warm disease, based on the degree of fever, there are several solutions to it: *Baihu Tang* (*White Tiger Decoction*) is used for treating the high fever, *Liangjie Tang* (*Cool Relieving Decoction*) and *Hanjie Tang* (*Cold Relieving Decoction*) are used for treating the common fever. Furthermore, even with the single drug, *Shigao* (*Gypsum Fibrosum*), the fever still can be cured, which had been illustrated and proven for several times in the article talking about *Shigao* in Zhang's book.

Zhāng Xīchún (张锡纯) did not know the side effects of aspirin at his era. However, aspirin which is not the solution to the cause of disease, can only make people sweat excessively. Excessive sweating leads to the deficiency of the exterior. When the exterior is deficient, the defensive ability of the exterior will be weakened. In TCM, the defensive ability of the exterior is equal to the immunity in Western Medicine. That is to say, the immunity system will be weakened. Moreover, there is an old saying in TCM, 'skin and body hair (the exterior) originating from the kidney'. It means the deficiency of the exterior results in the deficiency of the kidney, which is the innate foundation. All in all, we can come to the conclusion that excessive sweating by taking aspirin can harm the kidney. This is the general knowledge that every TCM doctor should know. How can we benefit from it? As the master of TCM, for supporting his own theory of integrating TCM and Western Medicine, he created *Asipilin Jia Shigao Tang* (*Aspirin and Gypsum Decoction*). It is unnecessary for him to do that. We should not believe in this.

Of course, *Asipilin Jia Shigao Tang* (*Aspirin and Gypsum Decoction*) is only one of more than 160 formulas created by Zhāng Xīchún (张锡纯), which can be described as a small defect. However, it set a bad precedent in the TCM circle — involving western drugs into Chinese medicinals when prescribing. Nowadays, there are numerous hospitals and clinics adding western drugs into Chinese medicinals, especially hormones and claimed them as pure Chinese medicinal preparation, that could seriously harm patient's health.

This small defect caused by Zhāng Xīchún (张锡纯) has now become the 'big flaw' in the westernization of TCM, which he might never foresee before.

However, no one is perfect, so did Zhāng Xīchún (张锡纯). As the master doctor of TCM, he was a man instead of a god. We point out his error with no offense.

There is no perfect medicine system in the world, Traditional Chinese Medicine included.

Traditional Chinese Medicine with a long history has plenty of famous doctors and various schools through different dynasties, but there is no miracle doctor that have the ability to cure all diseases.

Zhāng Zhòngjǐng (张仲景), with the reputation of 'medical sage', was the precedent of syndrome differentiation and treatment. In his *Treatise on Cold Damage Diseases* (*Shāng hán lùn*, 伤寒论), the concepts of three yin and three yang, yin and yang, exterior and interior, cold and heat, deficiency and excess are all described precisely; 113 formulas and 397 therapeutic methods are all recorded including sweating method, emetic method, purgation method, harmonizing method, warming method, clearing method, tonifying method, and resolving method. Even the original therapeutic method of releasing the exterior with pungent-cool created by the school of warm disease are also based on this irreplaceable masterpiece.

However, in the preface of *Treatise on Cold Damage Diseases* (*Shāng hán lùn*, 伤寒论), Zhāng Zhòngjǐng (张仲景) told us that even the readers had studied this book attentively and had perfectly understood the applications of these formulas, they could only cure more than half of these diseases in the book. As a result, in the premise of inheriting the theoretical and clinical thoughts of Zhāng Zhòngjǐng (张仲景), four eminent physicians in Jin and Yuan dynasties (known as *Jinyuan Sida Jia*) further developed one aspect of these thoughts and built up their own theory respectively.

But the words of Zhāng Zhòngjǐng (张仲景), 'observe the pulse and symptoms carefully and treat the patient accordingly', leads to the right path for learning TCM. Although thousands of new formulas have been created since then, obeying these words is still the only path for curing diseases. This is a highly summarized guideline both for all theories of *Internal Classic* (*Nèi jīng*, 内经) applying to the clinical treatment and for the scientific attribute of TCM. Therefore, these words can be regarded as bible for all TCM doctors to save people's lives, and Zhāng Zhòngjǐng (张仲景) was worthy of an exemplary master for all ages and to be honored as the 'medical sage'.

The book written by Zhāng Xīchún (张锡纯) has a wealth of benefits for clinical experience for later generations, with a high reputation, which is indeed a great masterpiece.

However, he brought a wrong way for TCM by integrating TCM with modern Western Medicine, leading the development of TCM to a wrong path for more than one hundred years.

Nowadays, this phenomenon is called the westernization of TCM that, as is known to all, results in the overall medical level of TCM falling behind.

Certainly, the westernization of TCM in the past 100 years cannot fully be attributed to Zhāng Xīchún (张锡纯), though he was the root after all.

In the praises to Zhāng Xīchún (张锡纯) today, he is extolled as the man who broke through the previous inherited theory, abandoned the worship to ancient habits, accepted the modern experimental science, created a new academic style, and set a good example for future generations. He is honored as 'the master for the combination of TCM and Western Medicine', 'the first one to advocate the academic opinion for the combination of TCM and Western Medicine', and 'the person who firstly advocated that the principle of combining TCM with Western Medicine should be through the process of theoretical practice'. All of the above seem like the praise to Zhāng Xīchún (张锡纯), but they actually play a role of fueling the westernization of TCM. What is worse, these words far from general praise are actually the puffery to the distortion of the contents of *Records of Traditional Chinese and Western Medicine in Combination* (*Yī xué zhōng zhōng cān xī lù*, 医学衷中参西录). Such absurdity is spreading seriously not due to Zhāng Xīchún (张锡纯) but the descendants.

In fact, *Records of Traditional Chinese and Western Medicine in Combination* (*Yī xué zhōng zhōng cān xī lù*, 医学衷中参西录) is just the title of this book. With an overview of the book, the author's clinical experience only sticks to TCM without any western medical skills. As an authentic TCM doctor, he did not break through the previous inherited theory or abandon the worship to ancient habits, which can be proven in his words created when climbing the Yellow Crane Tower.

Considering myself would lead an extraordinary life.
Unfortunately, being a good doctor or an excellent chancellor is still a dream.
Frustrations never defeat my spirit.
However, the reality I suffered makes me sympathize with my scarred and battered motherland.
Never have I been so strongly concerned about the fate of my nation since many failures.
To understand the theories of saving lives, concentrating is needed.
The profound truth of Qihuang lies in the book of Internal Classic (Neijing).
Studying and mastering the truth, then I should dedicate to saving lives.

Did he actually break through the previous inherited theory or abandon the worship to ancient habits? Absolutely not! His worship to the ancient habits is not equal to the copy of ancient habits.

His worship means respect; ancient habits refer to the ancient Chinese Medicine.

TCM, as the intangible science, is characterized for its *Tao-like medical knowledge* and the science based on its universal principle. An independent and thorough theoretical system had been formed called 'the profound truth of Qihuang' two thousand years ago. The worship and the respect of this science is the essential point to master it.

Just like no one can learn the science well without advocating it, there is not a person mastering TCM without the respect to the ancients.

Only to advocate the science can a person study the science and make inventions and creations, so does the worship to the ancients. According to Zhāng Xīchún (张锡纯), the development of the medical science depends on the inspiration from the ancient intelligence. In addition, the old saying, 'seeking for the ancient lessons diligently', from Zhāng Zhòngjǐng (张仲景), holds the same meaning as concentrating on studying the profound truth of Qihuang.

Shengxian Tang (*Raising the Dropping Decoction*) created by Zhāng Xīchún (张锡纯) is based on the theories from *Internal Classic* (*Nèi jīng*, 内经). In the book, he wrote that, 'Through the examination, I found that the patient's pulse at left Guan position was too weak. Therefore, the patient was diagnosed with the syndrome of liver yang deficiency. I prescribed the patient 1 liang of *Huangqi* (*Radix Astragali*) and 3 qian of *Guizhi jian* (*Ramulus Cinnamomi(tip)*). After several doses, the patient was cured.' The therapeutic method of warming and tonifying liver-qi was created in this way. He also wrote that, 'Although the anatomical position of liver is at the right side of the body, the movement of liver-qi is at the left. Thus, the pulse reflecting the state of liver is at left Guan position; although the anatomical position of spleen is at the left side of the body, the movement of spleen-qi is at the right. Therefore, the pulse reflecting the state of spleen is at right Guan position.' Through this part, Zhāng Xīchún (张锡纯) pointed out the difference between the theories of TCM's visceral manifestation and Western Medicine's anatomy.

He has always been regarded as the person who accepted the modern experimental science. However, what he accepted is just some compositions of Chinese medicinals detected by Modern Science. Just like what he wrote in the chapter talking about *Shigao*, '*Shigao* (*Gypsum Fibrosum*), one mineral with hydro calcium sulfate fibriform crystallized polymeric.' This is far from creating a new academic style, and setting a good example for future generations.

There is a widespread phenomenon that an increasing number of people, in order to indicate their scientific nature, fully copy the chemical compositions of the western medical studies detected by the modern scientific methods when describing Chinese medicinals. This however misleads the public and blurs the real scientific attribute of the properties (four natures and five flavors) of Chinese medicinals, which should be regarded as a kind of unhealthy trend instead of a 'new style'. In terms of 'the master for the combination of TCM and Western Medicine', in my opinion, after reading the book, *Asipilin Jia Shigao Tang* (*Aspirin and Gypsum Decoction*) is only one failed formula among his more than 160 prescriptions, except that he never did any practical experiments again.

Someone may wonder that Zhāng Xīchún (张锡纯) used to claim that everything would be known after the experiment.

Actually, this 'experiment' stated by Zhāng Xīchún (张锡纯) refers to the practical spirit, rather than the laboratory experiment. In his book, he once wrote that, 'All medicinals should be personally tasted first and then can be prescribed to the others. Even when facing the toxic medicinal like *Gansui* (*Radix Euphorbiae Kansui*), *Mahuang* (*Radix Cannabis*), *Liuhuang* (*Sulfur*), and *Huajiao* (*Pericarpium Zanthoxyli*), we should still taste them first to know the degree of the toxicity.' Therefore, he fully understood the properties and functions of Chinese medicinals. From his book, we know that *Shanzhuyu* (*Fructus Corni*) can save the patient from the syndrome of collapse, *Huangqi* (*Radix Astragali*) accompanied with *Renshen* (*Radix Ginseng*) can promote urination. These theories were all deduced from his clinical practice. Through his clinical practice, he summarized and created lots of excellent formulas which have benefited us so much. As a result, that's why we should regard Zhāng Xīchún (张锡纯) as an authentic clinical master of TCM.

The belief of Zhāng Xīchún (张锡纯) for 'sticking to Traditional Chinese Medicine' lays his status as a great master.

Honoring Zhāng Xīchún (张锡纯) as the representative of 'combining Chinese Medicine with Western Medicine' is the extreme distortion of this master as well as being misleading for the followers.

As for his words of 'having no views for territory between TCM and Western Medicine' only indicate that he did not exclude Western Medicine.

We nowadays advocate the authentic TCM, but it does not mean that Western Medicine should be totally denied. Instead, we need to develop the unique features of Traditional Chinese Medicine, i.e. the scientific attribute of TCM.

Moreover, although we point out the errors in the ideas and methods of the treatment of Western Medicine, it does not mean we fully negate that science.

Analyzing the global health care situation comprehensively, instead of the westernization of TCM, Western Medicine should learn from Chinese Medicine. Otherwise, the crisis of the health care faced by the whole society cannot be solved.

In fact, this book should be named as *'Sticking to Traditional Chinese Medicine without the Combination of Modern Western Medicine'*. The original book title was not consistent with the content.

Now we learn from this book by focusing on and benefiting from the part sticking to the authentic TCM instead of the combination of Western Medicine.

Due to my decades of clinical experience rather than theories, Traditional Chinese Medicine and Western Medicine are on two opposite sides that can never be integrated together.

However, some experts nowadays claim that TCM should focus more on the scientific attribute and modernization. All these are affected by the wrong idea of the combination of TCM and Western Medicine. In order to test its validity, clinical experience is enough.

The old saying goes, 'one word can both flourish and endanger a country', and this is what happens to the combination of TCM and Western Medicine.

It is unknown how those people were to crazily abandon the tradition when the movement of the eastward transmission of western sciences dominated the culture at the era of Zhāng Xīchún (张锡纯), or why he used 'the combination of TCM and Western Medicine' as the key words of his book even if he only copied a few sentences from western medical knowledge and added aspirin in his prescription. Maybe he just wanted to follow the trend at that time, or for some other reasons we never know.

All is all, although he was a master, he was still a human being instead of a god. We should not blame him.

Anyway, TCM has been misled for more than 100 years so far due to his book title being irrelevant to the subject. If he knew and witnessed TCM struggling and losing itself in the immense combination with Western Medicine, he would be in deep sorrow.

This is supposed to be the conclusion of this case, but I have some words of digression which are my personal inspiration after the treatment for this aplastic anemia patient.

One of my university mates, Mr. Zhang, also suffered from this disease. His body was much stronger than Mr. Han. He only took two doses of my prescription before his son, a senior official, said: "Father, we could find more professional specialists instead of this non-famous doctor of TCM. Let me take you to high-level experts."

The filial piety was commendable, so his son then asked the famous blood disease specialists in Beijing for treatment, taking imported medicines that cost more than RMB 10,000 every month. Unfortunately, after spending hundreds of thousands yuan of money, Mr. Zhang passed away in less than two years.

Hearing of the sad news, I made haste to his home to offer my condolence. I was in great sadness when seeing his remains. Even till now, I still cannot get over it and fell regrettable.

I do not know what the result would be if Mr. Zhang asked me for prescription. However, there is no way back.

With great sadness, the only thing I want to emphasize is that it is vital to select the right doctor, for it is a matter of life and death.

We often say that learning TCM requires perception. It now seems that choosing the appropriate treatment also need the perception.

Disease differentiation and treatment has been mistakenly used for treating again and again

— Discussing TCM practitioners must get out of the misunderstanding of disease differentiation and treatment by taking the example of curing bladder cancer

Mr. Ren, over 70 years old, was my classmate at Jiexiu Middle School. Around ten years ago, we met each other again when both were attending the wedding ceremony of the son of our classmate, Ms Zhao, previous bank president in Shanxi Province. Since we had not met each other for over 30 years, we were very excited to get together again in a distant land and had a very pleasant talk.

After the wedding ceremony, I invited Mr. Ren to my home to talk more about our old days. I then realized that after graduated from high school in 1963, he did not attend the university entrance exam due to poverty, instead, he was engaged in farming at home. During the reform and opening up, he founded a construction company in Jiexiu Town. Thanks to his honest and reliable personality, he contracted plenty of projects and started to live a well-off life.

During our conversation, I knew that there was only one thing that kept disturbing him, i.e. he had suffered from lumbar disc herniation for many years and received no effective treatment for such a long term.

At that time, he still did not know that I had already switched career to TCM for a long time. I smiled, saying I have cured this kind of disease for many cases.

I told him: "Ms. Zhao also suffered from this disease and could not walk unless with the support of wall or table, but she was cured by me and can walk easily like healthy people."

Having heard my words, Mr. Ren was very delighted and asked for my treatment immediately.

Less than one month later, he called me from Jiexiu, saying it was incredible that he did not have backache anymore after taking the medicinals for several days and expressed his appreciation to me.

After that, he continuously introduced over 20 patients from Jiexiu suffering from lumbar disc herniation and they were all cured by me. Therefore, he trusted me very much and all his family members and relatives came to Taiyuan for prescriptions every time they felt ill.

Unexpectedly, on September 2, 2009, Mr. Ren called me from Beijing, saying that he used to suffer from bladder cancer in 2007 and had received electro-excision in the General Hospital of Chinese People's Liberation Army; however, he was diagnosed with the recurrence of bladder cancer in that hospital and the doctor suggested that he excise the whole bladder. He had no idea and asked me for advice.

I told him not to receive this surgery but take Chinese medicinals from me.

He held the same view that he was not willing to accept that surgery.

At that time, I was in Weihai for business. I returned to Taiyuan in the middle of October, and Mr. Ren came to me specially from Jiexiu with his case report on October 25. From his case report, I knew that he took Color Doppler ultrasound (CDUS) examination on August 14, 2008, at the First Affiliated Hospital of Shanxi Medical University, and the result showed: 'Bladder: normal bladder capacity, well internal acoustic permeability, rough bladder wall, a heterogeneous and hypoechoic mass of 4.4 cm × 2.8 cm in size can be found on the left front bladder wall; the mass: blurry boundary, no capsule, a small amount of blood streams in the shape of strips and spots visible inside.' The hospital diagnosed it as the space-occupying lesion, and thought it might be the relapse of bladder cancer.

Having known the result, he went to Beijing General Hospital of Chinese People's Liberation Army where he received the surgery for further examination. The ultrasonic diagnosis report of this hospital on August 28 shows: 'Normal bladder capacity, echoic tubercles on the left front and left rear of the bladder wall with 3.2 cm × 2.3 cm and 2.5 cm × 2.2 cm respectively in size, clear boundary, blood stream signals visible inside the masses.' The diagnose is the multiple echoic nodules on bladder wall, with a great possibility of the relapse of bladder cancer.

He also took the cystoscopy examination in this hospital on August 31 and the report was: 'Proper bladder capacity, a cauliflower-like neoplasm of 3 cm × 3 cm in size outside the left ureterostoma, a neoplasm of 3 cm × 3 cm in size near to the top of the left side of bladder wall and several cauliflower-like neoplasms in different sizes visible surrounding the mucous membrane of this neoplasm.' The microscopic diagnosis and treatment: The relapse of bladder cancer and a surgery should be advised for further treatment.

After returning to Jiexiu, Shanxi Province, Mr. Ren suffered the lower abdominal pain and excreted urine blood on October 1.

On October 5, he went to Shanxi Boda Urinary Surgery Hospital, one of the China's Top Ten Urinary Special Hospitals, and took the urinalysis: 'pyocyte of full view under microscope.' He also took the ultrasound examination once again and the report was: 'normal bladder capacity, rough bladder wall, heterogeneous incrassation, many hyperechoic nodules inside, of which the maximum is on the left side in the angle area of bladder with 2.4 cm × 2.1 cm in scope and the echo inside is heterogeneous. CDFI: abundant arterial blood stream signals visible inside.'

The diagnosis indicated that the multiple nodules inside the bladder lumen and the recrudescence of bladder cancer, and the therapeutic suggestion was to receive the surgical treatment in hospital. At the request of the patient, the doctors gave him intravenous transfusion temporarily to control the inflammation and stop the bleeding. After a three-day treatment, he still refused to have the surgery.

On November 1, 2009, Mr. Ren came to my clinic.

At the clinic, I saw that he had a yellow dull face, eyes without lustre and a dull expression. After the query, I realized that he had a poor appetite, limb weakness, difficult urination and lower abdominal pain. He had no other sufferings except for urine blood with occasional blood clots. He had a pale and slight dull purple tongue with a white and a little greasy coating. His pulse was huge on both hands beating 5 times in a cycle of breath.

Synopsis of the Golden Chamber (*Jīn kuì yào luè*, 金匮要略) records: 'A man who looks healthy but has a huge pulse is suffering from a consumptive disease (general debility). When the pulse is extremely deficient, it also indicates a consumptive disease.'

And: 'When a man is suffering from a consumptive disease, the pulse is floating-huge.'

And: 'The pulse of a patient at the age of fifty or sixty is huge [...] Such cases all indicate the exhaustion of the vital energy.'

And: 'The pulse is wiry and huge. When pressed deeply, it is not as strong as a true wiry pulse. Though huge, it is hollow within. Such pulse is called 'hollow-wiry' pulse. Wiry pulse of reduced strength indicates prevalence of pathogenetic cold. Hollow pulse reflects interior deficiency. When hollow-wiry pulse occurs in female patients, this indicates premature delivery or mild, chronic bloody vaginal discharge. In male patients, it indicates loss of blood and sperm.'

In conclusion, this weak and huge pulse was the sign of qi deficiency and blood stasis. Given his pulse and symptoms, although the blood urine came from the bladder, it didn't mean that the illness was only restricted to his bladder. The real reason of his blood urine was not that simple: aging and debility, weakness of five organs led to the disorder of qi movement; thus resulting in the blood stasis and qi stagnation in three energizers which brought about the dampness turbidity originating from interior; this dampness turbidity then moved into the bladder; the accumulation of dampness turbidity in the bladder could originate heat which would damage the blood vessels; as a result, the blood urine appeared due to the broken blood vessels.

Therefore, the treatment should primarily focus on tonifying qi-blood, invigorating spleen and tonifying kidney, resolving dampness turbidity, and regulating three energizers. What's more, the treatment should also secondarily focus on clearing heat, cooling blood, and resolving phlegm. We should treat both root cause and symptoms, and here were the ingredients of the formula:

Yedangshen (Radix Codonopsis) 60g
Cangzhu (Rhizoma Atractylodis) 10g
Chuanpu (Cortex Maganoliae) 10g
Chenpi (Pericarpium Citri Reticulatae) 10g
Zhuling (Polyporus) 15g
Zexie (Rhizoma Alismatis) 15g
Fuling (Poria) 15g
Baizhu (Rhizoma Atractylodis Macrocephalae) 10g
Guizhi (Ramulus Cinnamòmi) 10g
Baishao (Radix Paeoniae Alba) 10g
Shengdihuang (Radix Rehmanniae) 15g
Danpi (Cortex Moutan) 15g
Taoren (Semen Persicae) 10g
Chuanniuxi (Radix Cyathulae) 15g
Baimaogen (Rhizoma Imperatae) 30g
Danggui (Radix Angelicae Sinensis) 15g
Gancaoshao (Radix Glycyrrhizae(root)) 15g

Since then, the patient came to my clinic for five times and I just added or reduced some medicinals based on the above prescription every time. This prescription was successively added with *Xianhecao (Herba Agrimoniae)*, *Huashifen (Chinese talc powder)*, *Jinqiancao (Herba Lysimachiae)*, *Muli (concha ostreae)*, and *Zhizi (Fructus Gardeniae)*. *Yedangshen (Radix Codonopsis)* and *Baimaogen (Rhizoma Imperatae)* were once added with a maximum dosage of 100g and 120g, respectively.

The reasons of prescribing large dosages of *Yedangshen (Radix Codonopsis)* and *Baimaogen (Rhizoma Imperatae)* were as follows: the former medicinal can tonify five organs; when the five organs are tonified, then qi movement will be normal, and that is the therapeutic method of eliminating pathogen by reinforcing healthy qi; the latter one can tonify the middle and replenish qi, expell blood stasis, and diuresis. It's the proper treatment for the patient's pathogenesis of blood urine.

After several months of recuperation and taking the formula for over 60 doses, the patient had gradually recovered from the blood urine.

On April 11, 2010, Mr. Ren specially came to Taiyuan from Jiexiu for the ultrasonic medical imaging in Shanxi Boda Urinary Surgery Hospital, and the report presented: 'Normal bladder capacity, rough bladder wall, bladder wall thickening of about 10mm, fine acoustic permeability of emiction inside the bladder, no cauliflower-like neoplasms.' He was only diagnosed with the bladder wall thickening.

Mr. Ren was very excited when seeing the test report. However, I told him not to relax too early and exhorted him to continue to take Chinese medicinals in case of relapse. Prescription this time: drinking the water decocted by 10g of *Yedangshen* (*Radix Codonopsis*) and 60g of *Baimaogen* (*Rhizoma Imperatae*) everytime, and 2 times a day.

When he came to my clinic on September 26, he said he was very fine. Due to the coming of the late autumn, I prescribed him *Guifu Dihuang Wan* (*Six-Ingredient Rehmannia Pill* plus *Ramulus Cinnamomi* and *Radix Aconiti Lateralis Praeparata*) with a little of *hairy deerhorn* and told him to continue taking these pills (one pill twice a day) until the Beginning of Spring of next year. I also told him that the effect of nourishing tonic in winter will be shown in the coming year.

In the view of TCM, kidney is externally and internally related to the bladder, which means the bladder can hardly be damaged if the kidney is in good condition.

On November 28, Mr. Ren introduced his relatives and friends to my clinic. I could tell that he was very healthy with a rosy face and bright eyes that I had not seen for several years. He told me he was in good spirit without blood urine or any other difficulties in urination anymore.

Mr. Ren thanked me a lot and I also showed my appreciation to him.

He was confused about my appreciation, asking, "I thank you because you saved my life, but why do you appreciate me?"

"I appreciate you for your trust in me and insisting on taking the Chinese medicinals according to my prescriptions; otherwise I would not cure you even if I am the God," answered me, "it is both of us that should share this 'military medal'."

After hearing my words, he burst into laughter and left my clinic.

Actually, I was not joking at that moment.

According to what *Internal Classic* (*Nèi jīng,* 内经) records, 'To those who devoutly believe in the gods and the spirit, explanation of the noblest art of healing is unnecessary; to those who speak evil of acupuncture and stone-needle, explanation of the finest skill will be futile. Patients refusing doctor's treatment will never be cured and treatment by force will never achieve good results.' We know that the patients' trust and their insistence on taking medicinals are two vital premises.

Someone may wonder, "Cancer is a disease name from modern medicine. TCM nowadays focuses on the disease differentiation and treatment which has already substituted the traditional concept of syndrome differentiation and treatment. Why don't you keep up with the times?"

In my opinion, this is a good question. How dare I not keep up with the times though I am a conventional TCM doctor? The only purpose I learn TCM is to cure diseases and save people's lives. Therefore, I also believe that 'a black plum is as sweet as a white'.

Regardless of the people either in ancient times or at present and regardless of the concepts being either traditional or modern, I only learn from what can teach me to cure people, and will never be limited to one circle! Therefore, I have also purchased several books about modern disease differentiation and treatment and especially attached importance to the volume about cancer treatment. Despite reading those books for many times, I found them useless in practice.

I was very confused at first, but gradually had some enlightenment after years of clinical practice, knowing that I entered the wrong zone of disease differentiation and treatment.

Without any question, the modern disease names are given based on the scientific instrument examinations with strong evidence; moreover, half of this kind of books describe Western Medicine doctors' understandings about diseases and the contents related to the surgeries, chemotherapy, radiotherapy and even medicine taking details, misleading readers to believe that this is the only way to cure the cancers.

If the diseases can all be cured in this way, why should I learn TCM? On the contrary, TCM simply identifies diseases based on their symptoms and offers prescriptions due to different disease syndromes. TCM doctors offer the prescriptions according to disease syndromes, which can be seen as 'sitting in the right seat'.

Is this the disease differentiation and treatment? I do not think so. Instead, this is 'curing the disease by following up the clue' or we say 'sitting in the right seat'.

Some may think that even the topic of every chapter in the book of *Treatise on Cold Damage Diseases* (*Shāng hán lùn,* 伤寒论) is 'Differentiation of the Pulse, Syndrome Complex, and Treatment of XX Disease'. Why is disease differentiation and treatment a wrong direction?

In my opinion, although TCM and Western Medicine both use the word 'disease', they refer to totally different meanings. The disease of six meridians mentioned in *Treatise on Cold Damage Diseases* (*Shāng hán lùn,* 伤寒论) indicates different syndromes like exterior and interior, cold and heat, deficiency and excess, i.e. syndrome differentiation and treatment, which does not refer to the disease in Western Medicine. Don't you notice 'according to both the pulse manifestations and disease patterns' in the phrase 'curing the disease according to both the pulse manifestations and disease patterns'? Moreover, the disease mentioned in the *Treatise on Cold Damage Diseases* (*Shāng hán lùn,* 伤寒论) cannot be detected by any modern scientific instruments for it is intangible science; the diseases in modern medicine, on the contrary, are all proved by modern scientific instruments and belong to tangible science. Therefore, the diseases in TCM and Western Medicine are very different that should not be confused.

Syndrome differentiation and treatment can be greatly dissimilar to disease differentiation and treatment though there is only one word difference.

Depending on which kind of cancer, the anticancer methods must be chosen according to the categories of syndromes. This kind of 'matching' is the western medical thought that leads TCM to be inflexible, falling in the metaphysical idea of treatment based on disease differentiation.

People live through four different seasons; the land has different regions; there are males and females who may be strong or weak; disease conditions may be acute or chronic. Similar diseases may have different syndromes and should be treated with different methods; different diseases may have the same syndromes and can be treated in the same way.

Although TCM has some basic principles to follow, it treats diseases flexibly with the thinking pattern of syndrome differentiation. This is the dialectics of TCM.

The reason why TCM can be passed down to generations is that it can cure incurable diseases in the view of Western Medicine with the application of syndrome differentiation and treatment. This makes TCM unique.

The national-level master of TCM, Lù Guǎngxīn (陆广莘) once said: "The contemporary confusion in the combination of TCM and Western Medicine lies in the 'identity crisis', mainly in 'the syndrome being subject to the disease'." And this is indeed the point.

He introduced a great figure, Yuè Měizhōng (岳美中), and created two poems. One is as follows,

Although Kampo Medicine learns from Zhāng Zhòngjǐng (张仲景),
one prescription is made for one disease in their theory.
How do they know the TCM theory is based on the syndrome differentiation?
The profound essence of it should be pondered repeatedly.

This poem means the disease differentiation and treatment lost the 'essential principle' of syndrome differentiation and treatment in TCM!

The other one is as follows:

We pursue to differentiate the syndrome of a disease,
without differentiating the category of a disease.
There are countless treasures in the splendid medical world,
the point is whether we can recognize them?

This means the 'disease category' in the disease differentiation and treatment approach ignored the 'treasure' of TCM, that is, syndrome differentiation and treatment!

In the last century, in Japan *Sho-Saiko-to (Xiao Chaihu Tang) granules* were used to treat hepatitis and liver cirrhosis, causing 22 deaths in the early 1990s. Couldn't this wake up our stiff mind of disease differentiation and treatment?

Never go astray in the combination of TCM and Western Medicine

— The discussion on the reconciliation of TCM and Western Medicine by taking the example of curing severe rheumatoid arthritis

On July 10, 2010, a director from the Tsinghua University Science Park told me that a patient was badly suffering from the rheumatoid disease, and he asked me to help that patient.

Therefore, I went to the Tsinghua University Science Park with my wife and knew that Ms Xu, the mother of the patient, was a cleaner in that park. She was from Anhui Province and had made a living in Beijing for a long time though she was nearly sixty years old.

The patient Ms Sun was Ms Xu's daughter and was 29 years old. She could hardly walk even with her mother and her husband's help.

When we met each other, the poor daughter and her mother immediately burst into tears before I asked about her disease.

Ms Sun then sobbed out her state of disease to me.

In January, 2007, she started to suffer from the arthralgia in fingers, and then the pain spread to all the joints in her body. It was diagnosed as the rheumatoid disease by a major hospital.

Within the next three years, she sought for treatments from all specialized hospitals and well-known specialists in the field of rheumatoid disease. However, the pain could only be eliminated every time after taking medicines which made her disease more and more serious.

At the moment I met her, she just suffered from arthralgia in the whole body and could not walk unless with two people holding her arms.

What's worse, after taking those medicines, Ms Sun started to have a better appetite and sometimes could eat up a pot of rice for one meal; even pickles tasted good for her. Therefore, she became overweight: 1.7 meters tall and weighed more than 90kg; her fingers looked like small carrots, and her body, face included, was full of black hairs, especially on her back, which turned her into a 'hairy-women'; her belly bulged with lines like stretch marks, and a slight move could make her tremble.

I asked her what medicines she had taken.

She said that the specialists in rheumatoid disease prescribed her prednisone (6 pills per time) with Chinese medicinals together. Besides, the capsules of Chinese medicinals, which were prescribed by the so-called specialists in rheumatoid disease of TCM, took effect immediately by one dose, and the reason turned out to be that all those capsules had hormone. Those specialists said that the relief of the symptoms could only rely on the combination of TCM and Western Medicine. Therefore, they treated her with cupping, Gua Sha and Chinese medicinals at the same time, as well as gave her injection with so-called imported medicine that cost over one thousand yuan each.

In order to afford the treatment fees, her poor and old mother had to take a part-time job as a housekeeper after finishing her cleaning work. Her husband had no job but to look after her, and borrowed money from everywhere, without any ability to repay those debts.

Under this circumstance, Ms Sun thought suicide was the only way to get rid of those adversities.

She asked her 7-year-old daughter to buy the rat poison twice and was fortunately found out by her neighbors. The kindhearted old ladies were on duty at her home in turn to prevent her from committing suicide.

Having heard of this situation, the kind director of the science park not only provided the financial assistance for the patient, but also invited me to cure her disease.

I had cured patients with rheumatoid disease before, but it would be the first time for me to treat a patient in such a serious condition. And I am pretty clear that the rheumatoid disease is called 'the cancer not causing death' by modern medicine.

The data of modern medicine defines the rheumatoid arthritis (RA) as that, 'It is an autoimmune disease without the known cause and specificity diagnosis index. This disease is a chronic, systemic and multivariate inflammatory disorder that primarily affects small joints and may also have signs and symptoms in organs other than small joints (pericarditis, pleurisy, pneumonia, peripheral neuritis, and subcutaneous nodule).' It also says that the rate of deformity is 50% in two years and 70% in three years, etc.

The RA had tortured Ms Sun to be disabled and made her feel painful both physically and mentally. It was really pathetic.

Her hands kept trembling all along while I felt her pulse. After feeling her pulse, I found that her pulse was slippery, rapid, and tight on both hands, beating 7 times in a cycle of breath. Besides the ankylosis, thickness and malformation of the joints of hands and feet, she also suffered from the pain and stiffness of all the joints in her body, which made her easily break into cold sweat. The situation was more serious in the morning and less in the afternoon, and aggravated in cloudy days. Her face not only had hairs, but also was a typical moon shaped face emerging after taking hormones.

After analyzing her pulse and symptoms, I considered that she was attacked by the pathogens of wind, cold, dampness, heat, and blood stasis. What's more, due to the long-term hormonal therapy, she had aggravated into a complicated medical condition, which could not be treated merely with a single herbal formula or a small amount of medicinals. Then I comforted her that her disease was curable if she stopped taking hormones and bore the pain while taking Chinese medicinals, and told her I would compose the formula and send the medicinal powder to her after returning to Taiyuan. If she adhered to my medicinals, she would get better gradually.

After half a month, I sent someone to deliver the capsules made from authentic Chinese medicinals chosen by myself. The capsule was 0.5g for each one, and the patient should take 6 capsules once and 3 times each day with lukewarm water.

Unexpectedly, after one month, Ms Sun called me, saying that her pain was alleviated. I encouraged her to keep taking the medicinals without intermission.

Three months later, I went to the science park with my wife again and found that Ms Sun looked totally different. She greeted us with a smile and made tea in person without the help of others. She said that she had lost 20kg in weight, and there were no black hairs on her body anymore and the pain and ankylosis of her joints were also significantly alleviated.

One year later, she called to tell me that she only suffered slight pain and ankylosis in fingers in the morning and could do some light housework, and she had completely restored the confidence.

When I wrote this article, I called her specially to know about her recent condition.

I was told that she could look after herself and prepare a simple meal for herself when her husband worked outside for a week. Although she had not completely recovered, she had become a totally different person from one we met for the first time.

On December 4, 2012, Ms Sun called me again and said the ankylosis in the morning had disappeared and she merely felt a slight pain in her back and arms sometimes. I encouraged her to keep taking the medicinals.

The ingredients of the formula I made for her were as follows:

"Paofuzi (Radix Aconiti Lateralis Preparata), Tubiechong (eupolyphaga seu steleophaga), Baijiangcan (Bombyx Baytryticatus), Dilong (Pheretima Lumbricus), Chuanniuxi (Radix Cyathula), Guizhi (Ramulus Cinnamomi), Sangjisheng (Herba Taxilli), Zushima (Daphne giraldii Nitsche), Qiannianjian (Homalomenae Rhizoma), Luxiancao (Herba Pyrolae), Yedanshen (Radix Salviae Miltiorrhizae), Tianma (Gastrodia elata), Duzhong (Cortex Eucommiae), Qianghuo (Rhizoma et Radix Notopterygii), Duhuo (Radix Angelicae), Zhiruxiang (Olibanum), Zhimoyao (Myrrha), Fuling (Poria), Chuanduan (Radix Dipsaci), Gouji (Rhizoma Cibotii), Qinjiao (Radix Gentianea Macrophyllae), Danggui (Radix Angelicae Sinensis), Baishao (Radix Paeoniae Alba), Mugua (Fructus Chaenomelis), Muxiang (Radix Aucklandiae), Gancao (Radix Glycyrrhizae), Weilingxian (Radix Clematidis)."

All the medicinlas should be grounded into a fine powder in proportion for capsules. I advised her to stick to take the formula patiently and should not stop before it took effect. And told her about the principle that, 'Diseases come on horseback, but go away on foot'.

The treatment for Ms Sun through the combination of TCM and Western Medicine was the abuse of hormone with the use of regular prescription without analyzing the pulse and symptoms, which led to strange syndromes, making her life worse than death. I focused on her pulse and symptoms for treatment, and my therapeutic methods included restoring yang to stop collapse, releasing exterior and dissipating cold, clearing heat and removing toxin, draining dampness and dispersing swelling, activating blood and resolving stasis, relaxing sinew and activating collaterals, dissipating mass and relieving pain, nourishing liver and kidney, strengthening bones and muscles and facilitating joints. I advised her to stop taking western medicines that contained hormones gradually, or my prescription would not take effect even if I had differentiated the syndrome accurately.

There are more patients suffering the same tragedy as Ms Sun. As doctors, we should rethink the combination of TCM and Western Medicine.

From the perspective of the medical circle, the idea of the combination of TCM and Western Medicine originates from Táng Róngchuān (唐容川) in the late Qing Dynasty, who wrote five medical books, including the *Medical Essence of Chinese and Western Reconciliation* (*Zhōng xī huì tōng yī jīng jīng yì*, 中西汇通医经精义).

One of his famous sayings about the combination of TCM and Western Medicine is that, 'seeing no boundaries between TCM and Western Medicine, but compromising the meaning of Chinese and Western Medicine into one thing'.

The first half of the sentence is right, while the other half is wrong.

Through nearly half a century, there have been various opinions about the combination of TCM and Western Medicine, and their level of 'scientificity' is incomparable with those in the past, but it is merely the continuous renewal of nouns without great difference in the general concept. Therefore, Táng Róngchuān (唐容川) is called as the 'pioneer' of the combination of TCM and Western Medicine in the medical circle.

If we want to make it clear, I have to talk about my teacher to begin with. The grandfather and maternal grandfather of my teacher, Huáng Jiéxī (黄杰熙), who was born in Neijiang City, Sichuan Province, were exactly the brilliant disciples of Táng Róngchuān (唐容川).

Mr. Huang's father passed away at an early age, so my teacher was brought up by his late grandfather, honored as Master Zhi Ping (a title of renowned member of Traditional Chinese Medical Center of Kuomintang party at that time.) Master Zhi Ping was very famous so he was often captured by bandits to cure their chiefs living in the mountains.

He was a doctor from Sichuan Province and got famous around the country in the early post-liberation period in China, and some of his disciples were also celebrated doctors.

The deceased grandfather liked Mr. Huang because he was more perspicacious than others in his childhood. Ever since he was five, he was taught to read numerous books about TCM including classic theory and clinic aspects. His grandfather gave earnest exhortations to him even while treating a patient at his or her home.

My teacher Mr. Huang remembered that once when he was a child his grandfather was invited to treat Wāng Jīngwèi (汪精卫) at his home. Wang's wife Chén Bìjūn (陈璧君) thought my teacher was very lovely then and would like to have him as their godson. However, she was refused by my teacher's grandfather. Mr. Huang later talked about this with a smile, "Thanks to my grandfather's wisdom, I could get rid of their notoriety!"

In the 1980s, I was lucky to meet Mr. Huang, who then imparted his knowledge to me for years. However, he never talked about the principle of the reconciliation of Chinese and Western Medicine; instead, he spoke highly of the thought of TCM proposed by Mr. Táng Róngchuān (唐容川).

Take a simple case as an example:

In *Questions and Answers on Materia Medica* (*Běn cǎo wèn dá*, 本草问答) written by Táng Róngchuān (唐容川), there is a saying of his disciple, "Medicinals are made from such matters as insects, earth materials, grass roots and barks, which can cure human diseases even if they are different from human beings. Why?"

Táng Róngchuān (唐容川) answered: "There is nothing but yin and yang in the universe, which form the five circuits (metal, wood, water, fire, and earth circuit) and six qi (wind, coldness, dampness, dryness, fire, and heat) through motion. Human life adheres to the heaven and earth, that is to say, the five zang-organs and six fu-organs are formed from five circuits and six qi. Although all matters are different from human beings, they are also formed by adhering to the qi from heaven and earth. Every kind of qi possess a special nature, while human beings get all kinds of qi from the heaven and earth. The deficiency and excess of qi in human body will lead to diseases. The special nature of qi in Chinese medicinals (matters) can regulate the deficiency and excess of human body to a harmonious situation, so there will not be diseases! Because yin and yang of matters can change yin and yang of human beings. That's the reason why Shénnóng (神农) cured diseases with medicinals."

These words point out the pharmacology of treatment based on TCM. TCM treats a disease by using the special natures of Chinese medicinals originating from five circuits and six qi, rectify to imbalances.

One cannot understand TCM without understanding this truth. In spite of a simple sentence, Mr. Huang evaluated it as: "Establishing the fundamental principle for medicinals to cure diseases and approaching a higher level than other medical methods, which becomes the general principle and golden rule in pharmacology."

Besides, as for anatomy, some students may ask: "It is accurate and detailed that Shénnóng (神农) matched five circuits and six qi with five zang-organs and six fu-organs, and differentiated their properties and flavors to cure all diseases after tasting herbs. But the present western medical method, depending on analysis and observation of anatomy, thinks that the Chinese cannot see the internal organs and make prescriptions without academic basis. Is this reasonable or not?"

Táng Róngchuān (唐容川) answered: "No! When the westerners originally establish the medical methods, they cannot know the internal organs without dissecting, the body. The ancient Chinese saints defined items of five zang-organs and six fu-organs clearly, what's the use of anatomy at present? When Shénnóng (神农) established pharmacology, he may observe through anatomy or actually perceive the internal organs, but there is no need to discuss this. Now that the items of five zang-organs and six fu-organs have been defined and they actually exist, don't those who have to see the internal organs in person believe that the ancient saints had seen the internal organs by themselves? *Miraculous Pivot* (*Líng shū jīng,* 灵枢经) records, 'five zang-organs and six fu-organs can be observed through anatomy.' It can be concluded from this, that the ancient saints had observed them through anatomy. Besides, the western anatomy only knows the anatomical layers rather than the meridians and collaterals; it only knows the shapes and traces rather than qi transformation. Comparing with the modern medicine in China, they both have their own advantages and disadvantages. But if compared with *Huangdi's Internal Classic* (*Nèi jīng*, 内经) or *Shennong's Classic of Materia Medica* (*Shén nóng běn cǎo jīng*, 神农本草经), Western Medicine is inferior to TCM."

This indicates that Táng Róngchuān (唐容川) also regarded TCM and Western Medicine as two totally different medicine systems.

As for the human body, Western Medicine focuses on the anatomical layers, shape, and trace, i.e. tangibility; while TCM stresses meridians, collaterals, and qi transformation, i.e. intangibility. However, Western Medicine is inferior to TCM in the understanding of somatic science, namely, it is the 'blind zone' of Western Medicine.

How can reconciliation be achieved between TCM and the 'blind zone'? In order to reach the reconciliation, TCM has to copy the terminologies from Western Medicine without flexibility in use, merely giving strained interpretations and drawing farfetched analogies.

Very similar to the idea of integrating TCM and Western Medicine suggested by Zhāng Xīchún (张锡纯), Táng Róngchuān (唐容川)'s reconciliation of Chinese and Western Medicine is nothing but some literal words; however, he himself was an authentic doctor of TCM. In his early years, he put his heart and soul in studying *Huangdi's Internal Classic* (*Nèi jīng*, 内经) and the books written by Zhāng Zhòngjǐng (张仲景). He was a great clinical master of TCM in his generation, known as 'Grand master' at that time. Although his writings contain the terms of Western Medicine in the aspects of pharmacology, anatomy and experimentation, the defects still cannot obscure the virtues. I just dismiss those terms when I read his books. I always think about his enlightening opinions on TCM and place all his books on my desk for me to read from time to time.

Xí Shíxī (席时熙), who modestly called himself as 'Mr. Tang's younger brother', wrote a Chinese poem as the postscript for Mr. Tang's book of *Questions and Answers on Materia Medica* (*Běn cǎo wèn dá,*

本草问答). I appreciate that poem very much. Sharing it with you, the meaning of which is like:

'Postscript:

Human body is of one's own little world that qi and blood is divided into yin and yang. Regardless of normal life rhythm, people will get sick for the excess state. Yellow Emperor and his official Qibo showed solicitude for his people about their illness. Besides talking over the national governance, they also discussed five elements, six qi, five-zang and six-fu organs in detail. They brought the benefit to the people everywhere, their moral principle just like the sunlight and moonlight. Shénnóng (神农) gathered and tasted more than three hundred kinds of Chinese medicinals personally. He selected herbs to treat diseases and could really cure them. Since then, there were many more kinds of herbs arising in the later ages but none of them were effective as before. After Zhāng Zhòngjǐng (张仲景) carried forward the principle of decoction, TCM doctors have always been sticking to it. Doctors would possess superb medical skills after seeking for the truth from the classic books of TCM. Most of the famous sages appeared in the Han and Tang dynasties. At that time, academic ideas flourished but most of them were ambiguous. What's more, all sages argued with each other for proving their academic ideas. Later generations have to consider numerous ideas, but what they have learned from them may be very little. Táng Róngchuān (唐容川) from Tianpeng in the Qing Dynasty serves the country worthily with his words. He is so good at medicine that he can compare with the famous doctor. He has read many volumes of books and learned *Huangdi's Internal Classic* (*Nèi jīng,* 内经) by heart. His house is full of medical books and his clinical thoughts can come up to the level of Zhāng Zhòngjǐng (张仲景). His writing of *Questions and Answers on Materia Medica* gives a detailed exposition of Chinese medicine. It covers everything about TCM and the famous remarks in it last forever. Reading it will make you truly enlightened and will make you a good doctor. Every word in it is sparkling when you read it aloud.'

This postscript is not only catchy but also concise and comprehensive. It highly praises the contribution of Táng Róngchuān (唐容川) to TCM and Chinese materia medica and highly summarizes the scientific attributes of TCM and Chinese materia medica, as well as points out the way forward of studying TCM.

Every time I read it, I feel so impressed that I put all my heart to it. I am significantly proud of this intangible science — TCM invented by Chinese ancestors.

Speaking of academic family tree, Huáng Jiéxī (黄杰熙) was Táng Róngchuān (唐容川)'s disciple, and as a student of Mr. Huang, I am surely a disciple of Táng Róngchuān (唐容川). Therefore, the works of Táng Róngchuān (唐容川) are also with me every day, especially the *Questions and Answers on Materia Medica* (*Běn cǎo wèn dá*, 本草问答) which I peruse from time to time. From that book, I begin to understand the principle of curing diseases with TCM and learn some methods to both save people's lives and my soul. Because of that book, I deeply believe that TCM is an intangible science. All the knowledge I acquire depends on the teachings from my respected teacher as well as the virtues bestowed by Táng Róngchuān (唐容川), which can be seen as 'inheriting the previous works can make known the preciousness of the ancients, opening up the future for our successors.'

The knowledge of TCM is extensive and profound and of long standing. The famous doctors are coming forth in large numbers from various schools for thousands of years. There are so many works as numerous as stars.

However, why do TCM doctors only regard *Huangdi's Internal Classic* (*Nèi jīng*, 内经) and the works by Zhāng Zhòngjǐng (张仲景) as the classics? As said by Mr. Huang: "The previous saints made comprehensive concepts while the subsequent masters only focused on specific points; comprehensive concepts can cover the specific points, and specific points were deduced from those comprehensive concepts. This is the difference between saints and masters."

The works of Saints are the classics; the comprehensive concepts are the source. The masters are the famous doctors in all previous dynasties; the specific points constitute various schools.

Huangdi's Internal Classic (*Nèi jīng*, 内经) is the origin of TCM theory. Only by understanding this source can people get to know its different schools and can a deep-rooted tree be luxuriant.

Treatise on Cold Damage Diseases (*Shāng hán lùn,* 伤寒论) by Zhāng Zhòngjǐng (张仲景) is the first book that points out the thinking pattern of syndrome differentiation and treatment. It will be eternal and if we imitate this pattern, we will grasp the key method to cure diseases.

I have nearly dedicated my lifetime to researching and proving it, which shows "Good books reward reading for hundreds of times". Therefore, I am always surprised by its profound knowledge! Moreover, although the works of subsequent masters are about specific points, they have their own advantages. After I read them extensively, I realize their ingenuity to cure diseases. I can't help to sigh with emotion that specific points have their own schools.

However, similar to Zhāng Xīchún (张锡纯)'s *Records of Traditional Chinese and Western Medicine in Combination,* the *Medical Essence of Chinese and Western Reconciliation* (*Zhōng xī huì tōng yī jīng jīng yì,* 中西汇通医经精义), written by Táng Róngchuān (唐容川), a grand master in TCM, offers a wrong principle for the combination of TCM and Western Medicine nowadays. Thus, although he is my ancestral teacher, I have to point out his mistakes, just like the old saying goes, 'Plato is dear to me, but dearest is still the truth'. Both Mr. Huang and Mr. Tang in the heaven will forgive me.

Talking about the combination of TCM and Western Medicine, people closely involved in it cannot see it as clearly as those from outside.

At the end of 2009, the *Chinese Journal of Traditional Chinese Medicine* published an article about Qián Xuésēn (钱学森), the most famous scientist of atomic and hydrogen bombs and man-made satellites in China. Mr. Qian said in the article: "In the early years after the P.R. China was founded, the country has already given the importance to TCM; moreover it made the requirements for the modernization of TCM. However, the issue of how to achieve the modernization of TCM then seemingly became the so-called combination of Chinese and Western Medicine, that is to say, TCM is treated as an unscientific subject and it needs to use the science of Western Medicine to achieve the modernization of TCM. However, it is now worth considering whether such a method can succeed."

At a meeting a few years ago, I met professor Kuàng Ānkūn (邝安坤), a famous expert in the integration of TCM and Western Medicine. We had a pleasant conversation in that evening.

I told him that I am afraid that the combination of TCM and Western Medicine could not be reached by using the science of Western Medicine to achieve the modernization of TCM, because the guiding ideology of TCM is quite different from that of the Western Medicine. TCM is good at viewing the issue from the system as a whole.

Having heard my concerns, Professor Kuang said that he had studied the combination of TCM and Western Medicine for 30 years, but he also felt he couldn't go any further.

Therefore he was happy when he heard the other direction suggested by me. We had that conversation four or five years ago. In other words, he had studied the modernization of TCM in the way of combination of TCM and Western Medicine for 30 years, but still felt confused about it. His experience indicates that the problem is not a simple issue.

Yán Fù (严复) once said that only those who do research can know the truth of academic knowledge.

TCM is just a typical case. As an intangible science, it is hard for ordinary people, or even intelligent scientists, writers, philosophers or thinkers who never have experience in learning TCM to catch its points. Therefore, it is extremely valuable and great for Qián Xuésēn (钱学森) to have such a view on the combination of TCM and Western Medicine.

As for Professor Kuàng Ānkūn (邝安坤), I admire him a lot because he dares to speak out the truth and admit his failure. This kind of spirit of seeking the truth is the true scientific spirit.

I also remember the thing that taught me a lesson.

Since I began to learn medicine in the 1970s when the combination of TCM and Western Medicine sprang up, it seemed that the new medicine and pharmacology of Chinese and Western combination was to come into being which, according to some experts, was above both TCM and Western Medicine.

I remember that in addition to studying hard on the classic medical books, I devoted more to catching up with the new development of TCM as well. I not only bought TCM textbooks for university students and all books about TCM in the Xinhua Bookstore, but also subscribed to almost all TCM magazines which were available at that time. All those maga-zines would like to emphasize the word 'new' before 'TCM', for example, the *Journal of Traditional Chinese Medicine* in the 1950s omitted

'Traditional Chinese Medicine' and changed its title to the *Journal of New Medicine and Pharmacology*. At that time, I had only one belief that it would be worthy if I subscribed to ten magazines and only learned one useful prescription.

Therefore, I desperately recorded and memorized every formula and medicinal ingredients with their functions, using up dozens of notebooks.

When I sat in the consulting room, although I felt the pulse of each patient, I still wore a stethoscope and could only be at ease after hearing the lung sound of the patient, using a sphygmomanometer to take the patient's blood pressure, giving the patient a series of blood tests and an X-ray. Then I could decide the corresponding prescription and Chinese medicinals. Patients praised me a lot when they saw I was so responsible for them. I also enjoyed it very much!

I had experienced such a 'busy medical service' for almost 10 years. Then I found that no matter how I crazily master the most updated prescription researched by the modernization of TCM, I still felt difficult to have a nice match in the clinic. Even if I could occasionally cure some patients suffering from usual diseases in that way, the same prescription would not be suitable for other similar patients. Besides, all those prescriptions were useless when dealing with more serious diseases.

I rethought why I could not go any further even if I have spent so much time and efforts on TCM, and have been willing to devote all my lifetime to it.

Now I figure out the reason was that I was misled by those so-called experts in the combination of TCM and Western Medicine. Yáng Wànlǐ (杨万里), a famous poet in the Southern Song Dynasty, had a poem describing the natural scenery, 'Never say that the climbers will have no difficulties before they go down the hills, for they will rejoice too soon for it; They have a long way to go, because they are still surrounded by thousands of mountains.' I think that the combination of TCM and Western Medicine brings a new field of medicine and pharmacology that can cure no matter what kind of diseases without syndrome differentiation. It just leads me to be 'surrounded by thousands of mountains'.

With time passing by, I have grown old with my hair grey, but I still could hear the announcements from many experts. They said the combination of TCM and Western Medicine had made great progress on the aspects of the primary theory and microcosmic molecules, they talked about the new theory being formed; some experts even listed a time schedule for the era of that new medicine and pharmacology — around '2050s'. All the things they've done are vague with nothing in it for me, just as the old saying goes, 'it is said there is a Mount Heaven, but it locates at somewhere illusory'.

When talking about integrating TCM and Western Medicine, people at first mention TCM which means adhering to the thinking pattern of syndrome differentiation and treatment; as for integrating with Western Medicine, it indicates that modern science and medical knowledge should be regarded as the references to make the prescription during the treatment.

There is a saying in TCM, 'Inferior doctor cares about the form, superior doctor cares about the spirit'. TCM, as an intangible science, emphasizes the spirit, which means its therapeutic goal is to seek the original cause.

However, Western Medicine, as a tangible science, focuses more on the form and treats what can be observed.

During the treatment, it is hard to emphasize the spirit, but it is easier for the form. The problem is that TCM makes a big somersault in the endless process of referring to the thinking pattern of Western Medicine. By doing so, it will enter the wrong approach of curing head if there is a headache and foot if there is foot pain. Taking the case of *Asipilin Jia Shigao Tang* (*Aspirin and Gypsum Decoction*) as an example, the clinical application of it lacks the thinking pattern of syndrome differentiation and treatment, which makes it completely deviate from Chinese Medicine. If every treatment is so, then every treatment would lose this thinking pattern, entering the wrong region with no curative effect.

When walking onto the wrong path, a wise person can rethink it to find the way back to the right path. However, only those conventional TCM doctors with rich experience in TCM can find the right path, but for those acquiring surface knowledge from books, how can they find the way back?

Initially, for those who believe in the reconciliation of Chinese and Western Medicine, instead of just combining the knowledge of Chinese and Western Medicine, the intention was to see no boundaries for Western

Medicine, to make Chinese and Western Medicine co-exist. The author himself was not out of the thinking of TCM. *Medical Essence of Chinese and Western Reconciliation* (*Zhōng xī huì tōng yī jīng jīng yì*, 中西汇通 医经精义) by Táng Róngchuān (唐容川) points out the 'essence' of Chinese Medicine by simply comparing the anatomy of Western Medicine and the theory of viscera of TCM! However, this wording of 'Chinese and Western Reconciliation' quite easily to mislead the later learners to promote westernized TCM today, regarding Táng Róngchuān (唐容川) as a pioneer of the combination of TCM and Western Medicine. However, there is an essential difference between Táng Róngchuān (唐容川) and the persons supporting the combination of Chinese and Western Medicine today.

For the present situation of the combination of Chinese and Western Medicine, Qián Xuésēn (钱学森) once pointed out that some experts treated TCM as unscientific and tried to achieve the modernization of TCM by using the science of Western Medicine. In my opinion, what they have done completely denies the scientific attribute of TCM. Some experts regard extracting the herb ingredients through modern scientific methods as a new development of the study of the combination of TCM and Western Medicine, and even announce that only in this way can we rejuvenate TCM. However, if TCM loses its soul of syndrome differentiation and treatment, how can TCM be developed?

The combination of TCM and Western Medicine not only does not rejuvenate TCM, but indeed will lead the true TCM to merely exist in name.

An article entitled '*TCM as a Canadian Scholar Sees It*' was published in *Chinese National Geography* in July 2003, and was written by Ms Hu Biling (Brenda Hood) who studied in China.

"Every time I get sick, I will go to see doctors in a very famous TCM hospital in Beijing. However, they always make the prescription with the western medicines", says Hu, "When I stress that I must take Chinese medicinals, they feel very surprised. It is not because I am a foreigner so they treat me like that; even if my Chinese friends go to see TCM doctors, they still prefer to prescribe the western medicines."

She also presents a case she witnessed as an example. "Five years ago, I was having my internship in a TCM hospital", says Hu, "One day there was an old lady suffering from hyperacidity coming to see a doctor. After carrying out four examinations of inspection, listening and smelling, inquiry, pulse taking and palpation, the doctor told us that there were 7 Chinese medicinals that can control the gastric acid. Then, he used all those 7 medicinals in the prescription which only had 12 ingredients!"

Even this young female scholar who knows little about TCM feels very shocked by our Chinese doctors using the Chinese medicinals in such a way!

She says, "The thinking mode of TCM shouldn't be like this. Only one or two medicinals are enough to control the gastric acid, and the rest can be used to treat the causes of her gastric acidity. Obviously, the thinking mode of this doctor is the one of a Western Medicine doctor, that is 'treating the stomach when the stomach aches'."

The biggest problem of such seemingly modern TCM is that it cannot cure the disease. "Not surprisingly, in the next week, the old lady came again. Obviously, the prescription didn't work", Hu says.

Hu thinks a lot about this phenomenon and says, "The combination of TCM and Western Medicine can only develop Western Medicine but weaken TCM at the end, and the great TCM will become dependent on Western Medicine."

She straightly points out, "I think the thinking mode and the effect of the combination of TCM and Western Medicine hide the destruction of TCM."

In that article, she also talks about her understanding of current situation of the development of medicine in the western world. She says, "In recent decades, the mainstream Western Medicine has undertaken a quiet but profound change. Alternative medicine (the way the western world talks about TCM due to their little understanding of it — noted by the author) begins to be popular due to its capacity of curing diseases both from physical and mental aspects. TCM is the fastest growing one in the dozens of alternative medicines. The westerners have found that the mode of Western Medicine is hard to make progress in the field of mind and body, because the western medical doctors are only good at treating the human being's body. Therefore, when the western scholars think the 21st century should be the century for curing mental illness, the part of 'deficiency' and 'superstition' that we think in TCM perhaps can just remove the curtain covering the science and Western Medicine, so as to make TCM to be treated more objectively and comprehensively."

This Canadian lady Hu Biling had hoped to learn Traditional Chinese Medicine in the birthplace of TCM in China.

She says, "Although I am a foreigner, I love TCM very much for the reason I don't know. I hope it can enrich the wisdom of human being and everyone, regardless of their race and nationality, can be healthier both physically and mentally due to TCM." However, the things she had heard and seen in China these years made her very disappointed and she decided to leave.

She also says, "For thousands of years, TCM has applied its own unique theory and methods to cure countless people. It itself is a complete and effective medicine system so that there is no need to use other knowledge to correct the 'shortcomings of TCM'."

She also says, "Perhaps, Chinese people always think of Western Medicine in a wrong way, because the west in reality is not what the Chinese think it is. In the western world, the so-called Western Medicine that the Chinese people think of is only one mainstream medicine among other medicines. Another thing is that in the wast people no longer equate 'science' with 'correctness' or 'uniqueness'. However, Chinese people today still treat the word 'science' as a good adjective. The difference on such understandings results in different medical situations in China and the west. Traditional Chinese Medicine is easier to be passed down in the west than in China."

What Ms Hu criticizes is exactly the 'crux' of the combination of TCM and Western Medicine.

The great scientist Newton had a very famous saying that, 'I do not frame hypotheses'. When explaining its meaning, Newton said: "I have not as yet been able to discover the reason for these properties of gravity from phenomena, and I do not frame hypotheses. For whatever is not deduced from the phenomena must be called a hypothesis; and hypotheses, whether metaphysical or physical, or based on occult qualities, or mechanical, have no place in experimental philosophy (*Newton's Philosophy of Nature Selections From His Writings*, Shanghai People's Publishing House, 1974:7–8)."

Thus it can be seen that the saying 'I do not frame hypotheses' does not mean that he opposes the 'hypothesis' that is put forward after researching known scientific facts and is based on scientific principle. The 'hypothesis' he objected to refers to the 'assumption or conjecture' that has no relation that has all experimental phenomena.

As for the combination of Chinese and Western Medicine today, isn't it the type of 'hypothesis' that Newton was against at that time? However, such thought is popular till now and has gained more followers. Isn't it leading TCM astray?

Syndrome differentiation and treatment is the key to solve difficult medical problems worldwide

— Discussing that the way of revitalizing and developing TCM should focus back on the origin of TCM by taking the example of curing an 87-year-old colon cancer patient

On March 1, 2012, Mr. Wang, the general manager assistant from a science and technology company in Beijing, called me and said that her 87-year-old grandmother Ms. Zhang started to have a stomachache from March, 2011 and the symptoms became more serious with time passing by. She was hospitalized in the People's Hospital of Weichang County at Chengde, Hebei Province in October. Because she was old and weak, she could not bear the proctoscopy examination. After CT scanning, a raised mass was found in the colon under the gallbladder, which blocked 3/4 of the enteric cavity, so she was diagnosed as having colon cancer. However, taking nutrition medicines and anticancer drugs in the hospital did not result in any positive effect.

After the Chinese New Year, she was hospitalized in that hospital again due to the intensified abdominal pain in March, 2012. Her medical record was No. 441712. Because it was an advanced-stage colon cancer, there was no alternative but to receive Dolantin injection treatment. Although the injection could take the pain away for a while, the adverse reaction was very severe.

Every time after the treatment, the patient would vomit whatever she ate. She thought the feeling of severe vomiting was much worse than the pain, and she would have died from vomiting, needless to say curing the cancer.

During that period of time, the patient lied in bed and couldn't move or eat anything. She was almost at her last breath.

Since she was suffering from the incurable disease in her eighties, all her families knew that it was hopeless to cure the disease, so they had bought the coffin and got her affairs in order.

However, having witnessed his grandmother's condition suffering from deadly pain, Mr. Wang was so grieved that he decided to call me for some treatment that could simply relieve his grandmother's pain.

I knew that once a malignant tumor was found, almost all the hospitals would suggest having a surgical removal with chemotherapy and radiotherapy. Thus I asked Mr. Wang why his grandmother did not receive the surgery since she had such a serious disease.

He said that he had seen so many patients who suffered from cancer had the chemotherapy and radiotherapy; the treatment cost large amounts of money, even the family fortune and the patient had to suffer a lot, but the result was still not satisfactory. In addition, his grandmother was always in poor health. Two decades ago, she had cholecystectomy due to gall stones; when she was in her sixties, because of myoma of uterus, she had received another surgery, which caused her to suffer a lot before the wound healed.

His grandmother was already 87 years old and was in a worse health condition than before. He worried that the wound would not heal and his grandmother might not survive the surgery.

His grandmother had been found with congestive heart failure after the examination in the hospital and could not bear the surgery. He begged me that it would be very much appreciated as long as his grandmother could suffer less from the pain and get rid of the Dolantin injection. They were not willing to see the patient dying of the pain.

Having heard his words, I was very depressed. What a tragedy it was! However, studying TCM would be meaningless for me if I could not cure this disease which could not be handled by Western Medicine. After deep thought, I dictated him a formula to have his grandmother taken immediately.

Here were the ingredients of the prescription:

Huangqi (*Radix Astragali*) 60g
Danggui (*Radix Angelicae Sinensis*) 30g
Taizishen (*Radix Pseudostellariae*) 45g
Yuanhu (*Corydalis yanhusuo*) 90g
Gancao (*Radix Glycyrrhizae*) 30g

All ingredients should be decocted with water for oral administration, and one dose should be taken each day.

On March 26, Mr. Wang called back and said that his grandmother's pain was alleviated the day she took my medicinals and she could bear it without Dolantin injection.

3 days later, the pain was much more relieved. Although she had a little blood in the stool, she did not feel uncomfortable. Since she did not take Dolantin injection any more, she no long vomited. Therefore, she had a better condition and would like to have meals, which made her family very pleased. However, she still suffered from abdominal pain.

I speculated that the hemafecia may be caused by the rupture of the tumor, and the resolving method was the only way to relieve the pain. Moreover, there was a large dosage of tonic and nourishing medicinals in the prescription so it was fine to continue to take the medicinals and the dosages needed to be increased. Therefore, I changed the prescription as follows:

Huangqi (*Radix Astragali*) *90g*
Danggui (*Radix Angelicae Sinensis*) *40g*
Taizishen (*Radix Pseudostellariae*) *60g*
Yuanhu (*Corydalis yanhusuo*) *120g*
Gancao (*Radix Glycyrrhizae*) *40g*

All medicinals should be decocted with water for oral administration, and one dose should be taken each day.

I told him not to let his grandmother stop taking the medicinals until the pain was all gone.

On April 20, Mr. Wang called me again and said that the prescription was more effective, and his grandmother had stopped taking the medicinals as requested after the pain was gone.

He just called to tell me that the stool blood was more serious after the increase of dosages, and she slept for 3 days after taking the medicinals for ten days (This old lady was always in poor health, and had a physique of qi-blood deficiency. The reaction after taking medicine this time perfectly matched what was said in the book of *Huangdi's Internal Classic* (*Nèi jīng,* 内经) that, 'If a person's condition does not get worse temporarily after taking medicine, then the disease wound not be cured (Translator note: this sentence is quoted from The Book of History (Shàng shū, 尚书)).'). However, when she woke up 3 days later, there was no blood in faces and her stomach did not ache anymore; she also had a better appetite; her bowel movement was also finally back to normal after so many years of illness.

When I heard that, I finally felt relieved.

The old lady had taken the medicinals for a month and a half, by a rough calculation, she had taken 3300g of *Huangqi* (*Radix Astragali*); 1100g of *Danggui* (*Radix Angelicae Sinensis*); 2250g of *Taizishen* (*Radix Pseudostellariae*); 4500g of *Yuanhu* (*Corydalis yanhusuo*); 1500g of *Gancao* (*Radix Glycyrrhizae*).

Thereafter, Mr. Wang called me several times to tell me that his grandmother was getting better and better after stopping taking the medicinals and had a healthy diet.

When I was writing this article in the evening on September 28, I specifically called Mr. Wang, inquiring about his grandmother's current condition.

He said that his grandmother did not feel uncomfortable anymore, and had a good appetite. She even wanted to eat pig trotter and roast chicken. The family met all her requirements, buying whatever she wanted to eat. She was in a better condition than before, and was capable to sit up by herself, sometimes talking and laughing. His four aunts took shifts to go to the hospital to look after her. All the family members felt relieved since she did not suffer from the disease any more.

I asked why his grandmother was not discharged from the hospital. He said that she was unwilling to leave, because she would receive a nutrient solution transfusion every 4 to 5 days. The only thing mattered was that her blood vessels were too thin to be injected.

I asked whether his grandmother had another CT examination.

He told me that she had quite a good health condition now and was at such an old age, so she did not want to have any examinations.

The reason I tell readers this case is to prove that it will be difficult to solve the medical problems in the world without adopting the thinking pattern of syndrome differentiation and treatment of TCM.

I remember that someone wrote to question me, saying, "is the authentic Chinese Medicine leading the modern Chinese Medicine to the starting point of the *Internal Classic* (*Nèi jīng*, 内经) two thousand years ago?"

In my opinion, it is right to regard the *Internal Classic* (*Nèi jīng*, 内经) as the starting point of TCM, while the 'humoralism' of Hippocrates, the founder of Western Medicine, is the starting point of Western Medicine.

The development of both two medicinal systems has their own 'starting point' respectively, but their successors treat them with totally different attitudes. Western Medicine is a tangible science, so the medical skill keeps being updated and no one comes back to the starting point, while TCM is an intangible science, which can also be regarded as a natural rule, everlasting like stars and eternal as the diamond. Although famous doctors come forth in large numbers in every generation, all of them still deeply study the starting point, acquire knowledge and make good use of it, so no new theory can substitute the start point. Only in this way can TCM deal with complex diseases.

Just like this case I treated, *Huangqi* (*Radix Astragali*), *Danggui* (*Radix Angelicae Sinensis*), *Taizishen* (*Radix Pseudostellariae*), and *Gancao* (*Radix Glycyrrhizae*) that I used were to tonify and nourish qi-blood, which indicates the therapeutic principle of treating deficiency with tonification.

Using *Yuanhu* (*Corydalis yanhusuo*) was to utilize its functions of activating blood and moving qi, so as to remove the blood of abdominal mass, which indicates the therapeutic principle of treating excess with purgation.

For the dosages I prescribed were ten times the safety dosages of the pharmacopoeia, indicating the flexible therapeutic principles of treating serious deficiency with significant tonification, treating huge pain with significant purgation.

Herbal Classic (*Shén nóng běn cǎo jīng*, 神农本草经) states that when treating abscess, carbuncle, and long-term sore, using *Huangqi* (*Radix Astragali*) not only can strengthen the body resistance to eliminate pathogenic factors, but also can rectify the deviation to get a balance state of the body.

After the patient took the medicinals, I was not anxious when hearing that she had hemafecia, because I knew she was relieved from the pain and the hemafeica was due to the congestion of the tumor but not a disease.

If the blood stasis is not drained out from the body, is there any Chinese traditional anticancer medicinal that can cure the cancer? Is there any Chinese traditional pain-killer medicinal that is more effective than Dolantin?

Although the old lady's blood stasis was drained out from the body, I still increased the dosages of the medicinals. Because I knew that her pain was reduced, but not diminished, which means that the efficacy of the medicinals was not enough. This old lady suffered the intense pain caused by the tumor. At this critical moment, only removing the pathogen completely can relieve the pain and save her life in an instant.

The reason why she was in a coma for three days is because that although the old blood can be drained out of the body in a short period of time, the new blood cannot generate instantly, which needs a period of time.

Her revival after 3 days' coma indicates the removal of the pathogen and the recovery of the healthy qi. That's the reason why she could have a good appetite and could communicate with other people shortly after waking up.

Just a mere five usual medicinals made significant contribution to curing the disease, and the therapeutic method was enlightened from *Miraculous Pivot* (*Líng shū*, 灵枢) and *Plain Questions* (*Sù wèn*, 素问). The therapeutic method was based on Qi-Huang, and the medicinals were from *Herbal Classic* (*Shén nóng běn cǎo jīng*, 神农本草经). Only reverently following the old maxim from Zhāng Zhòngjǐng (张仲景), which is 'observe the pulse and symptoms carefully and treat the patient accordingly', can achieve such an effect.

Nevertheless, the 'starting point' of TCM the person mentioned above is really extensive and profound. My therapeutic principles and methods are all obtained from this 'starting point'.

The famous saying from Newton, 'If I have seen further it is by standing on the shoulders of giants', is worldwide famous. As for TCM doctors, the 'starting point' is equivalent to the 'giants'. Only by studying the 'starting point' all my life can I see farther than others, and treat the diseases that Western Medicine doctors cannot cure.

Therefore, only syndrome differentiation and treatment is the precious key to unlock medical problems in the world. I have decided to study it without any other option in my whole lifetime.

A sensible person once said: "Our suffering is not having no choice, but the opposite. These choices are from this developing world. It is because that people become confused faced with too many choices that the more knowledge we have, the more blind we are." What a penetrating insight it is! This is also the disadvantage of modern TCM education!

One person named Dù Yàn (杜艳) once said: "According to the five-year undergraduate degree course of TCM in a university of TCM in 2000, the time for TCM course accounts for only 33.8%, while the Western Medicine course accounts for 39.38%; English, computer studies and other general courses account for 26.7%. This leads to a vague idea of TCM, and an unversed idea of Western Medicine."

However, the percentage of TCM course time is only part of the problem. Actually, all the knowledge we gain from middle school and high school, such as math, physics and chemistry has laid a great foundation for learning Western Medicine; in order to learn TCM, one has to completely change the thinking mode, and must establish a new way of thinking that TCM is an intangible science at the first place; however, the most difficult thing in the world is to change one's mind.

Though equipped with lots of modern medical knowledge, in the view of the TCM learners, modern medical knowledge is just like a magic illusion potion, a chaos. As a result learners merely acquire the most superficial knowledge of TCM, but lose the 'judgment' of the essence of TCM — syndrome differentiation and treatment. No wonder those who honor themselves as modern TCM learners look down upon the ancients, often talking about the scientificity and modernization of TCM, but failing to mention what TCM would be like through scientification and modernization, and how to treat the disease with that kind of method. Isn't it what the scholar Zhū Xī (朱熹) of the Song Dynasty said: "The concern about the learners is that they are often addicted to speaking highly of some theories, but never take practical actions?"

There are only unknown diseases but no incurable ones

— Discussing that TCM is the new approach of developing medical science by taking the example of curing myelofibrosis

In recent years, I often take a morning flight back to Taiyuan from Beijing. Since I live far away from the capital airport, I always make a taxi reservation to pick me up at five in the morning. Coincidently, a taxi driver Mr. Huang picked me up twice, so we become familiar with each other and I often take his taxi if I go somewhere further.

Mr. Huang is from Badaling Town, Yanqing County in Beijing. Having known I am a TCM doctor, he told me that his father was badly ill and a major hospital in Beijing confirmed it as myelofibrosis. His father relied on blood transfusion to sustain life. Huang and his brother were both taxi drivers, so they could not afford the expensive treatment fees with their limited income. Besides, relying only on the blood transfusion was unlikely to save his father's life. Therefore, he asked me if I could make some prescription of Chinese medicinals, and I told him that I could have a try.

On November 19, 2010, Huang drove his father to my clinic. Since his father was weak and out of breath if going upstairs, I felt the pulse and prescribed for him in his car.

The patient Senior Huang was 56 years old. He showed me all kinds of test reports and X-rays plates of the People's Hospital of Yanqing County, but I only took a glimpse at the diagnosis result — myelofibrosis.

Myelofibrosis, as the name implies, means the bone marrow has become the fiber, losing the function of hematogenesis, which must be an incurable disease of modern medicine; therefore, he would not survive only by relying on the blood transfusion.

His father was pale and skinny with a low breathing, seemingly no strength to talk. Junior Huang told me his father's condition, and I knew that he had to receive blood transfusion of 400 ml once a week.

Sometimes, he had to have blood transfusion twice a week, that is 800 ml. It had lasted for over a year.

After the pulse diagnosis, I found that although his pulses beat 5 times in a cycle of breath, the pulses were extremely deep and weak, especially at Cun and Guan positions. What's more, his right pulse was in an even worse situation.

After inquiring, he told me that he had extreme fatigue, lying in bed all day long, feeling numbness in the hands and feet, tightness in chest, with dysuria. He also had a dry and tasteless mouth, and sighed frequently.

The symptoms were caused by asthenia of qi-blood leading to the exhaustion of both yin-yang. His father was a bricklayer in the village, living a humble life for his lifetime; his two sons made a living by driving taxis. However, he had to save his life through blood transfusion with high treatment fees. How could the old man be relieved facing such a hopeless situation? Greatly tonifying qi-blood, nourishing yin and invigorating yang, as well as soothing the liver and elevating the spleen-qi were needed. Here were the ingredients of the formula:

Huangqi (Radix Astragali) 50g
Dangshen (Radix Codonopsis) 30g
Danggui (Radix Angelicae Sinensis) 20g
Baizhu (Rhizoma Atractylodis Macrocephalae) 15g
Fuling (Poria) 15g
Guizhi (Ramulus Cinnamomi) 10g
Maidong (Radix Ophiopogonis) 20g
Wuweizi (Fructus Schisandrae) 6g
Shengma (Rhizoma Cimicifugae) 10g
Chaihu (Radix Bupleuri) 10g
Baishao (Radix Paeoniae Alba) 15g

Fuzi (*Radix Aconiti Lateralis Preparata*) *10g*
Zhigancao (*Radix Glycyrrhizae Preparata*) *10g*
Shengjiang (*Zingiber officinale*) *3 slices*
Dazao (*Fructus Zizyphi Jujubae*) *5 pieces*

All the ingredients should be decocted with water for oral administration and 10 doses should be taken.

On December 1, 2010, the patient came to my clinic for the second time. He told me that all symptoms had been relieved, and he himself felt a little bit recovered. However, the ulcer in his mouth made it inconvenient for him to have meals. Thus, based on the previous prescription, I reduced the dosage of *Huangqi* (*Radix Astragali*) to 30g, and added 30g *Pugongying* (*Herba Taraxaci*) and 10g *Tianhuafen* (*Radix Trichosanthis*). This time, 30 doses should be taken.

The third treatment on February 2, 2011: He told me that his hands were not numb, but the strength was still not enough; he was easy to have short of breath, a dry mouth and lip, abdominal distension even with reduced food intake. His pulses beat 6 times in a cycle of breath; though more powerful compared with the previous one, the pulses at Cun and Guan positions were still not powerful enough. It was not only because of asthenia of qi-blood, but also because of asthenia of spleen yin and spleen yang. The therapeutic methods should include tonifying qi and nourishing blood, tonifying spleen yin and spleen yang, promoting digestion and removing food stagnation. Prescription:

Huangqi (*Radix Astragali*) *30g*
Dangshen (*Radix Codonopsis*) *30g*
Baizhu (*Rhizoma Atractylodis Macrocephalae*) *10g*
Fuling (*Poria*) *10g*
Maidong (*Radix Ophiopogonis*) *15g*
Wuweizi (*Fructus Schisandrae*) *6g*
Shanyao (*Rhizoma Dioscoreae*) *30g*
Danggui (*Radix Angelicae Sinensis*) *20g*
Shengdihuang (*Radix Rehmanniae*) *15g*
Tianhuafen (*Radix Trichosanthis*) *20g*

Shashen (Radix Glehniae) 20g
Taizishen (Radix Pseudostellariae) 15g
Gouqizi (Fructus Lycii) 15g
Juhua (Flos Chrysanthemi) 10g
Muxiang (Radix Aucklandiae) 6g
Guya (Fructus Setariae Germinatus) 10g
Maiya (Fructus Hordei Germinatus) 10g

All the ingredients should be decocted with water for oral administration and 15 doses should be taken.

The fourth treatment on March 6, 2011: Dry mouth was less serious, abdominal distention was reduced, eating was normal, but only with shortness of breath and poor sleep all the time. His pulses were the same as before. This time, the therapeutic methods included greatly tonifying qi and nourishing blood, invigorating spleen and tonifying kidney, nourishing blood and calming mind. Prescription:

Huangqi (Radix Astragali) 50g
Dangshen (Radix Codonopsis) 30g
Baizhu (Rhizoma Atractylodis Macrocephalae) 20g
Fuling (Poria) 15g
Danggui (Radix Angelicae Sinensis) 20g
Chuanxiong (Rhizoma Chuanxiong) 10g
Muxiang (Radix Aucklandiae) 6g
Buguzhi (Fructus Psoraleae) 30g
Longyanrou (Arillus Longan) 30g
Hehuanpi (Cortex Albiziae) 30g
Yuanzhi (Radix Polygalae) 15g
Gancao zhi (Radix Glycyrrhizae Preparata) 10g

All the medicinals should be decocted with water for oral administration and 20 doses should be taken.

On April 5, 2011, the fifth treatment: He had no short of breath. Although he was more spirited than before, the strength was still not enough. Both hands and feet were not numb any more, instead they were cold. He also had weak legs, and tasteless mouth. His pulse was deep on both hands. According to the previous prescription continuously, the treatment should focus on greatly tonifying qi and blood, restoring yang, as well as elevating the spleen-qi slightly. Prescription:

Huangqi (Radix Astragali) 50g
Dangshen (Radix Codonopsis) 30g
Shudihuang (Radix Rehmanniae Preparata) 20g
Guizhi (Ramulus Cinnamomi) 10g
Baizhu (Rhizoma Atractylodis Macrocephalae) 15g
Shanyao (Rhizoma Dioscoreae) 30g
Yujin (Radix Curcumae) 15g
Huainiuxi (Radix Achyranthis Bidentatae) 15g
Shihu (Herba Dendrobii) 15g
Danggui (Radix Angelicae Sinensis) 15g
Fuzi (Radix Aconiti Lateralis) 10g
Buguzhi (Fructus Psoraleae) 30g
Hehuanpi (Cortex Albiziae) 30g
Longyanrou (Arillus Longan) 30g
Chenpi (Pericarpium Citri Reticulatae) 10g
Gancao zhi (Radix Glycyrrhizae Preparata) 15g

All the medicinals should be decocted with water for oral administration and 30 doses should be taken.

On August 11, 2011, the patient came to my clinic for the sixth time. He said that since taking Chinese medicinals, not only did he have a better health condition, but also the times of blood transfusion were reduced. Till then, only a blood transfusion of 400 ml was needed in one and a half month. He also told me that he could do some farming. His hands and feet were not cold, and defecation was back to normal. In spite of no shortness of breath, he still gasped when walking fast, had a low sleep quality (he had suffered from it for many years) and had no appetite. Though the pulses were more powerful compared with the previous one, they were still a little deep. Therefore, according to the previous prescription,

I reduced the dosage of *Shudihuang* (*Radix Rehmanniae Preparata*), and the dosage of *Danggui* (*Radix Angelicae Sinensis*) was changed to 20g, I also added 60g *Zaoren* (*Semen Ziziphi Spinosae*) and 15g *Maiya* (*Fructus Hordei Germinatus*). The ingredients were to be decocted in water for oral administration, and 30 doses should be taken.

On October 30, 2011, he called me for the seventh treatment. I was in Taiyuan at that time, and Junior Huang told me that his father was in a very good condition, and he only needed blood transfusion once every two months. After blood test in hospital, the doctor said everything was fine on the whole in spite of some indexes being lower than the normal standard. Now he just often sweat on forehead when having a meal, and was easy to catch a cold. It was still because of asthenia of qi-blood. Thus, this time, the therapeutic methods included tonifying qi-blood, yin-yang, and invigorating kidney yang. Prescription:

Huangqi (*Radix Astragali*) *60g*
Dangshen (*Radix Codonopsis*) *30g*
Guizhi (*Ramulus Cinnamomi*) *10g*
Baishao (*Radix Paeoniae Alba*) *10g*
Danggui (*Radix Angelicae Sinensis*) *30g*
Maidong (*Radix Ophiopogonis*) *15g*
Chenpi (*Pericarpium Citri Reticulatae*) *6g*
Shengma (*Rhizoma Cimicifugae*) *6g*
Chaihu (*Radix Bupleuri*) *6g*
Shihu (*Herba Dendrobii*) *15g*
Zhimu (*Rhizoma Anemarrhenae*) *15g*
Huainiuxi (*Radix Achyranthis Bidentatae*) *15g*
Fuzi (*Radix Aconiti Lateralis*) *10g*
Ganjiang (*Rhizoma Zingiberis*) *6g*
Baizhu (*Rhizoma Atractylodis Macrocephalae*) *15g*
Fuxiaomai (*Fructus Tritici Levis*) *30g*
Gouqizi (*Fructus Lycii*) *15g*
Xianlingpi (*Epimedium brevicornu Maxim*) *10g*
Buguzhi (*Fructus Psoraleae*) *30g*
Tusizi (*Semen Cuscutae*) *15g*

Honghua (*Flos Carthami*) 5g
Gancao zhi (*Radix Glycyrrhizae Preparata*) 10g

All the medicinals should be decocted in water for oral administration, and 30 doses should be taken.

On August 6, 2012, I was in Weihai at that time. Junior Huang told me by phone that his father had no blood transfusion for eight months since a blood transfusion before the Spring Festival. On October 12, hearing that I would come to Beijing for business trip, Junior Huang drove his father to see me specially. His father, with a rosy complexion, told me that he felt energetic now, and was not even tired when busy with the autumn harvest every day. Hospital tests showed that except that the hemoglobin level was low (10.6, normal is 11 ~ 30), the rest of indicators such as the platelets and white blood cells were normal. On April 7, 2013, when I saw his father again, he even had some black hair.

Zhū Liángchūn (朱良春), a leading authority in TCM once said: "There are only unknown diseases but no incurable one." This sentence combines all his experience and feelings in his lifetime, and is an irrefutable truth.

I would like to remind younger doctors of modern TCM that the 'unknown disease' refers to the 'ignorance' to TCM, instead of the 'ignorance' to Western Medicine.

On the contrary, this incurable disease refers to a disease that cannot be cured by TCM, and also refers to the various difficult and complicated cases in Western Medicine.

I think this is the only correct understanding to that sentence.

Why? Because Western Medicine both as the modern medicine and the mainstream medicine at present relies on the modern high-tech methods to observe the tangible aspects of the human body and disease but ignores those intangible ones. However, Western Medicine has made a huge mistake, which is being trapped into a dead end of tedious philosophy, unable to extricate itself, or it can be known as 'missing the wood for the trees'.

If a TCM doctor does not understand the above and does not study the ancient TCM with efforts to solve the 'incurable disease' of Western

Medicine, instead, he or she only studies Western Medicine with great efforts to master the modern scientific knowledge, this will lead to a 'dead end'. These TCM doctors cannot be more scientific than doctors of Western Medicine, so the incurable disease for doctors of Western Medicine will always be their 'incurable disease'.

Someone may ask: since I do not have any scientific knowledge of myelofibrosis, how can I cure such a disease?

Actually, I cure the disease relying on my superficial knowledge of the theory of TCM, that is, as Wáng Qīngrèn (王清任) once said: "The key for treatment of diseases is to have a good understanding of qi and blood, whether external or internal diseases[...] what is injured is always qi and blood."

About my treatment of myelofibrosis, for each treatment, I would consider selecting medicinals according to the symptoms on the premise of greatly tonifying qi and blood, which seems to have nothing to do with this 'bone marrow' of myelofibrosis. Fibrosis, however, had reversed; the patient could generate blood on his own and didn't have to sustain life by a blood transfusion. If the myelofibrosis didn't reverse, could he sustain life without a blood transfusion? Because the overall pattern of human body is changed, so the local areas will repair and change by itself automatically. TCM is a medical science focusing on the overall picture without the shortcoming of 'missing the wood for the trees'.

Wáng Qīngrèn (王清任) (1768–1831), also known as Quán Rèn (全任), courtesy name Xūnchén (勋臣), lived in Yutian County of Hebei in the Qing Dynasty. He was an innovative medical practitioner in the Chinese medical history. His book *Corrections of the Errors of Medical Works* (*Yī lín gǎi cùo*, 医林改错) had great influence on Chinese TCM and was acclaimed as 'essentials of old knowledge, unique and unprecedented.' Especially, he personally went to the graveyard and execution ground to observe human viscera, which ordinary people were unable to do, so his spirit of practice deserves to be commended.

Nonetheless, people in the later generations have also evaluated his book as 'correct the errors of medical works; the more he corrects, the more errors there are', which is also reasonable.

Wáng Qīngrèn (王清任) had said: "When a professional doctor treats the disease, he should have a good knowledge of viscera firstly. Otherwise, everything he concerns about would be wrong for losing the origin." He also said: "Writing a book without knowing viscera, isn't it insane? Treating diseases without having a good knowledge of viscera is similar to a blind person walking at night."

However, in the same book, he also said: "The key for treatment of diseases is to have a good understanding of qi and blood." That is a self-contradiction. What matters is that what he emphasized of viscera was not viscera-state doctrine, but the form and shape of viscera. He even criticized the predecessors: "What they said seems to be right, but they never saw the viscera; so they deceived others in order to gain reputation, which indeed harms people's health."

He strongly repudiated the predecessors. His rhetosic was not only fierce, but also deviates from the treatment principle of 'superior doctor cares about the spirit' from the book of *Internal Classic* (*Nèi jīng*, 内经). The 25 pieces of 'viscera graphics' that he drew cannot be compared with the modern human body anatomy. He definitely exposed himself to ridicule.

Changing his words to 'Writing a book only with the knowledge of viscera but without viscera-state doctrine is an idiotic nonsense. Treating diseases only with the knowledge of viscera but without viscera-state doctrine is similar to a blind person walking in the night.' would be impeccable.

Such a famous doctor who had gained considerable fame in Beijing with his unrivalled spirit of practice could have such a wrong understanding of TCM that misled the successors. It shows the difficulty of being a doctor.

However, some experts of TCM in modern times still evaluated Wáng Qīngrèn (王清任) as such: 'He is a complete inspiration in TCM, marking the stage that scholars of TCM have begun to set foot on the forefront of experimental research through practice'. This evaluation is even more misleading.

However, Wáng Qīngrèn (王清任) pointed out sharply in the same book that 'the key for treatment of diseases is to have a good understanding of qi and blood', 'people's movement is based on the original qi', 'what the channels and collaterals have is nothing but qi and blood', 'no qi and spirit in the brain for a moment, one will die for a moment; no qi and spirit in the brain for a quarter hour, then one will die for a quarter hour', 'what lies in the body is nothing but yin and yang, which is the same as fire and water; and fire and water is the same as qi and blood', 'what transports blood is qi, and what guards qi is blood', 'qi leads blood and promotes circulation of blood; while blood guards qi, enabling qi to be quiet; stagnation of qi will lead to blood stasis, deficiency of qi will lead to bleeding, qi pushing will lead to blood circulation' and so on. Aren't his views inconsistent with the previous one, 'practicing medicine and treating diseases should have a good knowledge of viscera firstly'?

Had he noticed qi since he had seen viscera of so many cadavers? Qi is intangible, so how can one see or feel it from a dead body?

If he couldn't see it, why was he proposing the theory of 'qi deficiency leads to blood stasis'?

The 25 formulas invented by him for treating blood stasis not only include medicinals that activate blood and resolve stasis, instead, they also include medicinals to regulate and tonify qi. Especially how different the dosages of qi-tonifying medicinals and blood-activating medicinals are in the formula of *Buyang Huanwu Tang* (*Yang-Tonifying Five-Returning Decoction*)!

Behind this contradiction lies a reasonable connotation, that is, after all, he was a veteran TCM doctor, and also a profound and pure TCM doctor. After making so many detours, he finally came back to the thinking mode of authentic TCM when treating diseases, and back to the ideological level of 'superior doctor cares about the spirit'. Therefore, the prescriptions he invented have an enlightening effect on the successors. This cannot be compared with those who have just learned a little knowledge of TCM and then begin to westernize TCM vigorously.

The knowledge of human anatomy among those experts westernizing TCM also cannot be compared with that of Wáng Qīngrèn (王清任). They are more profound. However, the theory of 'qi deficiency leads to blood stasis' of Wáng Qīngrèn (王清任) is more intelligent than those experts who only study blood stasis by integrating TCM with Western Medicine. Those experts are far behind to catch up with Wáng Qīngrèn (王清任).

Although the students in universities of TCM have mastered the knowledge of human anatomy and learnt it by heart, it is still useless to help them make prescriptions of TCM to cure diseases, because there is no viscera-state doctrine with regard to modern human body anatomy.

Those experts in the strategic development of TCM often earnestly warned us on newspaper that TCM can only survive by being 'in line' with the international world. The phrase 'in line' was used very ridiculously here; actually, there is no line for connecting at all!

If this phrase must be used, since there is no line for us to connect, it would be better to say that we 'create a line' to help them eliminate illiteracy of TCM. Let them gradually go out of the 'blind area' and know that, there is not only tangible science but also intangible science in the body science. Moreover, the intangible science may be the truth of the body science.

I also notice that many groups of western experts come to China to explore a new treatment approach with relevant experts in China because their medical research has already entered a dead end.

Our experts often tell them, "The long-term practice and experience of TCM will provide effective help to explore new therapies."

Actually, why aren't we bold and straight enough to tell them that there is no need to discuss this issue: only the ancient and eternal TCM with a history of thousands of years is the new way to conquer diseases, and there is no other way besides it?

Taking my treatment of the myelofibrosis case as an example, except for adopting the therapeutic principle of syndrome differentiation and treatment from authentic TCM seriously and earnestly, is there any other way to cure it?

What Chinese medicinals treat is to readjust imbalance

— Discussing the TCM therapeutic theory by taking the example of curing a patient with a history of trigeminal neuralgia for 20 years

In recent years, I often go to Weihai in Shandong Province and get to know Doctor Yang of the local naval hospital through my friend. Mr. Yang is a doctor of Western Medicine, but he loves TCM. What's more, he is also from Qingxu in Shanxi Province, so we become very good friends. He then introduced me to Doctor Zhou, an experienced TCM doctor in a local clinic. Mr. Zhou used to be a doctor of Western Medicine in the army, but after he was cured by a TCM doctor, he started to believe in TCM and also found a TCM master to study TCM. Due to the same belief, we are both very pleased to talk with each other and visit each other for many times.

On February 2, 2009, Mr. Zhou called and invited me to his clinic to treat a patient. The 53-year-old patient Mr. Bi was from Shidao in Shandong Province and worked in an oilfield at Dongying City.

He told me that his disease was caused by overworking and depression. In the autumn of 1990, he started to have left-side toothache and was not cured after many treatments. Afterwards, he was diagnosed with trigeminal neuralgia, and then he visited many experts of trigeminal neuralgia in major hospitals in Qingdao, Jinan and Beijing, but the ache was still not relieved.

He was then treated by small needle knife, and got a little relieved.

However, he fell ill again in the autumn of 2008. He had violent tic and pain on his left face like electric shock. The face convulsed every 10 minutes when the condition went serious. The symptoms were mild during the day time and became worse at night, so he could hardly asleep. What is worse, he felt painful as long as he spoke, drank water or even was touched, so he could not wash his face and brush his teeth for over four months.

He took innumerable Chinese medicinals for treatment year after year, which were found to be the medicinals with functions of expelling wind, activating blood and clearing heat, as well as stopping convulsions, such as *Mahuang* (*Radix Cannabis*), *Guizhi* (*Ramulus Cinnamomi*), *Chuanxiong* (*Rhizoma Chuanxiong*), *Fangfeng* (*Radix Saposhnikoviae*), *Baifuzi* (*Radix Aconiti Lateralis*), *Quanxie* (*Scorpio*), *Wugong* (*Scolopendra*), *Shigao* (*Gypsum Fibrosum*), *Niubangzi* (*Fructus Arctii*), *Jiangcan* (*Bombyx Batryticatus*), *Baizhi* (*Radix Angelicae Dahuricae*), *Baishao* (*Radix Paeoniae Alba*), *Taoren* (*Semen Persicae*), *Honghua* (*Flos Carthami*), *Gancao* (*Radix Glycyrrhizae*).

He was found to have very painful facial expression, a red face, a red tongue with a yellow coating, and a bitter taste. His pulses beat 10 times in a cycle of breath, his left Guan pulse was wiry, huge, and rapid.

From his pulse and symptoms, his illness was caused by the syndrome of liver yang transforming into wind, not by the syndrome of external wind attacking exterior or the syndrome of cold congealing in meridians. Therefore, the therapeutic method should focus on pacifying liver and subduing yang, extinguishing wind and stopping convulsions. Here were the ingredients of the formula:

Shijueming (*Concha Haliotidis*) *30g*
Muli (*Concha Ostreae*) *60g*
Danshen (*Radix Salviae Miltiorrhizae*) *30g*
Baishao (*Radix Paeoniae Alba*) *40g*
Gancao (*Radix Glycyrrhizae*) *30g*
Gouteng (*Ramulus Uncariae cum Uncis*) *30g*
Dilong (*Lumbricus*) *10g*

Decoct with water for oral administration, and 3 doses should be taken.

On 11, February, the second treatment: He said that the pain was effectively relieved, so I asked him to take 5 more doses.

On 16, February, the third treatment: He said that he no longer felt painful, and he just felt slightly uncomfortable on his left face when chewing the food. He had no bitter taste, but had a slightly red tongue, dry lips and poor sleep. His pulse was wiry and thready on both hands, beating 7 times in a cycle of breath. This time, for the better prognosis, the therapeutic methods included smoothing liver, nourishing yin and blood, and cooling blood. Here were the ingredients of the formula:

Danggui (Radix Angelicae Sinensis) 15g
Shengdi (Radix Rehmanniae Recens) 30g
Baishao (Radix Paeoniae Alba) 30g
Gancao (Radix Glycyrrhizae) 15g
Danshen (Radix Salviae Miltiorrhizae) 30g
Muli (Concha Ostreae) 60g
Guiban (Carapax et Plastrum Testudinis) 15g
Biejia (Carapax Trionycis) 15g
Danpi (Cortex Moutan Radicis) 20g
Yuanshen (Radix Scrophulariae) 15g
Yejiaoteng (Caulis Polygoni Multiflori) 30g

Decocted with water for oral administration, and 10 doses should be taken.

On May 7, Mr. Bi specially came to appreciate me from Dongying, saying that he was finally relieved from the pain that had tortured him for more than 20 years.

In August 2010, his wife came to Shidao from Dongying, telling me that her husband never got ill again since then.

Trigeminal neuralgia is a term in Western Medicine, and it is a neuropathic disorder characterized by episodes of intense pain in the face, originating from the trigeminal nerve. Its pain is like electric shock, knife cutting, or fire burning, therefore the patient is very painful.

I know nothing about the etiology and pathology of the trigeminal neuralgia in modern medicine, nor am I an expert in treating trigeminal neuralgia.

Mr. Bi had visited all the major hospitals in Qingdao, Jinan and Beijing and found numerous experts in treating trigeminal neuralgia, but still he was not cured.

Meanwhile, he also had taken various Chinese medicinals but they had no effect. It is not that TCM was not effective, but because those doctors failed to differentiate the correct syndromes.

The key that I can cure the patient who had suffered from the disease for over twenty years is that I made prescriptions based on his pulse. Besides, I was also inspired by a TCM theory of 'treating dynamic syndrome with static-natured medicine' proposed by a famous TCM doctor Xià Dùhéng (夏度衡) in Hunan Province, to treat primary trigeminal neuralgia.

When treating this kind of disease, Dr. Xia only prescribes four medicinals, namely, *Baishao* (*Radix Paeoniae Alba*), *Muli* (*Radix Paeoniae Alba*), *Danshen* (*Radix Salviae Miltiorrhizae*), and *Gancao* (*Radix Glycyrrhizae*). In this case, I followed Xia's prescription and added some medicinals according to the patient's condition, using *Shijueming* (*Concha Haliotidis*) and *Muli* (*Concha Ostreae*) to pacify liver and subdue yang, using *Danshen* (*Radix Salviae Miltiorrhizae*) and *Dilong* (*Lumbricus*) to activate blood circulation and dredge collaterals, using *Baishao* (*Radix Paeoniae Alba*) and *Gancao* (*Radix Glycyrrhizae*) to relax spasm and relieve pain, using *Gouteng* (*Ramulus Uncariae cum Uncis*) to extinguish wind and stop convulsions. As a result, the curative effect was rapid.

Although the meaning of treating dynamic syndrome with static-natured medicine is not the same as treating cold syndrome with hot-natured medicine, treating heat syndrome with cold-natured medicine, asthenia requiring tonification, and excess requiring purgation, but the principle is the same. All are using the properties of medicinals to readjust the imbalance state (disease), balancing yin and yang of the body. This is the principle for TCM to make prescriptions to cure diseases; in TCM, it is called the origin of TCM.

It should be stressed that in this 'treating dynamic syndrome with static-natured medicine', dynamic syndrome refers to the disease syndrome caused by internal problems instead of external reasons.

The pulse manifestation of this case was a wiry, huge, and rapid pulse at left Guan position. This pulse manifestation was like what Yè Tiānshì

(叶天士) wrote in his writing, 'Medicinals calm in nature are suitable for dynamic syndrome caused by internal stirring of liver wind.' If it was mistreated as external wind syndrome using medicinals such as *Mahuang* (*Herba Ephedrae*), *Guizhi* (*Ramulus Cinnamomi*), *Qianghuo* (*Rhizoma et Radix Notopterygii*), *Fangfeng* (*Radix Saposhnikoviae*), then the illness would get worse.

That is because such exterior releasing medicinals are pungent-warm and they are dynamic in nature. Treating a dynamic syndrome with dynamic-natured medicinals will result in a worse dynamic syndrome. It is the misuse of those medicinals that caused this patient to suffer from the disease for more than 20 years with the condition getting more serious. Chinese medicinals cure diseases through readjusting imbalances of patients. How can balance be achieved without readjusting? How can diseases be cured without balance? Balance is the major principle for TCM to cure diseases.

No matter how Western Medicine defines a disease, the therapeutic methods should include pacifying liver and subduing yang, stopping convulsions and extinguishing wind, as long as it is diagnosed with liver yang transforming into wind and ascendant harassing of liver wind.

Zhāng Shānléi (张山雷) once said: "When subduing yang, medicine of shell category is the first choice." This is indeed the insights of such an expert in clinic treatment. These medicinals are *Shenglonggu* (*Os Draconis*), *Shengmuli* (*Concha Ostreae*), *Shijueming* (*Concha Haliotidis*), *Zibeichi* (*Mauritia arabica*), *Guiban* (*Carapax et Plastrum Testudinis*), *Biejia* (*Carapax Trionycis*), *Zhenzhumu* (*Concha Margaritifera*), etc., which can be selected and used based on the patient's condition. The key and the essential issue of curing diseases in TCM is 'observing complexion and taking pulse, differentiating yin and yang first'. As long as the doctor takes the right principle and makes the proper prescription, the effect can be easily achieved.

No fixed therapeutic regimes, formulas, or fixed dosages

— Discussing the core of TCM clinic is the comprehensive analysis of the pulse and symptoms by taking the example of curing an 80-year-old cerebral thrombosis patient

Mr. Lu, a retired manager from Shanxi Construction Engineering Corporation, suddenly had cerebral thrombosis on November 7, 2007, when he was 80 years old. After being hospitalized for a month in Chinese People's Liberation Army 264 Hospital, he came to my clinic on December 12 after leaving the hospital.

After the examination, I found that he had facial paralysis, right hemiplegia, an unmovable right hand, a stiff tongue, slurred speech. He had a slight red tongue with a thin and white coating. The pulse at his left Cun and Guan positions was floating, slightly tight and rapid. Although he was diagnosed with cerebral thrombosis in Western Medicine, from the pulse and symptoms, he belonged to stroke in TCM. The treatment should primarily focus on dispelling pathogenic wind, then on activating blood and dredging collaterals. Here were the ingredients of the formula:

Mahuang (Herba Ephedrae) 10g
Fangji (Radix Stephaniae Tetrandrae) 10g
Yedangshen (Radix Codonopsis) 30g
Guizhi (Ramulus Cinnamomi) 10g

Huangqin (Radix Scutellariae) 10g
Chishao (Radix Paeoniae Rubra) 10g
Chuanxiong (Rhizoma Ligustici Chuanxiong) 10g
Xingren (Semen Armeniacae Amarum) 10g
Fangfeng (Radix Saposhnikoviae) 15g
Fuzi (Radix Aconiti Lateralis Preparata) 10g
Xixin (Herba Asari) 5g
Shengma (Rhizoma Cimicifugae) 10g
Baizhi (Radix Angelicae Dahuricae) 10g
Sumu (Lignum Sappan) 10g
Honghua (Flos Carthami) 10g
Gancao (Radix Glycyrrhizae) 10g

All the medicinals should be decocted with water for oral administration, and 6 doses should be taken.

The patient was advised to take the formula three times in the daytime and once at night and to live in the room with no wind from outside.

On December 27, 2007, the second treatment. The patient said that after taking the formulas for 4 days, all symptoms were effectively decreased and that his brother looked after him and boiled medicinals for him; he took the formula strictly according to my advice and lived in the wind-proof room. Therefore, he was cured after four days.

I said that I was enlightened by the oral administration method of *Xiao Xuming Tang* (*Minor Life-Prolonging Decoction*) mentioned in the book *Prescriptions Worth a Thousand Pieces of Gold for Emergencies* (*Qiān jīn fāng,* 千金方) written by Sūn Sīmiǎo (孙思邈). The words 'only living in a wind-proof room can cure this disease' was also proposed by this great doctor and not me.

Although there is a statement of 'To treat wind syndromes, the blood shall be treated first, and the wind syndromes would disappear with smooth blood circulation' in TCM, in this specific case, dispelling wind shall be emphasized, or it can be said that 'To treat blood, pathogenic wind shall be treated first, and the blood will be back to normal with the leaving of wind'. How can cerebral thrombosis be cured only with activating blood and resolving stasis? This is the case of making the prescription based on the pulse manifestation.

When asked about the reason for coming to my clinic this time, Mr. Lu said that he had felt fullness in head, dizziness, heaviness at the front of his head, dry mouth and bitter taste, so he was afraid it was the sign of the cerebral thrombus again; therefore, he came to me immediately.

After the examination, the pulse at his left Cun and Guan positions was wiry and huge, which obviously indicated the syndromes of ascendant hyperactivity of liver yang and liver yang transforming into up-disturbing wind. Therefore, the treatment should primary focus on settling liver and extinguishing wind with large doses of medicinals, then on resolving phlegm and dredging collaterals. Prescription:

Daizheshi (Hematite) 50g
Huainiuxi (Radix Cyathulae) 30g
Longgu (Os Draconis) 30g
Muli (Concha Ostreae) 30g
Baishao (Radix Paeoniae Alba) 15g
Yuanshen (Radix Paeoniae Alba) 30g
Tiandong (Radix Asparagi) 30g
Chuanlianzi (Fructus Meliae Toosendan) 20g
Maiya (Fructus Hordei Germinatus) 15g
Yinchen (Herba Artemisiae Scopariae) 30g
Banxia Sheng (Rhizoma Pinelliae) 20g
Tiannanxing Sheng (Rhizoma Arisaematis) 20g
Baifuzi Sheng (Tuber Typhonii) 20g
Yemingshao (Feaces Vespertilio) 15g
Wugong (Scolopendra) 10 pieces
Quanxie (Scorpio) 5 pieces

All the medicinals should be decocted with water for oral administration, and 10 doses should be taken.

On March 16, 2008, the patient came to me for the third treatment. All symptoms were eliminated. However, he still had fullness in head, dizziness, dry mouth and bitter taste, and chest distress. I found that the pulse at his left Cun and Guan positions was wiry and huge. This indicated the relapse of liver yang transforming into wind. What's more, he also suffered from blood stasis. Treatment should primarily focus on settling liver and extinguishing wind, and then on activating blood and resolving stasis, smoothing chest and regulating qi, and dredging collaterals. Prescription:

Daizheshi (Hematite) 60g
Huainiuxi (Radix Cyathulae) 30g
Longgu (Os Draconis) 30g
Muli (Concha Ostreae) 30g
Baishao (Radix Paeoniae Alba) 30g
Yuanshen (Radix Paeoniae Alba) 30g
Tiandong (Radix Asparagi) 30g
Jiegeng (Radix Platycodonis) 10g
Zhiqiao (Fructus Aurantii) 10g
Gualou (Fructus Trichosanthis) 20g
Xiebai (Bulbus Allii Macrostemonis) 10g
Yinchen (Herba Artemisiae Scopariae) 30g
Yedanshen (Radix Salviae Miltiorrhizae) 30g
Yemingshao (Feaces Vespertilio) 30g
Maiya (Fructus Hordei Germinatus) 15g
Juhua (Flos Chrysanthemi) 10g
Dilong (Lumbricus) 10g
Wugong (Scolopendra) 5 pieces
Quanxie (Scorpio) 10g

All the medicinals should be decocted with water for oral administration, and 10 doses should be taken.

On April 30, 2008, he came to me for the fourth treatment. He said that he was cured after taking the formula; he also gained a better sleep quality and a good appetite. The only problem was that his eyes were often with tears, and he felt exhausted and unstable for a long walk. The pulse beat 6 times in a cycle of breath. The pulse at his left Guan position was slightly floating, huge, and slippery. The therapeutic methods included smoothing triple energizer, activating blood and resolving stasis, harmonizing exterior and interior, invigorating spleen and draining dampness, and clearing liver and improving vision. Prescription:

Cangzhu (Rhizoma Atractylodis) 10g
Chuanpo (Cortex Magnoliae Officinalis) 10g
Chenpi (Pericarpium Citri Reticulatae) 10g
Gancao (Radix Glycyrrhizae) 10g
Sangye (Radix Glycyrrhizae) 10g
Juhua (Flos Chrysanthemi) 10g
Fangfeng (Radix Saposhnikoviae) 10g
Danggui (Radix Saposhnikoviae) 15g
Chishao (Radix Paeoniae Rubra) 15g
Jinyinhua (Radix Paeoniae Rubra) 15g
Gualou (Fructus Trichosanthis) 10g
Xiebai (Bulbus Allii Macrostemonis) 10g
Zhishi (Bulbus Allii Macrostemonis) 10g
Chaihu (Radix Bupleuri) 10g
Huanglian (Rhizoma Coptidis) 10g
Yedanshen (Radix Salviae Miltiorrhizae) 40g
Fuling (Poria) 10g
Zhuling (Polyporus) 10g
*Zexie (Rhizoma Alismatis)*10g
Baizhu (Rhizoma Atractylodis Macrocephalae) 10g
Guizhi (Ramulus Cinnamomi) 10g
Shengdi (Radix Rehmanniae Recens) 15g
Huanglian (Rhizoma Coptidis) 5g
Danpi (Cortex Moutan Radicis) 10g
Shengjiang (Rhizoma Zingiberis Recens) 3 slices
Dazao (Fructus Jujubae) 3 pieces *(guiding herb)*

All the medicinals should be decocted with water for oral administration, and 10 doses should be taken.

On July 23, 2008, he came to me for the fifth treatment. He said that his condition was much better, but he still felt easily exhausted. I found that he had a red tongue with a thin and slight yellow coating. His pulses at his Cun and Guan positions were weak under heavy pressure, beating 5 times in a cycle of breath. This old and feeble man shall be primarily treated with qi and blood tonifying medicinals. Though he had weak legs which belong to the lower part of the body, its treatment area should focus on the upper part — replenishing and uplifting qi. Moreover, activating blood and resolving stasis, clearing heat and cooling blood were also needed in the treatment. Prescription:

Huangqi (Radix Astragali seu Hedysari) 60g
Yedangshen (Radix Codonopsis) 30g
Baizhu (Radix Codonopsis) 10g
Chenpi (Radix Codonopsis) 10g
Shengma (Radix Codonopsisn) 6g
Chaihu (Radix Bupleuri) 10g
Danggui (Radix Angelicae Sinensis) 15g
Danpi (Cortex Moutan Radicis) 20g
Dihuang Sheng (Radix Rehmanniae Recens) 30g
Shanyao Sheng (Rhizoma Dioscoreae) 30g
Huainiuxi (Radix Cyathulae) 30g
Yedanshen (Radix Salviae Miltiorrhizae) 30g
Fuling (Poria) 15g
Chishao (Radix Paeoniae Rubra) 15g
Juhua (Flos Chrysanthemi) 10g
Xianlingpi (Herba Epimedii)10g
Gancao (Herba Epimedii) 10g

All the medicinals should be decocted with water for oral administration, and 10 doses should be taken.

On October 21, 2008, he came to me for the sixth time. He said that the medicinals were very effective, but he walked with unsteady steps and easily shed tears. Therefore, I advised him to take the fourth prescription for 10 doses.

On November 30, 2008, he came to me for the seventh treatment. He said that his eyes had not shed tears any more, but he had fatigue in the legs and numbness in the feet. His pulse was wiry and slightly rapid on both hands. The therapeutic methods included replenishing qi, smoothing triple energizer, activating blood and dredging collaterals. Prescription:

Huangqi (Radix Astragali seu Hedysari) 60g
Cangzhu (Rhizoma Atractylodis) 10g
Yedanshen (Radix Salviae Miltiorrhizae) 30g
Chuanpo (Cortex Magnoliae Officinalis) 10g
Chenpi (Radix Codonopsis) 10g
Huainiuxi (Radix Cyathulae) 30g
Shihu (Herba Dendrobii) 15g
Gualou (Fructus Trichosanthis) 10g
Xiebai (Bulbus Allii Macrostemonis) 10g
Zhishi (Fructus Aurantii Immaturus) 10g
Fuling (Poria) 10g
Chaihu (Radix Bupleuri) 10g
Zexie (Rhizoma Alismatis) 10g
Zhuling (Polyporus) 10g
Baizhu (Rhizoma Atractylodis Macrocephalae) 10g
Dihuang Sheng (Radix Rehmanniae Recens) 10g
Danpi (Cortex Moutan Radicis) 10g
Guizhi (Ramulus Cinnamomi) 10g
Baishao (Radix Paeoniae Alba) 10g
Muxiang (Radix Aucklandiae) 10g
Shuizhi (Hirudo) 10g
Gancao (Radix Glycyrrhizae) 10g

All the medicinals should be decocted with water for oral administration, and 10 doses should be taken.

On January 18, 2009, he came to me for the eighth treatment. He said that he was in good condition and had a good appetite, but only felt cold feet recently. The pulses beat 5 times in a cycle of breath. His left pulse was deep and huge, while right pulse was deficient. His symptoms were caused by the syndromes of stomach qi ascending counterflow and both yin and yang deficiency in kidney. Therefore, the treatment should firstly focus on invigorating spleen, harmonizing stomach and descending adverse qi, then focus on tonifying kidney yang and nourishing kidney yin. Prescription:

Yedangshen (Radix Codonopsis) 30g
Baizhu (Rhizoma Atractylodis Macrocephalae) 15g
Fuling (Poria) 30g
Gancao (Radix Glycyrrhizae) 10g
Chenpi (Pericarpium Citri Reticulatae) 10g
Banxia Sheng (Rhizoma Pinelliae) 15g
Zhuru (Caulis Bambusae in Taenia) 10g
Yedanshen (Radix Salviae Miltiorrhizae) 30g
Xianlingpi (Herba Epimedii) 10g
Dingxiang (Herba Epimedii) 3g
Shidi (Herba Epimedii) 10g
Guibanjiao (Chinemys reevesii(Gray)) 10g
Lujiaojiao (Colla Corni Cervi) 10g

All the medicinals should be decocted with water for oral administration, and 10 doses should be taken.

On April 5, 2009, he came to me for the ninth time. He said that he was healthy except for hiccupping in recent days. This time, he had a red tongue and a dry mouth. His pulse was wiry and huge on both hands, beating 7 times in a cycle of breath. The treatment should focus on pacifying liver and harmonizing stomach, descending counterflow of qi and nourishing yin. Prescription:

Longgu (Os Draconis) 30g
Muli (Concha Ostreae) 30g
Daizheshi (Hematite) 30g
Baishao (Radix Paeoniae Alba) 15g
Huainiuxi (Radix Paeoniae Alba) 30g
Yuanshen (Radix Scrophulariae) 15g
Tiandong (Radix Asparagi) 15g
Guiban (Carapax et Plastrum Testudinis) 15g
Chuanlianzi (Fructus Meliae Toosendan) 10g

Maiya (Fructus Hordei Germinatus) 10g
Chenpi (Pericarpium Citri Reticulatae) 10g
Zhuru (Caulis Bambusae in Taenia) 6g
Yinchen (Herba Artemisiae Scopariae) 30g
Gancao (Radix Glycyrrhizae) 10g

All the medicinals should be decocted with water for oral administration, and 10 doses should be taken.

On November 8, 2009, he came to me for the tenth treatment. He said that he had been in good condition for half a year. However, he felt a little dizzy and had fatigued legs again. After the examination, I found that his tongue had a thin and yellow coating; his pulse beat 5 times in a cycle of breath; the pulse at his right Cun and Guan positions was deficient, while at left Cun position was floating. This indicated the recurrence of wind stroke, therefore the the wind should be dispelled. Since he had serious qi deficiency, the qi and blood shall be greatly tonified, assisted with activating blood and resolving stasis. Prescription:

Huangqi (Radix Astragali seu Hedysari) 70g
Yedangshen (Radix Codonopsis) 60g
Mahuang (Herba Ephedrae) 10g
Fangfeng (Radix Saposhnikoviae) 10g
Fuzi (Radix Aconiti Lateralis Preparata) 10g
Guizhi (Ramulus Cinnamomi) 10g
Chuanxiong (Rhizoma Ligustici Chuanxiong) 10g
Baizhi (Radix Angelicae Dahuricae) 10g
Huangqin (Radix Scutellariae) 15g
Fangji (Radix Stephaniae Tetrandrae) 10g
Xingren (Semen Armeniacae Amarum) 10g
Yedanshen (Radix Salviae Miltiorrhizae) 30g
Gegen (Radix Puerariae) 15g
Shengma (Rhizoma Cimicifugae) 6g
Chaihu (Radix Bupleuri) 6g
Huainiuxi (Radix Cyathulae) 20g

Juhua (Flos Chrysanthemi) 10g
Gancao (Radix Glycyrrhizae) 10g

All the medicinals should be decocted with water for oral administration, and 10 doses should be taken.

On June 6, 2010, he came to me for the eleventh treatment. He said that he had been in a good condition, but felt a little dizzy recently. He had a red tongue and a dry mouth. His pulse was wiry, huge, and weak on both hands, beating 5 times in a cycle of breath. All his symptoms were still caused by the deficiency of qi and blood. He should be treated with tonifying qi and blood, assisted with activating and cooling blood, clearing head and vision. Prescription:

Huangqi (Radix Astragali seu Hedysari) 30g
Yedangshen (Radix Codonopsis) 60g
Yedanshen (Radix Salviae Miltiorrhizae) 30g
Gegen (Radix Puerariae) 30g
Juhua (Flos Chrysanthemi) 10g
Xianlingpi (Herba Epimedii) 15g
Chuanniuxi (Radix Cyathulae) 15g
Shihu (Herba Dendrobii) 20g
Dihuang Sheng (Radix Rehmanniae Recens) 30g
Baizhi (Radix Angelicae Dahuricae) 10g
Muxiang (Radix Aucklandiae) 10g
Shuizhi (Hirudo) 10g
Danpi (Cortex Moutan Radicis) 20g
Gancao (Radix Glycyrrhizae) 10g

All the medicinals should be decocted with water for oral administration, and 10 doses should be taken.

On November 7, 2010, he came to me for the twelfth treatment. He said that he had felt quite well over the past half a year with a good appetite, but suddenly the two legs were weak and fatigued recently. After the examination, I found that his pulse at left Cun, Guan positions was wiry, huge, and feeble, beating 5 times in a cycle of breath. Therefore, qi and blood should be greatly tonified again, assisted with activating blood and dredging collaterals. Prescription:

Huangqi (Radix Astragali seu Hedysari) 60g
Taizishen (Radix Pseudostellariae) 20g
Yedanshen (Radix Salviae Miltiorrhizae) 50g
Gegen (Radix Puerariae) 20g
Juhua (Flos Chrysanthemi) 10g
Xianlingpi (Herba Epimedii) 15g
Chuanniuxi (Radix Cyathulae) 15g
Baizhi (Radix Angelicae Dahuricae) 10g
Taoren (Semen Persicae) 10g
Honghua (Flos Carthami) 10g
Chishao (Radix Paeoniae Rubra) 10g
Chuanxiong (Rhizoma Ligustici Chuanxiong) 10g
Paofuzi (Radix Aconiti Lateralis Preparata) 10g
Dilong (Lumbricus) 15g
Shuizhi (Hirudo) 20g
Gancao (Radix Glycyrrhizae) 10g

All the medicinals should be decocted with water for oral administration, and 10 doses should be taken.

On November 14, 2010, the patient came to me for the 13th treatment. He had a flushing complexion and said that he did not have leg fatigue anymore. He even showed us he could stand up easily without the help of the armrests. In the past, he had to rely on the armrests to stand up slowly.

It can be seen from the examination that the pulse beat 5 times in a cycle of breath and was still slightly huge and feeble on both hands.

He was advised to continuously take the medicinals according to the last prescription for ten doses, changing *Taizishen (Radix Pseudostellariae)* into 60g of *Yedangshen (Radix Codonopsis)*, the dosage of *Yedanshen (Radix Salviae Miltiorrhizae)* changing into 60g, adding 30g *Gegen (Radix Puerariae)* and 15g *Shihu (Herba Dendrobii)*.

On December 12, 2010, the patient came to me for the 14th time. He said that he was quite healthy and in a very good condition. He even traveled to Xi'an for more than ten days by train. During the trip, he got a cold, his feet were cold, and he had leg cramps. The pulse beat 5 times in a cycle of breath. 30g *Paofuzi* (*Radix Aconiti Lateralis Preparata*) (be decocted first) was added to the previous prescription, and 10 doses should be taken this time.

I also warned him that although the cerebral thrombosis had been cured and he was in a very good condition, he had better not go travelling in midwinter since he was already 83.

I told him that TCM attaches importance to the harmony between human and the earth; people shall reduce the time outdoors in winter, sleeping early and getting up late, to avoid the wind. I also told him the theory that 'the old is afraid of cold damage syndrome, while the young is afraid of tuberculosis'. People should regard this seriously.

Mr. Lu had cerebral thrombosis in his eighties and had not been cured after receiving the transfusion treatment for a month in Western Medicine hospital; however, after 14 times of TCM treatment and taking more than one hundred doses of formulas, he was totally cured. In March 2012, I specially called him from Weihai in order to confirm his current condition. He picked up the phone by himself and talked to me with a loud and clear voice, saying that he was very fine and asked me not to worry about him.

On November 18, 2012, he came to my clinic in Taiyuan again. Although he was 85 years old, he could talk with me with a clear mind and a loud voice as a healthy person. I was very much impressed.

Someone may think that it is a doctor's duty to save people's lives and to ask about their conditions after several years. Why should I be so impressed?

Here is my answer: Actually, people may have no idea that curing a patient in such an old age is the most difficult thing according to my experience. The reason is pretty clear. It is recorded in *Internal Classic* (*Nèi jīng*, 内经) that, 'yin qi has died out a half when one's age is over forty'. That is to say, in the old age, the functions of each body system gradually decline, and the 'invasion of pathogen must be due to deficiency of essential qi'. Therefore, old people often have various illnesses, and they can hardly return to a healthy condition if suffering from diseases like cerebral thrombosis. Even if the old patients are temporarily cured, they tend to have the second and third recurrence leading to final death.

The cerebral thrombosis is called wind stroke or hemiplegia in TCM.

Since the wind is the primary pathogen, all medical books in the past dynasties regard wind stroke as the vital issue. The syndromes include genuine wind stroke, apoplectic stroke, wind striking meridians, wind striking zang-fu organs, and wind attacking blood vessels; its therapeutic methods included eliminating phlegm and extinguishing wind, nourishing blood and moistening dryness, nourishing yin and subduing yang, tonifying qi and banking up primordial qi. The more theories were devised, the more complex treating the disease is; the more difficult its principles are to be understood; the harder it is to be studied.

Therefore, wind stroke has been regarded as a serious disease that is hard to be cured since the ancient times. Different doctors and schools hold different opinions on it.

According to Zhū Dānxī (朱丹溪)'s viewpoint, the left hemiplegia belonged to blood deficiency and blood stasis which should be treated by *Siwu Tang* (*Four Ingredients Decoction*) added with *Taoren*(*Semen Persicae*), *Honghua*(*Flos Carthami*), *Jiangzhi*(*ginger juice*), *Zhuli*(*bamboo juice*), while the right hemiplegia belonged to qi deficiency and phlegm which should be treated by *Sijunzi Tang*(*Four Gentlemen Decoction*) added with *Jiangzhi*(*ginger juice*), *Zhuli*(*bamboo juice*). He simply and distinctly divided left and right by qi and blood.

However, this therapy had no effect and made people confused. Therefore, I suspect that it is not a clinical experience but an assumption of Zhū Dānxī (朱丹溪). Dating back to the Qing Dynasty, Wáng Qīngrèn (王清任) wrote the *Correction of the Errors of Medical Works* (*Yī lín gǎi cùo*, 医林改错), creating *Buyang Huanwu Tang* (*Yang-Tonifying Five-Returning Decoction*) that used a large dose of *Huangqi* (*Radix Astragali seu Hedysari*) with few medicinals having the effect of activating blood and dredging meridians to treat hemiplegia. This thereby initialized the treatment approach and received critical applause. However, the effect is remarkable when used in cerebral thrombosis patients with a deep and feeble or a huge and weak pulse on both hands, but still there is no effect on patients with a wiry, huge, and rapid pulse. Moreover, Wáng Qīngrèn (王清任) said that it was the primordial qi deficiency that caused the hemiplegia.

He said that if one person lost 50% primordial qi, then he will have 50% primordial qi left; therefore, Channels and Collaterals would have empty space; if there is an empty space, qi will inevitably concentrate to one side; if 25% qi of the right side is incorporated into the left side, the right side will have no qi; if 25% qi of the left side is incorporated into the right side, the left side will have no qi; one cannot move without qi; this immovability is called hemiplegia which means it cannot be used according to one's will.

What Wáng Qīngrèn (王清任) said seems reasonable, but it is actually also his conjecture.

If it is really the case, the side losing 25% primordial qi cannot move due to no qi, while the other side obtaining the extra 25% primordial qi will have 50% primordial qi, and this side shall feel more powerful, because its primordial qi is twice as much as before! Is there any patient with such a symptom?

Moreover, the book by Wáng Qīngrèn (王清任) emphasizes that 'the essential issue for TCM doctors to treat patients is to know about the viscera firstly', otherwise, it is 'talking idiotic nonsense' and 'a blind person walking at night'. Therefore, he observed the viscera of corpse in the grave and execution ground in person. Such a truth-seeking spirit with remarkable courage should indeed deserve our respect.

However, qi is intangible. How can one see qi by dissecting the corpse? How can one see that 25% qi of one side runs to the other side? Isn't it self-contradictory?

Viscera theory in TCM refers to the state of internal organs. It is 'inspecting exterior to predict interior' and is intangible. However, the state and position of internal organs studied by Wáng Qīngrèn (王清任) are tangible and belong to the human body anatomy, which is misleading for TCM.

However, he is praised as 'the milestone of ancient Chinese Medicine developing from yín-yang speculation to empirical dissection'. Giving such a high praise to his misleading theory is an even worse mistake.

The key problem is, the 'empirical dissection' by Wáng Qīngrèn (王清任) belongs to the basis of Western Medicine. He went away from the fundamental idea of yin-yang theory in TCM which is 'superior doctor cares about the spirit' and got involved in the work of 'inferior doctor cares about the form'. To what extent did he benefit TCM?

According to what Wáng Qīngrèn (王清任) said in his book, before he published the book, he spent 42 years studying the viscera from practice, and finally drew the pictures based on accurate details.

Wang once said that 'the essential issue for TCM doctors to treat patients is to know about the viscera firstly', but how could he treat diseases before he finally had a good knowledge of the viscera after 42 years? If he could not know how to treat diseases until 42 years later, how could he treat patients from Yutian County to Luanzhou (in Tangshan in Hebei Province) and Fengtian (Shenyang), and even ran a herbal medicine shop called Zhiyitang in Beijing? Isn't it self-contradictory again?

However, Wáng Qīngrèn (王清任) was an experienced TCM doctor after all. He only drew the internal organs that he saw and published it, but cared less about its utility. Later on, he started to say 'the key of the treatment of diseases is to have a good understanding of qi and blood', calling attention to 'examining the flourish and exhaustion of qi and blood, as well as distinguishing the stagnation of Channels and Collaterals', and returned to TCM thoughts. Thus, treating hemiplegia caused by qi deficiency and blood stasis with *Buyang Huanwu Tang* (*Yang-Tonifying Five-Returning Decoction*) is the highlight of the whole book and praised highly by the medical circle. Although the other prescriptions created by him, which emphasize curing blood stasis, can enlighten the later generations as well, little effect is achieved when verified in clinic.

Therefore, we shall distinguish the right from the wrong and only acquire that reasonable knowledge when reading TCM books instead of accepting all the principles they convey.

If people only rely on Wang's book and do empirical dissection, they will be misled and unable to understand the theory of TCM treating diseases.

This is like 'the letter kills, but the spirit gives life'.

Cerebral thrombosis is caused by thrombus blocking the blood vessel of a brain. The thrombus is tangible and visible. Western Medicine takes the transfusion treatment to achieve thrombolysis, while TCM promotes blood circulation to remove blood stasis. They all aim to eliminate the thrombus and the therapy has become a set pattern. Through this method the patient can be cured right after suffering from this disease, but the effect will be greatly affected with one or two days delay!

The reason I can cure the old-aged patient is that I benefit from much attention to the pulse and symptoms as the core. In spite of no fixed method, no fixed formula and no fixed quantity, the prescription and medication of each treatment do have a certain reason.

I would also like to emphasize that *Xiao Xuming Tang* (*Minor Life-Prolonging Decoction*) in the first treatment cannot be used simply by following the ordinary boiling method for Chinese medicinals, but needs to comply with Sūn Sīmiǎo (孙思邈)'s advice: firstly, the patient must live in a wind proof room to prevent any wind-cold attack; secondly, take the medicinals 3 times in the daytime and once in the nighttime to guarantee the effect and to drive the pathogen out of the body. Those who prescribe according to this prescription but see no effect may be due to not noticing the details in his books; however, sometimes the devil is in the detail, so please pay attention to details.

Every subject has its core knowledge. It is closely based on the core that one can quickly acquire the essence of the knowledge.

The core of TCM clinic is to differentiate pulse and symptoms. So to speak, the study of TCM is the study of differentiating pulse and symptoms.

The most distinguishing character between TCM and Western Medicine is that Western Medicine treats diseases based on diseases, while TCM treats diseases based on pulse and symptoms, which means finding the right disease syndrome through the analysis of pulse and symptoms. In other words, TCM is exactly the 'people oriented' science that cures the disease through eliminating all the symptoms causing people's discomfort and pain.

TCM cures the diseases that Western Medicine cannot treat through entirely different thoughts. People studying TCM, no matter smart or not, shall closely focus on the core of pulse and symptoms to study, comprehend and practice. Only by entering this core domain can one reach a higher level and become a master in treating diseases.

Above is the reason why Zhāng Zhòngjǐng (张仲景) is crowned with eternal glory and honored as the 'Medical Sage' or the 'Second Sage' (after Confucius).

Both *Treatise on Cold Damage Diseases* (*Shāng hán lùn*, 伤寒论) and *Synopsis of the Golden Chamber* (*Jīn kuì yào luè*, 金匮要略) focus on differentiating the pulse, the symptoms, and the treatment at the beginning. This proves the importance of the pulse and symptoms.

In Qing Dynasty, the rise of the school of warm diseases was not to go against the Medical Sage; instead, they had a deeply understanding of the essence of treating diseases.

As we can see in Taiyang disease outline of *Treatise on Cold Damage Diseases* (*Shāng hán lùn*, 伤寒论): 'A floating pulse, headache, stiff neck, and a feeling of aversion to cold are always the general symptoms and signs of the Taiyang (greater yang) syndrome', 'The greater yang syndrome with symptoms and signs of fever, perspiration, aversion to wind and moderate pulse is termed wind damage disease', 'The greater yang syndrome with or without fever, but with aversion to cold and pain in the body, nausea, vomiting and pulse tight both in yin and yang, is termed cold damage disease'.

Due to different pulse and symptoms, there are differences between wind stroke and cold damage diseases. It is said in *Systematized Identification of Warm* (*Pathogen*) *Diseases* (*Wēn bìng tíao biàn*, 温病条辨) that, 'Greater yin syndrome, with the symptoms of neither moderate nor tight pulse but stirred and rapid pulse, or huge pulses at Cun positions, forearm skin fever, headache, slight aversion to wind-cold, fever and spontaneous sweating, coughing with thirst or not thirst, afternoon fever, is called warm disease.' Since it has different pulse and symptoms from 'cold damage disease' and 'wind stroke', it is called warm disease.

There is no superiority or inferiority between the school of cold damage disease and the school of warm disease. *Medical Records for Clinical Guidance* (*Lín zhèng zhǐ nán yī àn*, 临证指南医案) by Yè Tiānshì (叶天士) also used a large amount of classic formulas. Someone has calculated that, in 5598 cases left by Yè Tiānshì (叶天士), among 70% were treated by the formulas modified from the classics of Zhāng Zhòngjǐng (张仲景). Therefore, a famous modern doctor, Cheng Menxue once said: "When treating diseases, Yè Tiānshì (叶天士) took advantage of prescriptions from many famous doctors, especially from Zhāng Zhòngjǐng (张仲景)." At the beginning of *Systematized Identification of Warm* (*Pathogen*) *Diseases* (*Wēn bìng tíao biàn*, 温病条辨), it says that, 'The patient with the syndromes of greater yin wind-heat, warm febrile, pestilence, winter-warmth and initial aversion to wind-cold, shall be treated with *Guizhi*

Tang (*Cinnamon Twig Decoction*); the patient who has thirst with fever without chills, shall be treated with pungent-cool and moderate formula — *Yin Qiao San* (*Lonicera and Forsythia Powder*).' That is to say, no matter what the name of disease is in TCM, the disease shall be treated based on syndrome differentiation. If the syndrome can be treated by *Guizhi Tang* (*Cinnamon Twig Decoction*), *Guizhi Tang* (*Cinnamon Twig Decoction*) shall be used; if the syndrome can be treated by *Yin Qiao San* (*Lonicera and Forsythia Powder*), then *Yin Qiao San* (*Lonicera and Forsythia Powder*) shall be used.

In the preface of *Systematized Identification of Warm* (*Pathogen*) *Diseases* (*Wēn bìng tíao biàn,* 温病条辨), Zhēng Bǎo (征保) wrote: "The treatment method for cold damage diseases lies in saving yang; the treatment method for warm febrile diseases lies in saving yin." Two different methods are used due to the difference of pulse and symptoms. Ignoring the pulse and symptoms and only directly using cold damage diseases prescription to treat warm disease is 'inflexible', 'confused' and 'incompatible'.

Páng Ānshi (庞安时) always said: "If warm diseases such as wind-warm syndrome and damp-warm syndrome are misdiagnosed as cold damage diseases and the therapeutic method is sweating, then the patient will die without any exception." The severity of the problem can be seen. Therefore, Zhēng Bǎo (征保) also said: "If fever rises again, the treatment method for cold damage disease must not be used to treat warm diseases." Why? Because what Zhāng Zhòngjǐng (张仲景) advocates is 'observe the pulse and symptoms carefully and treat the patient accordingly'. How can he use the treatment method for cold damage diseases to treat warm diseases?

In the preface of *Systematized Identification of Warm* (*Pathogen*) *Diseases* (*Wēn bìng tíao biàn,* 温病条辨), Zhū Bīn (朱彬) said: "After I made friend with Wú Jútōng (吴鞠通) in Beijing, I witnessed the way he treated diseases. He used the theories of Zhāng Zhòngjǐng (张仲景) as the basis, but made changes according to the symptoms and did not stick to one pattern. He often had talented treatment methods, all based on the core method of Zhāng Zhòngjǐng (张仲景) that he had a deep understanding of."

The former 'method' shall be understood as the method of the six-channel.

The latter 'method' shall be understood as the method of analyzing pulse and symptoms. And this 'method' is the core of Zhāng Zhòngjǐng (张仲景) and also is the core of TCM clinic.

Just as what Xǔ Shūwēi (许叔微) said in *Discussion on Cold Damage Diseases* (*Shāng hán fā wēi lùn*, 伤寒发微论), "I read Zhāng Zhòngjǐng (张仲景)'s books and use Zhāng Zhòngjǐng (张仲景)'s method, but do not stick to Zhāng Zhòngjǐng (张仲景)'s prescription, which can be seen as understanding the essence of the theory of Zhang."

This exactly emphasizes that learning from Zhāng Zhòngjǐng (张仲景) is not simply using Zhāng Zhòngjǐng (张仲景)'s prescription, but to use Zhāng Zhòngjǐng (张仲景)'s method which is the differentiation of the pulse and symptoms.

The ancients often said that 'Zhāng Zhòngjǐng (张仲景) had found out and understood the profound implication of Xuanyuan and Qibo', and the 'pulse and symptoms' is the 'implication'. They also expressed that *Treatise on Cold Damage Diseases* (*Shāng hán lùn*, 伤寒论) is like the sun in TCM and should be admired eternally.

Therefore, Zhū Bīn (朱彬) said: "The ancient people said Zhāng Zhòngjǐng (张仲景) is the meritorious man for the understanding of Xuanyuan and Qibo, but actually Wú Jútōng (吴鞠通) is also another one." TCM is about *Tao-like medical knowledge;* doctors use the same principle when making prescriptions through different methods.

Due to the different pulses and symptoms, the cold damage diseases are different according to six-channel syndrome differentiation.

Due to the different pulses and symptoms, the warm diseases are different according to defense-qi-nutrient-blood syndrome differentiation.

For the same disease, if the pulses and symptoms are different, they shall be treated differently.

For different diseases, if the pulses and symptoms are the same, they can be treated with the same method.

Knowing the pulse and symptoms, the ancient prescriptions can be used to treat contemporary diseases.

Otherwise, even the contemporary prescriptions cannot treat contemporary diseases.

The knowledge of TCM can be called the knowledge of pulse and symptoms.

Since TCM is the knowledge of pulse and symptoms, four medical schools in Jin-yuan Dynasty have their own emphases and their own achievements. We cannot tell them right or wrong.

Since TCM is the knowledge of pulse and symptoms, cold damage diseases and warm diseases have their own treatment, and there is no difference in superiority or inferiority.

Since TCM is the knowledge of pulse and symptoms, the 397 methods and 113 formulas in *Treatise on Cold Damage Diseases* (*Shāng hán lùn*, 伤寒论) not only can cure cold damage diseases, but also can cure thousands of complex diseases. Only pulse and symptoms is the gist and the core of intangible science in clinic. Is there anything else as the true essence for curing diseases?

Discussing that pulse diagnosis is more important than symptoms and prescribing should base on it

In the core of pulse and symptoms, pulse is more important than symptoms.

If pulse and symptoms are the core of TCM, then pulse is the key of the core.

"Observe the pulse and symptoms carefully and treat the patient accordingly", the Medical Sage Zhāng Zhòngjǐng (张仲景) tells the essence of TCM treating diseases. He emphasized the importance of pulse and symptoms.

Sūn Sīmiǎo (孙思邈) said: "Feeling the pulse is very important for doctors. How can one be a qualified doctor without a good skill of pulse feeling (*Valuable Prescriptions for Emergency* (*Bèijí qiān jīn yào fāng*, 备急千金要方))!"

TCM doctor diagnoses a disease according to inspection, listening and smelling, inquiry, pulse taking and palpation. Although pulse comes last, Sūn Sīmiǎo (孙思邈) gave an extremely high appraisal for it and believed that a doctor without a deep study of pulse is not a qualified TCM doctor. Why? Because feeling the pulse is the most important part, sometimes the key, in four examinations.

Máo Xiánglín (毛祥麟) from Qing Dynasty once said: "Feeling the pulse, analyzing the symptoms (differentiating the syndrome) and making the prescription are three essentials for TCM, among which, feeling the pulse is especially important. If knowing the pulse, syndrome differentiation and prescription making can be naturally done."

It appears that the key of treating diseases by a doctor of TCM lies in 'knowing the pulse' which directly affects the clinical effects.

In the book of *Internal Classic* (*Nèi jīng*, 内经), it records, 'A doctor who is good at diagnosis will observe complexion and take pulse, differentiating yin and yang first', 'If the doctor can combine the complexion with the pulse, there will be no mistake for treating disease.' It is clear that this is the key relating to the clinical effects of TCM. Thus we can understand why Sūn Sīmiǎo (孙思邈) thought pulse-feeling is 'very important for doctors'.

Although it seems very easy for TCM doctors to treat patients with 'three figures and one pillow', the skills cannot be easily mastered.

Just like what Wú Jútōng (吴鞠通) said before: "Among four ways of examinations, only pulse-feeling is the most difficult and also the most reliable one." Therefore, among 162 articles of *Internal Classic* (*Nèi jīng*, 内经), there are more than 30 ones talking about pulse condition. Among 81 questions in *Classic of questioning* (*Nàn jīng*, 难经), the first 20 questions also talk about pulse-feeling. One can well perceive that how important pulse-feeling is for a doctor of TCM!

In the past, the ordinary people asking a TCM doctor to treat diseases is commonly called as 'feeling pulse'. These two words can represent the whole diagnosis process and the knowledge and technical level of a doctor, which for thousands of years is the most immediate experience of ordinary people when they ask a TCM doctor to treat diseases. In fact, a good TCM doctor must be good at pulse-feeling; in other words, only be good at pulse-feeling can a doctor be regarded as an excellent doctor.

At this moment, I suddenly think of a story read from a book *Views on Extending Medical Knowledge* (*Gé zhì yú lùn*, 格致余论) by Zhū Dānxī (朱丹溪). He once visited and wanted to take Luó Zhītì (罗知悌) as his teacher, but the result was 'he was accepted after being scolded for five or seven times and lingering about in front of Luó Zhītì (罗知悌)'s home for more than three months'.

Zhū Dānxī (朱丹溪), as one of four great masters in Jin and Yuan Dynasty, had gained considerable fame among his contemporaries. In terms of reputation, Luó Zhītì (罗知悌)'s reputation was far lower than that of Zhū Dānxī (朱丹溪). However, when Zhū Dānxī (朱丹溪) came to take him as his teacher, he scolded Zhu for several times, but Zhū Dānxī (朱丹溪) still embarrassedly waited for 3 months outside Luó Zhītì (罗知悌)'s home. Zhū Dānxī (朱丹溪) finally moved Luó Zhītì (罗知悌) with sincerity and was accepted.

What is the advantage of Luó Zhītì (罗知悌) that attracted Zhū Dānxī (朱丹溪) to be so persistent?

Zhū Dānxī (朱丹溪) said: "Every time when patients ask Luo for treatment, he would send his disciples to feel the patient's pulse and tell him. Luo just makes the prescription after hearing the pulse manifestation. Then he would tell the disciples the function of every medicinal. There was no fixed prescription in my one-and-a-half-year observation."

It turns out that the talent of Luó Zhītì (罗知悌) lies in his use of medicinals depending on the type of pulse (also can be understood as pulse and symptoms), and that he was especially good at pulse diagnosis. Afterward, Zhū Dānxī (朱丹溪) understood that 'it is effective to use the ancient prescription to cure diseases in modern society' as long as adopting the ancient prescription according to the pulse.

Adopting the ancient prescription according to the pulse also obeys 'observe the pulse and symptoms carefully and treat the patient accordingly' from Zhāng Zhòngjǐng (张仲景). This is why Zhū Dānxī (朱丹溪), who was so famous at that time, still acknowledged Luó Zhītì (罗知悌) as his master.

The example made by Zhōu Shēngyì (周声溢) in Qing Dynasty in *Jing'an's Opinion on Medicine* (*Jìng'ān shuō yī*, 靖庵说医) can also illustrate the issue. It is extracted as follows:

"My friend Dèng Chūnfǎng (邓春舫) always says that a doctor should master in feeling the pulse. Chūnfǎng (春舫) is from Jinzhou, Hubei Province and lives in Shashi. He is proficient in medicine and good at making classic formulas. It is obvious that his medical experience is proficient because his classic formulas can be used directly by other doctors. At the time when I did not begin to learn medicine, he told me that people studying medicine must firstly feel the pulse proficiently enough before making the prescription. He said that at the beginning of studying medicine, he explored and researched the method of pulse-feeling and diagnosed patients following his teacher. He felt the pulse and told the type of the pulse to his teacher.

His teacher would then feel the pulse and decide whether his pulse-feeling was correct. After lots of practice, he could make the prescription. Then he gave his prescription to his teacher, who would correct his prescription. Three months later when his pulse-feeling and prescription conform to those of his teacher, he started to read crucial and essential books at home without interruption, and then could cure all his patients without failure one year later."

Dèng Chūnfǎng (邓春舫) became a proficient doctor in a short time because he seized the main point, pulse-feeling, and learned it from his teacher.

It can be concluded that pulse-feeling is a key issue that directly relates to the clinical level of TCM. If Chinese pharmacological science is a great treasury, then pulse-feeling is the most valuable and important one of it. With it, one can see and think clearly in front of symptoms, just as seeing the bright lighthouse during night cruise; while without it, it is just like the blind people walking.

There is a theoretical basis either for the classics of TCM or for the discussion about the importance of pulse-feeling made by famous doctors in the past ages. However, TCM studied today is westernized and is quite different from that proposed by ancient sages. The concern is always on the prescription and medicinals for diseases rather than for pulses; although modern TCM doctors feel the pulse, they can acquire nothing through the process. They have to diagnose through inquiring the symptoms and take advantage of the set prescriptions, and even diagnose the symptoms according to the prescriptions made by former doctors, which puts the cart before the horse and badly decreases the curative effect. And someone even criticized that TCM cannot merely satisfy with the diagnosis based on 'the three fingers and one pillow'. This seems full of creativity but was ridiculous.

Pulse-feeling of TCM seems simple, but it is in fact very difficult to master.

I have learnt Traditional Chinese Medicine from Liáng Xiùqīng (梁秀清), my first teacher of TCM in the 1970s. Mr. Liang's method of pulse-feeling is like that of *Classic of Questioning* (*Nàn Jīng*, 难经). For example, practicing to make the pulse beat 6 times in a cycle of breath for a long time can make one know something wrong through the times of pulse beating, namely, knowing where the disease is; practicing to take the pulse under light, moderate and heavy pressure is to stick beans to and gradually add strength on the three fingers according to *Classic of Questioning* (*Nàn Jīng*, 难经). Wiry pulse in spring, surging pulse in summer, weak and floating pulse in autumn, deep and tight pulse in winter are the normal pulses of four seasons.

Liang's father told him that only by obtaining the ability to feel the normal pulse could he feel the abnormal pulse.

At the beginning of learning the skill of feeling the pulse, however, his father did not let him feel the pulse of the people, instead, he let him touch the water in the river.

His father said that rivers are like the veins of the earth. They change in four seasons and four time periods (morning, afternoon, evening, night), just like the change of the pulse of human.

Mastering the changing of veins of river will help to master the changing of pulses of human body.

To master 'weak and floating pulse in autumn', he tried to touch the sparrow feathers in the wind. He mastered the Liang's pulse method after practicing for three years.

Liáng Xiùqīng (梁秀清), with his skill of feeling the pulse, not only could diagnose a tumor, but also could make prescriptions according to the differentiation of pulse and symptoms, rescuing many patients' lives.

The other teacher of mine, Sir Huáng Jiéxī (黄杰熙), also learnt and studied pulse diagnosis with lots of efforts, initially from *Internal Classic* (*Nèi jīng*, 内经), *Classic of questioning* (*Nàn jīng*, 难经), *Treatise on Cold Damage Diseases* (*Shāng hán lùn*, 伤寒论) and *Jīn Kui Yao Lüe* (*Synopsis of the Golden Chamber* (*Jīn kuì yào luè*, 金匮要略)), to the books related to pulse diagnosis and cases solved by famous doctors in various dynasties. After his sensible and careful verification, Huang finally mastered the skill of making prescriptions based on pulse diagnosis as the 'secret' of TCM, and became a clinic expert.

The fact that Sir Lǐ Kě (李可) is never obsessed with those disease names given by Western Medicine or never insisted on finding a specific name in TCM field every time he treated diseases also emphasizes the importance of pulse diagnosis.

The study of TCM would always remain on the surface and be stuck in making prescriptions based on disease names if the pulse and symptoms as the core were abandoned, in which situation, it would be very difficult to cure diseases effectively, faced with various diseases changing unpredictably!

Only focusing on the study of symptoms and ignoring the pulse is a serious imperfection in TCM, because symptoms sometimes can be false while pulse seldom lies to doctors. My teacher Huáng Jiéxī (黄杰熙) treated a male patient who was in his thirties and had had a prolonged high fever for more than 20 days and an extreme aversion to cold. Although it was in the mid-summer, he still wore a cotton-padded jacket. All these symptoms presented that he seemed to be yang deficient. His pulse was soggy under slight pressure, but was powerful under the heavy pressure. He had a thick and white tongue coating and the middle area was dry and yellow. Mr. Huang diagnosed him as the syndrome of serious summer-heat with dampness. Mr. Huang prescribed him formula which included 200g of *Shengshigao* (*Gypsum Fibrosum*) and 100g of *Huashifen* (*PULVIS TALCI*), with the purpose of clearing pathogenic summer-heat directly. In this formula, he also added *Dangshen* (*Radix Codonopsis*), *Xuanshen* (*Radix Scrophulariae*), *Peilan* (*Herba Eupatorii*), *Lianqiao* (*Fructus Forsythiae*), *Huafen* (*Radix Trichosanthis*), *Gancao* (*Radix Glycyrrhizae*) to eliminate turbid with aromatics, replenish qi and nourish yin, clear heat and remove toxin. After taking only two doses, the patient's fever was brought down.

In the summer of 2006, I was introduced to treat a patient in a major hospital in Shanxi Province who also got high fever for over 20 days with similar pulse and symptoms as the previous one. I made prescriptions based on Mr. Huang's with several changes: 150g of *Shengshigao* (*Gypsum Fibrosum*) and 60g of *Huashifen* (*PULVIS TALCI*). I advised him to take the dose every four hours and his fever was also brought down after only two doses.

Mr. Huang often applied *Shengshigao* (*Gypsum Fibrosum*) and *Huashifen* (*PULVIS TALCI*) together to bring down fever, that is, *Shengshigao* (*Gypsum Fibrosum*) with extreme cold nature can relief heat and *Huashifen* (*PULVIS TALCI*) with sweet flavor and cold nature can help to remove heat from the body through urination. This method is very effective and has successfully cured many patients.

I have treated a female patient in her fifties with massive uterus hemorrhage. She had a pale face and no strength to talk; her pulse was weak and feeble on both hands and her condition was badly in danger. I immediately advised her to cut one *Korean ginseng* into small pieces and take them all together with hot water. In a short while, she stopped bleeding.

Another case was a young female doctor who had her menstruation continuously for over 20 days with rectocele. Her pulse was weak and thready. I advised her to take a finger-sized piece of *ginseng* and the menstruation was over quickly, after which, she took half of one *ginseng* and then remained in a healthy condition.

The book does not tell that *ginseng* has the effect on hemostasis, but judging from the above cases, the two patients both belonged to qi deficiency. The reason why tonifying qi by *ginseng* can have the effect on hemostasis is that qi is the commander of blood.

The clinic application of *ginseng* should strictly base on the pulse manifestation which is deep, thready, feeble. If the patient reveals a floating or rapid pulse manifestation, then *ginseng* should not be taken. If taken in the wrong situation, it is just like adding fuel to the flame. If both Cun pulses are deep and feeble, *ginseng* can also be taken.

However, *ginseng* should be avoided if the pulses are huge at Guan and Chi positions, because it may cause up-flaming of liver fire and exacerbate the disease.

If both pulses are deep and thready, *ginseng* should be better considered in the prescription; if the patient has dry mouth symptom, *Tiandong* (*Radix Asparagi*), *Shengdi* (*Radix Rehmanniae Recens*) should also be added to produce a decoction called *San Cai Tang* (*Three Ingredients Decoction*) to treat the deficiency of yin.

When treating some difficult diseases, doctors should pay more attention to the pulse for making prescriptions.

Mr. Huáng Jiéxī (黄杰熙) used to treat a rare disease. The patient was a middle-aged woman who acted just like normal people except that she could not go upstairs or climb mountains, otherwise she would faint and fall. Whichever hospitals she had visited, no one could cure her disease. During the one-year time hospitalizing in a major hospital in Shanxi Province, she had been examined by various instruments, such as CT and Ultrasonic without any useful results. Some doctors treated her disease as a heart disease but still received no effects. The hospital finally refused to treat her with an excuse as 'unknown disease', so she had to go back and stay at home.

When Mr. Huang took her pulse, he found that both Cun pulses were huge and sufficient, while the pulses at Guan and Chi positions were deep, slow, thready, and short. Therefore, her symptoms were caused by qi-blood stagnated at upper-energizer which could hardly circulate through the middle and lower-energizer.

Every time she went upstairs or climbed mountains, the stagnated blood would go up and stimulate the brain and caused her to feel dizzy and faint; however, when she walked on the plain road or went down-stairs, there would be no stimulation, so she acted as normal people. Therefore, Mr. Huang prescribed some medicinals with effect of leading blood downward, such as *Huainiuxi* (*Radix Cyathulae*) and *Daizheshi* (*Hematite*). Having taking two doses, the patient was cured and then went to work after a two-year rest. Afterward, she would climb the mountain as easy as normal people with her family every Double Ninth Festival.

Were it not based on pulse diagnosis, how could the patient be diagnosed with qi-blood stagnated at upper-energizer and then be cured?

Western Medicine diagnoses diseases using the stethoscope, X-ray, Ultrasonic, the Doppler ultrasound and electrocardiogram and other examination data, which cannot be used by TCM to make prescriptions.

TCM diagnoses diseases according to pulse and symptoms. Without taking the pulse, the doctor cannot make a clear prescription, then how can the medicinals be effective?

There is plenty of knowledge involved in TCM doctor's 'three fingers and one pillow (for pulse taking)'.

Xú Chūnfù (徐春甫) from Ming Dynasty once said: "The pulse taking is the key of TCM. If a doctor fails to feel the pulse, there will be no other evidence to diagnose the disease and then no effective treatment. The doctor who is good at feeling the pulse is definitely a good doctor, otherwise he is a quack."

These words present the drawback in the modern TCM, i.e. the main cause of low cure rate of TCM.

Differentiating the syndrome based on pulse taking, together with other three examinations in clinic diagnosis, will help to figure out the patient's condition and grasp the general idea about prescription, which will produce better effects; moreover, this will also help doctors be skillful in treatment and even cure many difficult and rare diseases.

Therefore, when learning from teachers and memorizing those pre-scriptions, I would always firstly ask about the pulse of the patient and the reason of every medicinal in the prescription. In time, I was gradually enlightened by those prescriptions, and I would like to share and explain several cases about making prescriptions based on pulse as examples.

I. Prescribing should base on pulse when facing the same symptoms with different pulses

Most of the clinical cases are that the patients have the same disease or symptoms but with different pulses. In this situation, the prescription should be made based on their pulse in order to acquire positive effects.

Two male patients suffering from cerebral thrombosis, Mr. Lu and Mr. Li, were both in their eighties. They both had stiff tongues, could not speak clearly and their right-side body was stiff. After receiving thrombo-lytic drug transfusion treatment for over one month, there was still no effective results.

According to the pulse diagnosis, I found that the pulse was floating and slightly rapid at left Cun and Guan positions. Floating pulse indicates the pathogenic wind, and *Xiao Xuming Tang* (*Minor Life-Prolonging Decoction*), which contains large amounts of wind dispelling and extin-guishing medicinals, should better be prescribed for treating. I advised him to take the decoction slowly. After three doses, the patient was cured and did not relapse for more than one year.

By contrast, Mr Li's pulse was deep and feeble on both hands, espe-cially of the right hand. This indicated that he suffered from serious qi deficiency. I prescribed him with *Buyang Huanwu Tang* (*Yang-Tonifying Five-Returning Decoction*), including 150g of *Huangqi* (*Radix Astragali seu Hedysari*). The patient was also cured after three doses, and with three more doses for consolidation, he did not relapse in the next two years.

Treating patients suffering from cerebral thrombosis only with the prescription that promotes blood circulation and remove blood stasis without consideration of pulse would have little effect on the patient; what's worse, medical negligence may even occur if the patient having liver-yang hyperactivity takes *Buyang Huanwu Tang* (*Yang-Tonifying*

Five-Returning Decoction) by accident. Therefore, the doctor must be careful when making prescriptions!

Another 60-year-old patient, Mr Li suffered vomiting and diarrhea because of taking bad food last summer.

His right Guan pulse was soggy and slightly rapid and huge, so I knew that he suffered internal damage of dampness turbidity. I advised him to take *Huoxiang Zhengqi San* (*Patchouli Qi-Righting Powder*), and he felt much better after taking the prescription for one day and was cured the next day.

This summer, he relapsed after having bad food. According to the prescription last year, he himself took *Huoxiang Zhengqi San* (*Patchouli Qi-Righting Powder*) and some anti-inflammatory drugs like norfloxacin for four days without any positive effect. He vomited and had diarrhea for seven to eight times per day and often had stomachache and was sick. He was very exhausted and lay in bed. His family worried about dehydration and was going to send him to the hospital for transfusion. However, the patient insisted on inviting me to treat him.

I found that he was emaciated with a pale face and low voice. His right Guan pulse was deep, moderate, and feeble. He was diagnosed with cold deficiency. Thus, I advised him to take one dose of modified *Fuzi Lizhong Tang* (*Aconite Middle-Regulating Decoction*) at once, and his stomachache was relieved with no sick feeling and he began to have better complexion. After two doses, he could move like healthy people and stopped vomiting and having diarrhea. It is known that the symptoms of vomiting and diarrhea could be eliminated by *Huoxiang Zhengqi San* (*Patchouli Qi-Righting Powder*), but due to the ignorance of prescription based on pulse, seldom people know that many others also need *Fuzi Lizhong Tang* (*Aconite Middle-Regulating Decoction*).

Taking the treatment of constipation as another example, it seems that purgation was the only therapy. Western Medicine can use *phenolphthalein* and TCM has *Dahuang* (*Radix et Rhizoma Rhei*). However, people do not know that constipation as a symptom may be caused by different reasons and have different treatment methods based on pulse diagnosis.

I still remember how I treated a 65-year-old female patient three years ago. She excreted stool only once within three to four days with the help of her family members. The excrement was so dry that it made sound when dropped on the ground. No purgative drugs were effective to her disease. I took her pulse and found that the pulse was extremely deep and feeble at right Cun and Guan positions, so I diagnosed her with qi deficiency. I prescribed her with *Buzhong Yiqi Tang* (*Middle-Tonifying Qi-Replenishing Decoction*) with dosages of *Huangqi* (*Radix Astragali seu Hedysari*) added to 60g. After three doses, her excrement became soft and she kept a normal bowel movement, which made her family very pleased. This is 'treating obstructive syndrome with tonics'. If without taking the pulse, how could I dare to prescribe large dosages of *Huangqi* (*Radix Astragali seu Hedysari*) facing this serious constipation.

II. Prescribing should base on pulse when facing different symptoms with the same pulse

TCM often says that prescribing should base on the syndrome. Actually, this 'syndrome' here includes the pulse manifestation, i.e. prescribing should base on the pulse manifestation. Despite changing symptoms, every disease can be curable as long as the pulse is clearly taken.

(1) The case of recurrently having the bad cold

Mr. Sun was 41 years old. He said that he always had nasal obstruction, clear nasal discharge and sneezing. He had aversion to wind and cold with cold feet and hands, so he always wore coat even in summer time. The cold was sometimes released and sometimes advanced but never stopped. His pulse was wiry and feeble on both hands, and right Chi pulse was extremely deficient. I prescribed him with a small amount of *Guifu Dihuang Tang* (*Cassia Twig, Prepared Common Monkshood Daughter Root, Prepared Rehmannia Root Decoction*). After taking the medicinals for three months, the twenty-year bad cold was cured.

(2) The case of recurrent coughing

Mr. Zhang was 42 years old. He said that he easily coughed as long as he got a cold in recent years which often happened five to six times per year.

I found that, on both hands, his pulse was moderate, and right Chi pulse was extremely deficient. I prescribed him with modified *Guifu Dihuang Tang* (*Cassia Twig, Prepared Common Monkshood Daughter Root, Prepared Rehmannia Root Decoction*) for over twenty doses. This year, he told me excitedly: "I have not coughed for more than one year after taking the formula."

(3) The case of recurrent geographical tongue

Mr. Liu was 62 years old. He said that he had geographical tongue for over three years. I found that there were two one-penny-sized non-tongue coating circles in the centre of the tongue. He did not felt any illness except that he could not wear short sleeved clothes in summer because of aversion to cold. His pulse manifestation was normal except for the right Chi pulse was deficient. I advised him to take modified *Guifu Dihuang Tang* (*Cassia Twig, Prepared Common Monkshood Daughter Root, Prepared Rehmannia Root Decoction*). After one month, his tongue coating was back to normal. Last summer, he specially visited me in T-shirt.

(4) The case of the aversion to cold in the back

Ms. Wang was 32 years old. She said that her back was averse to cold and her menstruation was delayed and the amount reduced. Her pulse was moderate on both hands, except for the extremely deficient pulse at his right Chi position. I prescribed her with modified *Guifu Dihuang Wan* (*Cortex Cinnamomi, Radix Aconiti Lateralis Preparata, Radix Rehmanniae Preparata pills*). After taking fifteen doses, she was not afraid of cold in the back, the menstruation was back to normal and her face had flushing complexion.

(5) The case of recurrently having stomachache

Mr. Dong was 63 years old. He said that he had dull pain in stomach for many years, and the pain would be severe after he had some fruit or cold food. He was emaciated with a yellowish complexion. He had taken lots of medicines for stomach diseases but without any positive effect. He had a wiry, thready, and moderate pulse, and the pulse at his right Chi position was extremely deficient. Based on these, I figured out that the location of disease was his kidney. Therefore, I prescribed him with modified *Guifu Dihuang Tang* (*Cassia Twig, Prepared Common Monkshood Daughter Root, Prepared Rehmannia Root Decoction*) for twenty doses. Three years later, I encountered him on the street, and he said that he did not have stomachache anymore after taking the formula. He had a better appetite and could eat different fruits. I observed that he had a flushing complexion and was quite different from the person I met in 2005.

(6) The case of frequent urination

Mr. Wang was 32 years old. He said that he urinated for four to five times per night during sleep, and he had heavy pain in the waist. Both of his Chi pulses were deficient, especially of the right one. I prescribed him with modified *Guifu Dihuang Tang* (*Cassia Twig, Prepared Common Monkshood Daughter Root, Prepared Rehmannia Root Decoction*) for six doses, and he did not get up at night to urinate or have waist discomfort anymore after taking the prescription.

(7) The case of erectile dysfunction

Mr. Han was 42 years old. He said that he had erectile dysfunction and was so averse to cold and wind that he had to close the window near him when taking the bus even in summer. Both of his pulses were almost normal except for the deficient right Chi pulse, so I advised him to take modified *Guifu Dihuang Tang* (*Cassia Twig, Prepared Common Monkshood Daughter Root, Prepared Rehmannia Root Decoction*) for a long period. After taking the formula two doses a week for over two years, he was gradually cured and could do exercise in the park barebacked even in the bitter cold winter, which attracted much attention.

The pathogenesis of the above cases are all about the deficient right Chi pulse which indicates the deficiency of kidney-yang and the declined fire of life gate resulting in different diseases. Different as those diseases are, they can be cured by the same medicinals all due to the same pulse.

III. Prescribing should base on the pulse for the symptoms may have false appearance

The human body is complex. Due to different physical quality, the disease may have various symptoms which sometimes are in accordance with the disease nature while other times may have opposite appearance.

The truth can finally be figured out based on pulse taking.

Mr. Song was 43 years old. He easily had mouth ulcer from a very young age. In recent three years, he continuously had aphtha and could not be cured even though he took many anti-inflammatory drugs.

I found that he had a reddish tongue with many yellow ulcers around the tongue and on the oral mucosa. After observing and questioning him, I realized that he suffered from fire syndrome without any doubt. However, his pulse was deep, slow, and moderate on both hands, indicating that he suffered from deficiency cold. I advised him to take modified *Fuzi Lizhong Tang* (*Aconite Middle-Regulating Decoction*). He felt better after one dose and was cured after ten doses.

Mr. Jin was 74 years old. In recent three years, he was always extremely thirsty at night and had to drink one kettle of water at least.

He reminded me the first time he came to my clinic, "Although I had a deficient body, I dare not eat tonic because they make me get inflamed." His symptoms revealed that he suffered the syndrome of consumptive thirst, but both of his pulses were feeble and moderate, especially at right Chi position. Therefore, I knew that though his extreme thirst seemed like heat syndrome, he actually suffered from cold syndrome, which is upward reversal of deficiency-yang and should be treated by the method of returning fire to its origin. I prescribed him with modified *Guifu Dihuang Tang* (*Cassia Twig, Prepared Common Monkshood Daughter Root, Prepared Rehmannia Root Decoction*). After one month, his thirst was cured and did not relapse till now.

IV. Prescribing should base on the pulse when facing rare diseases with complex symptoms

There are sometimes rare diseases in clinical practice and it is difficult to figure out the mechanism of disease or effective treatment methods.

In this situation, taking the pulse carefully is the only way to find the key to those problems.

(1) The case of 10-year facial twitch

Mr. Sun was 38 years old. His face twitched at both sides and even to the ears every three to five minutes.

He said that he had suffered from this for ten years since he was only 27. Although he had visited many famous doctors from Beijing to various provincial capitals and spent more than one hundred thousand yuan, his condition still went worse and worse, such as developing extreme aversion to cold and wind. Most of the formulas he had taken were *Sini Tang* (*Cold-Extremities Decoction*) and *Wuzhuyu Tang* (*Evodia Decoction*). Those formulas could contain up to 100g *Fuzi* (*Radix Aconiti Lateralis Preparata*) and 45g *Xixin* (*Herba Asari*). However, the more formulas he had taken, the more serious the aversion to cold and the facial twitch he had. Therefore, he had no work ability and could only have a small bowl of porridge per meal, which made him have no persistence to survive. The mechanism of this disease was hard to analyze, but his pulses were wiry, and the right Chi pulse was deficient, thus I treated him as the deficiency of kidney-yang. I advised him to take large doses of modified *Guifu Dihuang Tang* (*Cassia Twig, Prepared Common Monkshood Daughter Root, Prepared Rehmannia Root Decoction*) for one dose every two days. Having taken the formula for half a year, he was released from all those symptoms and went back to work. Finally, he drew a period to his ten-year treatment experience.

(2) The case of recurrent perspiring of one side of the body

Mr. Chen was 44 years old. He said that every night when he lay on the right side, his left side would perspire and vice versa. He had to keep wiping perspiration every night when going to bed and this had lasted for three years without any effective treatment.

I found that he had a reddish tongue with a thin and yellow coating. Both of his pulses were deep and weak, especially at his Chi positions. The mechanism of this disease was unclear. Based on his pulse, I treated him from the point of kidney-yang deficiency and advised him to take modified *Guifu Dihuang Tang* (*Cassia Twig, Prepared Common Monkshood Daughter Root, Prepared Rehmannia Root Decoction*) for twelve doses till he recovered.

(3) The case of having 4-year aphtha

Ms. Tian was 31 years old. She said that in recent four years, as long as she had watermelon in summer, she would have oral ulcer. After the examination, I found that she had a slightly reddish tongue with no coating, a deep, thready, and rapid left Chi pulse. It was hard for me to tell the mechanism of this disease. However, based on the pulse, she suffers from yin deficiency. Therefore, I advised her to take *Liuwei Dihuang Tang* (*Six-Ingredient Rehmannia Pill*) for fifteen doses and then her pulse was back to normal.

Several years later, when she came to my clinic for treatment of another disease, she told me that she had no aphtha when having watermelon in summer after taking those medicinals.

V. Prescribing should base on the pulse when having no distinct symptoms

It is relative not absolute whether the disease exists or not.

People who feel comfortable and healthy can be examined to have disease by modern medical instruments sometimes. However, since TCM holds the view of syndrome differentiation and treatment, how can they face the situation with no apparent symptoms of the syndromes in six meridians or in urination and excretion?

Actually, the symptoms are not absolutely indiscernible. They can be found out as long as the pulse is felt carefully, after which the key to cure the disease can be figured out.

Mr. Xu was 42 years old. He said that in recent four years, his urine test result showed that there was a small amount of protein. Comfortable as he felt, he was still afraid that there might be something wrong with his kidney.

After the examinations, I realized that his complexion and tongue was normal as healthy people, nor did he have any symptoms, such as the soreness of waist or leg fatigue, to indicate that he suffered from kidney deficiency. His pulse was also in normal condition.

Facing the patient, I was very awkward because I could not tell whether he was healthy or sick for his urination contained protein while there were no symptoms to be analyzed. After a deep thought, I suddenly thought about the words that 'All internal changes of the body must have the corresponding manifestations which emerge on the exterior', so I took his pulse for the second time. Having carefully felt the pulse again, I finally found out that both of his Chi pulses were slightly hollow, which reminded me of 'people who has a hollow, stirred, faint, or tight pulse, would suffer seminal emission for male and suffer dreaming of intercourse for female.' in *Records of TCM* (*Yī xué zhèng zhuàn,* 医学正传).

Therefore, I mainly treated him with the medicinals that tonify kidney and increase semen. Considering that *Wuzhuyu* (*Fructus Evodiae*) was much milder than other medicinals with this function, I advised him to decoct and take 15g of *Wuzhuyu* (*Fructus Evodiae*) per day. One month later, the patient visited me excitedly, saying that there was no protein in his urination according to the latest check-up, and he felt much energetic than before. There has been no protein in his urination for five years.

Therefore, the scientific proof of TCM is the syndrome differentiation and treatment among which, the 'four examinations and eight principles' are the main outlines, especially four examinations as the precondition. In all ages, TCM always attaches the importance to four examinations, from which eight principles can be established and the prescription can be made. Most importantly, the pulse taking, in these four examinations, is the vital one. If there is any secret to learn TCM well, it must be mastering the pulse taking and prescribing based on the pulse which is also the key to curative effect. Every TCM learner must remember this by heart!

However, important as pulsing taking is, it only accounts for twenty class hours in a five-year university course. What is worse, teachers usually mention it roughly, causing students to have no practical experience in clinical practice. Despite memorizing lots of prescriptions, they are not able to prescribe one prescription to cure the disease, which results in many of them being confused of TCM and never being enlightened.

Treating serious cough with half dose of formula

— Discussing that 'thousands of medicinals cannot be equal to one correct pill' by taking the example of curing intractably intense cough in half dose of the formula

In the middle of October, 2011, I received a call from an editor of Shanxi Evening Newspaper after I came back to Taiyuan. He said that the newspaper office was going to hold a gratuitous medical treatment and would like to invite ten famous doctors, including five Western Medicine doctors and five TCM doctors, to participate. He asked me if I was willing to attend the activity, and I agreed with pleasure.

In the morning of October 22, the first 'Weekend Gratuitous Treatment by Famous Doctors' event was held on schedule at Fangzhi Neighborhood in Wanbailin District, Taiyuan Province. There were over three hundred residents attending the activity with the longest queue in front of TCM doctors.

When I was concentrated on feeling the pulse and making prescriptions, I accidentally noticed a middle-aged man at the back of the queue waving his hand and smiling at me. He looked familiar to me, so I nodded my head in response to him. However, I was too concentrated on treatment to remember where I had met him before.

It was not until the end of the activity did he come to me and shake my hand happily.

I suddenly realized that he was Mr. Huang from Malaysia.

Mr. Huang was introduced to me by Doctor Zhou five years ago. Although his major in university was physics, he was very fond of TCM. Therefore, after graduation, he went to Malaysia and worked on TCM. He was only 35, but had a very successful career in TCM.

After some small talk, Mr. Huang said he just arrived in Taiyuan from Malaysia. Having seen the information of this gratuitous service on newspaper, he specially came here to visit me.

Mr. Huang then called Doctor Zhou to have a dinner together in order to have a chat with each other.

Doctor Zhou was older than Mr. Huang, and also loved TCM very much. Every time he heard of a famous TCM doctor, he would pay a visit; every time he knew a good TCM book, he would purchase it immediately. Visiting famous doctors, buying books and doing treatment almost accounted for all his lifetime. More than a decade ago, he had taken a special trip to visit Sir Lǐ Kě (李可) at Lingshi County where he had heard about me. After coming back, he contacted me at once, and we became friends though we were of different generations. He used to treat patients in my clinic for a while.

We had our dinner at a restaurant near the Taiyuan Stadium. Not having seen each other for a long time, it was quite excited of us to meet again.

Mr. Huang talked a lot about the combined treatment of acupuncture and Chinese medicinal in Malaysia which had great effect on patients so that he was always over-scheduled. He said with deep feelings, "Leaning TCM is to be the authentic TCM doctor, and it is the authentic TCM doctor that can cure diseases."

During our conversation, I noticed that Doctor Zhou's eyes were drowned in tears, his face was in gloomy complexion and he kept coughing, so I asked, "Why don't you treat yourself since you have such a severe cough?"

Doctor Zhou frustratedly answered me: "I spend all my life on TCM but have no method to cure my own disease. I have been coughing without phlegm for over a month as long as I have itch in throat. I took medicinals prescribed by four TCM doctors separately without any effect! What about you giving me a treatment?"

Afterwards, he stretched his arm to me for a pulse diagnosis. I found that his right Cun pulse was floating, huge, slippery, rapid, and slightly tight, so I made a prescription as follows based on the pulse condition:

Mahuang (Herba Ephedrae) 10g
Guizhi (Ramulus Cinnamomi) 10g
Baishao (Radix Paeoniae Alba) 10g
Ganjiang (Rhizoma Zingiberis) 10g
Xixin (Herba Asari) 3g
Banxia (Rhizoma Pinelliae) 10g
Wuweizi (Fructus Schisandrae Chinensis) 10g
Xingren (Semen Armeniacae Amarum) 10g
Shengshigao (Gypsum Fibrosum) 30g
Houpo (Cortex Magnoliae Officinalis) 10g
Ziwan (Radix Asteris) 10g
Kuandonghua (Flos Farfarae) 10g
Sangbaipi (Cortex Mori) 15g
Chantui (Periostracum Cicadae) 6g
Gancao (Radix Glycyrrhizae) 10g
Shengjiang (Rhizoma Zingiberis Recens) 3 slices
Dazao (Fructus Jujubae) 3 pieces

He asked me for the reason of this prescription.

I told him: "Your right Cun pulse is slightly tight and your eyes are easily in tears, indicating that you have wind-cold fettering lung; your huge pulse presents you have been suffering from the syndrome of lung fire; your slippery pulse also presents you have phlegm and fluid retention; symptoms like dry cough without phlegm results from cold enveloping fire which congests your phlegm causing the severe cough; your pulse manifestations also include floating and slightly rapid pulse, your throat often feels itchy, and you have wind-warm symptoms. Based on above pulse manifestations and symptoms, I prescribe *Xiao Qinglong Tang (Minor Green-Blue Dragon Decoction)* to treat your disease."

The reason why prescriptions become increasingly complex nowadays is that the disease never shows up alone.

After making the prescription, I added, "I prescribe based on the pulse condition. You can have a try."

Having heard my words, Doctor Zhou showed me the prescriptions by other four doctors in his phone, most of which treated his disease as the dry cough caused by yin deficiency. Although someone also prescribed *Xiao Qinglong Tang* (*Minor Green-Blue Dragon Decoction*), he still added some medicinals to nourish yin and moisten dryness, such as *Tiandong* (*Radix Asparagi*), *Maidong* (*Radix Ophiopogonis*), and *Yuzhu* (*Rhizoma Polygonati Odorati*).

Unexpectedly, at eight o'clock in the next evening, Doctor Zhou called me excitedly, "Your prescription is so effective that I cough much less after only taking one dose!"

I said: "That's great. You can take one more dose to consolidate!"

After one day, we three gathered together in the same restaurant again for Mr. Huang would depart for Malaysia.

I noticed Doctor Zhou was in a very good condition this time without any cough or tears in eyes.

He said with emotions: "Your prescription is so effective. There was no effect of other medicinals on my disease after I took them for one month, but two doses of your prescription totally cured me. Pulse is indeed the core of TCM in clinic."

I answered: "It is fine you no longer cough. I thought it was really uncomfortable of you to keep coughing!"

Afterwards, we three drank and continued our chat about TCM happily.

Two days later, my phone rang at around 10 pm.

I am used to keeping early hours and I often go to bed at nine o'clock in the evening, so my close friends never call me after nine. I picked up the phone sleepily and heard the excited voice of Doctor Zhou, "How incredible your prescription is!"

I said: "What's going on?"

Then he told me the story below excitedly:

Actually, he worked as a contractor for a health service station in Taiyuan last year, and was busy with injections, transfusions and making prescriptions. Although he was cured after taking two doses of my prescriptions, he feared a lot after this incident, so he boiled another dose to consolidate. He boiled one set of medicinals twice and preserved them in two glass bottles separately so he could take them after returning home.

However, a 45-year-old female patient Ms. Zhao came to the station, asking for anti-inflammatory transfusion due to cough at that time.

Since Doctor Zhou was just cured from cough, he took her pulse (Doctor Zhou was the disciple of Mr. Zhang, a famous TCM doctor in Shanxi Province, so he was very good at feeling the pulse). He found that the patient had a similar pulse condition to his and her symptom was also dry cough which was much more severe than his. She continuously coughed for at least half an hour every time with tears and nasal mucus. Moreover, due to severe cough, she had to bend down for a long time. The cough was so severe that she had not gone to work for four months. She frequently received injection and transfusions, and also took numerous medicinals.

Doctor Zhou knew that transfusion could not solve the core problem. He suddenly thought of the decoction he left for himself and advised the patient to take it.

The patient was so frustrated so she took one bottle of the decoction and left.

Surprisingly, Ms. Zhao came to the station the next day specially to appreciate Doctor Zhou, saying that she stopped coughing after taking the decoction. It was so unexpected that half dose of the decoction could cure her four-month severe cough. She was pleased beyond imagination, saying that she finally could go back to work.

Seeing the patient's pleasant expression, Doctor Zhou was so surprised that he could not wait to share this story with me at 10 pm. He told me with emotions: "It seems that one shot of medicine is enough if the prescription matches the pulse condition; however, if it does not match the pulse, drinking a pint of medicine is still useless!"

"That's really something", I said, "but if the pulse is felt wrong, a pint of medicine cannot cure disease either. Isn't there a saying that 'one correct pill is worth more than one thousand other medicines'."

"That is like 'one enlightened word is worth a lot'", said Doctor Zhou, "I finally understand that the core of clinical TCM is pulse taking which needs to be focused on when learning TCM."

Although it was 10 pm, Doctor Zhou and I were still excited to continue our conversation.

About the prescription this time, he asked me more questions as follows:

Q: I have worked hard on TCM for almost two decades, it is hard to imagine that I am not able to cure such a small disease.

A: It is not shameful for a TCM doctor to be unable to cure his or her own disease, because every doctor has his or her specialties and drawbacks. It is even common for a TCM master not to be able to treat one's own disease and to ask others for help. The key is not to think that the disease that cannot be cured by you is also not curable by others or even by TCM. Though cough is not serious, it is not easy to be cured by mastering several related prescriptions. It needs to differentiate syndromes carefully. As an old saying goes, 'cough is an archenemy to doctors'. It is apparent that curing the cough is not simple, and may cause serious consequences, even death, after long periods of treatment without effect.

Q: I know that cough can be caused by any problems in internal organs or six excesses (wind, cold, summer-heat, dampness, dryness, fire). My symptom, however, was dry cough without phlegm caused by dryness, why did you prescribe me *Xiao Qinglong Tang* (*Minor Green-Blue Dragon Decoction*)?

A: The climate in Shanxi province is dry and rainless with severe air pollution. In autumn and winter, people easily have cough caused by dryness, whose symptom is dry cough. However, not all dry coughs are related to dryness; pathogenic dryness can be divided as warm dryness and cool dryness due to different properties.

Patient suffering from warm dryness must have a floating and rapid pulse with headache and fever. He or she will have dry cough with little or without phlegm, and have a red tongue with a thin and white coating. In this situation, *Sang Xing Tang* (*Mulberry Leaf and Apricot Kernel Decoction*) is a better choice.

By contrast, patients suffering from cool dryness will have a floating and wiry pulse, which can be cured by *Xing Su San* (*Apricot Kernel and Perilla Powder*).

If dryness damages lung-yin, patient will have a dry and sore throat which is the syndrome of lung dryness and fluid consumption. In this situation, *Maidong* (*Radix Ophiopogonis*), *Xuanshen* (*Radix Scrophulariae*), and *Chuanbeimu* (*Bulbus Fritillariae Cirrhosae*) should be prescribed in order to nourish yin and clear lung.

The four TCM doctors you mentioned above all focused on your dry cough symptom but ignored your pulse manifestation. They considered your dryness should be cured by moistening as they found you had dry cough. Therefore, they prescribed you with *Shashen* (*Radix Glehniae*), *Maidong* (*Radix Ophiopogonis*), and *Chuanbeimu* (*Bulbus Fritillariae Cirrhosae*). However, these medicinals have no effect on your illness due to the fact that they have no relation with your pulse.

Q: I understand that you prescribed me with *Xiao Qinglong Tang* (*Minor Green-Blue Dragon Decoction*), but this decoction is not to cure dry cough without phlegm due to its formula and symptoms.

A: That's true. According to *Treatise on Cold Damage Diseases* (*Shāng hán lùn*, 伤寒论), the formula and symptoms of *Xiao Qinglong Tang* (*Minor Green-Blue Dragon Decoction*) is 'Before the exterior syndrome is dispersed, *Xiao Qinglong Tang* suits the syndrome with the following symptoms and signs: nausea, fever and cough caused by water-fluid stagnancy in the chest (epigastrium). There might also be other symptoms like thirst for water, diarrhea, hiccuping, dysuria, asthma, or lower abdominal distention.' Certainly it doesn't include dry cough without phlegm.

Nevertheless, *Xiao Qinglong Tang* (*Minor Green-Blue Dragon Decoction*) is derived from *Daqinglong Tang* (*Major Blue Dragon Decoction*), both of which are the formula for treating greater yang syndrome.

'Cold damage disease caused by wind of the greater yang meridian: pulse floating and tight, fever and chill, and a general ache and restlessness without perspiration are the symptoms and signs of the syndrome for which *Daqinglong Tang* is suitable.' The key here is 'pulse floating and tight', which must be very easy to figure out at right Cun position, indicating the syndrome of water-cold attacking lung; the slightly rapid pulse indicates the syndrome of heat; these pulse manifestations represent that the lung has stagnated fire. In other words, it is 'cold covering the fire', causing the stagnation of cold and heat. The phlegm in the lung cannot be coughed out, so it transfers into nasal mucus and tears.

According to the mechanism of disease, *Xiao Qinglong Tang* (*Minor Green-Blue Dragon Decoction*), the elixir to cure syndrome of water-cold attacking lung, was the best choice to deal with your disease.

The slightly huge and rapid pulse indicated that stagnated heat was in the lung, so I added *Shigao* (*Gypsum Fibrosum*) and *Sangbaipi* (*Cortex Mori*) into the formula in order first to clear away pathogenic fire in the lung and stomach, as well as to dissipate pathogen out of the body through body hair and orifices due to the bitter flavor of *Shigao* (*Gypsum Fibrosum*); second to purge the lung of pathogenic fire which would be cleared away through urine.

The reason of adding *Houpo* (*Cortex Magnoliae Officinalis*) and *Kuxingren* (*Semen Armeniacae Amarum*) into the prescription was based on the greater yang Chapter from *Treatise on Cold Damage Diseases* (*Shāng hán lùn*, 伤寒论), 'When dyspnea appears, *Guizhi Tang* (*Cinnamon Twig Decoction*) with *Houpo* (*Cortex Magnoliae Officinalis*) and *Kuxingren* (*Semen Armeniacae Amarum*) is a better choice.' *Houpo* (*Cortex Magnoliae Officinalis*) can descend qi from spleen and stomach, and then qi from lung will also be descended, helping to resolve phlegm; *Kuxingren* (*Semen Armeniacae Amarum*) is the best medicinal to ventilate and descend qi from lung, which is the dominating organ of qi of whole body, so it will lead to the descending of qi from every organ in the body. These two medicinals not only can cure dyspnea caused by excessive phlegm but also can deal with cough due to the fact that cough is also caused by upward reversal of lung qi, and these medicinals can be beneficial to accelerate the descending of qi and the resolution of phlegm.

Ziwan (*Radix Asteris*) and *Kuandonghua* (*Flos Farfarae*) as the key medicinals to cure cough and resolve phlegm were also added into the prescription for quick results.

Every medicinal added in this prescription was based on the pulse and symptoms. Not precise as it was, it still had great and quick effect on the disease because of feeling of the pulse. However, this prescription is not the all-in-one drug for all cough syndromes.

Two months later, Mr. Huang unexpectedly called me from Malaysia, "I benefit a lot because of your words! Relying on your theory, I have highly improved my clinical effects, especially when treating fibroids. There are over 30 patients, half of whom are suffering from fibroids, asking for my treatment every day."

His words made me totally confused. I never had my own theory. All I knew is to move forward step by step in the world of TCM. Where is the theory I taught him coming from? I cannot help laughing. Afterwards, however, when I tried to remember what I had told him, I suddenly realized that I had indeed shared something with him.

Since we three are all TCM doctors, all things we had talked about relate to TCM and treatments. The following words are generally what I had said:

"The key principle for TCM doctors to cure patients is not to be influenced by western medical ideas, such as only focusing on anti-inflammation and anti-cancer aspects as long as there is one; it is hard for TCM doctors to cure diseases by prescribing based on the western medical ideas.

Above is what I said during our communication. How can this be any theory? This is only the real method for TCM doctors to cure patients. What I had done was to speak them out, and surprisingly Mr. Huang treated them as a theory!

During the Chinese New Year in 2012, Mr. Huang came back to Taiyuan again when I was in Beijing. He called me, excitedly sharing with me his experience of curing rare and stubborn diseases by authentic TCM ideas. I could tell his confidence of learning TCM from his excitement.

He also told me that he had seen Doctor Zhou several days earlier. Zhou mentioned again that I had cured his cough, saying I had saved his life.

I said I felt so flattered. As a TCM doctor however, we should treat every disease, serious or not, with our best effort. Common diseases should not be ignored because there are numerous serious diseases, such as trachitis, pulmonary heart disease, emphysema and even cardiovascular and cerebrovascular diseases causing death, that are transferred from a simple cough or a bad cold every year. How can we underestimate their seriousness?

Nonetheless, I stressed that the prescription I had made was only suitable for Doctor Zhou's cough but not for other various cough syndromes. Mr. Huang however said that Zhou had cured over 20 patients suffering from cough using the formula.

I said that it might be because this kind of cough was the epidemic disease in autumn and winter! Using this prescription would have great effect when dealing with similar pulse manifestation and syndrome, so every disease should be treated according to its syndrome.

In 2005, I visited Zhū Liángchūn (朱良春), one of the leading scholars in TCM field in Nantong, Jiangsu Province. Mr. Zhu gesticulated a small circle, saying, "I only learnt this little of TCM." However, it is such 'little' that has cured many patients and saved numerous lives!

Opportunity favors the prepared mind

— Discussing that 'treating fever without medicinals with sour flavor and cold nature is like fire fighting without water' and that 'TCM cures disease in coincidence' by taking the example of curing bilateral bronchial pneumonia

Hao was a two-year-old girl. She was sent to the hospital due to fever and cough on 11 December, 2010. According to the X-ray examination report (X-ray number: 918205) by Beijing Anda Hospital, she suffered bilateral bronchopneumonia. Having failed to cure by injection and transfusion, she was sent to me for treatment on 15 December.

After the examination, I found that this child had cough and shortness of breath, gurgled with sputum in the throat, reddish lips and face, nasal congestion and clear nasal discharge, a reddish tongue with a white coating. Her temperature was 39.7°C.

These symptoms revealed that the mechanism of her disease was exogenous wind-cold and stagnated lung qi transforming into heat which caused phlegm, leading to cough. The therapeutic methods should focus on releasing exterior with pungent-warm medicinals, dispersing wind and dissipating cold, and clearing heat and resolving phlegm in order to regain the ascent and descent function of lung. Here were the ingredients of the formula:

Mahuang (Herba Ephedrae) 5g
Shigao (Gypsum Fibrosum) 20g

Xingren (Semen Armeniacae Amarum) 6g
Qingbanxia (Rhizoma Pinelliae) 10g
Chenpi (Pericarpium Citri Reticulatae) 6g
Fuling (Poria) 10g
Jingjie (Herba Schizonepetae) 6g
Qianhu (Radix Peucedani) 6g
Huashifen (PULVIS TALCI) 10g
Machixian (Herba Portulacae) 20g
Wumei (Fructus Mume) 6g
Gancao (Radix Glycyrrhizae) 6g

All these drugs should be decocted with water for oral administration once every three hours.

The girl patient took the formula twice in the morning, and she brought down her fever and stopped coughing in the afternoon with other symptoms eliminated.

The above prescription combines *Mahuang Xingren Gancao Shigao Tang* (*Ephedra, Bitter Apricot Seed, Gypsum and Licorice Decoction*) and *Erchen Tang* (*Decoction of Two Old Ingredients*). In this prescription, pungent-warm *Mahuang* (*Herba Ephedrae*) was used to release exterior and ventilate lung qi. Considering the efficacy of *Mahuang* (*Herba Ephedrae*) was weak, *Jingjie* (*Herba Schizonepetae*) was added to enhance the efficacy; *Xingren* (*Semen Armeniacae Amarum*), as the key medicinal to relieve cough and dyspnea; *Erchen Tang* (*Decoction of Two Old Ingredients*) was added to dry dampness and resolve phlegm in order to descend lung qi. Adding *Qianhu* (*Radix Peucedani*) was because it can relieve phlegm both from the internal and the external, so that it could support the efficacy of *Erchen Tang* (*Decoction of Two Old Ingredients*); *Shigao* (*Gypsum Fibrosum*) as the crucial medicinal to clear away heat from the meridians of lung and stomach; adding *Huashifen* (*PULVIS TALCI*) was for draining water and expelling stone due to its sweet flavor and cold nature, helping to release heat from urination.

Machixian (*Herba Portulacae*) in the prescription has cold nature but little sour flavor while *Wumei* (*Fructus Mume*) has strong sour flavor and the combination of these two medicinals would produce sour flavor and cold nature so that I often add them in the prescription when dealing with externally-contracted febrile disease especially with high temperature (Hyperpyrexia).

Hyperpyrexia suffered by children not only made parents anxious but also may threaten children's lives due to pneumonia. As the main problem was solved, other symptoms would be eliminated and the pneumonia would be cured.

Mahuang Xingren Gancao Shigao Tang (*Ephedra, Bitter Apricot Seed, Gypsum and Licorice Decoction*) in *Treatise on Cold Damage Diseases*(*Shāng hán lùn,* 伤寒论) is to cure 'sweating and dyspnea patient without fever'. I was afraid this decoction was not able to have effect on fever, so I added these two medicinals. The method of bringing down the fever with sour flavor and cold nature medicinals was learnt from Jìn Wénqīng (靳文清).

Jìn Wénqīng (靳文清) (1915–1988) was a distinguished veteran TCM doctor and chief physician in Shanxi TCM Research Institution. He graduated from the Traditional Chinese Medical College of North China in 1930s. He learnt from famous doctors at that time, such as Shī Jīnmò (施今墨), Zhōu Jièrén (周介人), Zhū Húshān (朱壶山) and Zhào Xīwǔ (赵锡武), and had worked on the TCM clinic for over 50 years.

In 1984, I had my job transferred into Shanxi Science and Technology Press where I was introduced to Mr. Jin. Since then, I often visited him and asked questions about stubborn diseases. The first time that Mr. Jin applied sour flavor and cold nature medicinals to bring down the fever was in 1946 when he treated a 35-year-old male patient, Mr. Niu, who had been sick for over half a month. Initially, the patient had been averse to cold and had had a fever with head and body aches. He felt very exhausted. Later on, he got an even higher temperature than before with less aversion to cold and severe headache. Gradually, he turned from aversion to cold to aversion to hot temperature. Doctors treated him before had prescribed him with *Baihu Tang* (*White Tiger Decoction*) that failed to bring down his high fever. Therefore, he asked for treatment from Mr. Jin.

Having examined the patient, Mr. Jin thought the prescription used by previous doctors basically corresponded with his disease syndrome with little fault. So why did it had no effect on the disease?

Confused as he was, Mr. Jin suddenly remembered the words by ancient famous TCM doctors, 'treating fever without sour flavor and cold nature medicinals is like fire fighting without water'. Therefore, he added medicinals with sour flavor and cold nature into the previous prescription and increased the dosage of *Shigao* (*Gypsum Fibrosum*). The following was the prescription:

Shigao (*Gypsum Fibrosum*) 120g
Zhimu (*Rhizoma Anemarrhenae*) 15g
Jinyinhua (*Flos Lonicerae*) 25g
Lianqiao (*Fructus Forsythiae*) 25g
Daqingye (*Folium Isatidis*) 30g
Huangqin (*Radix Scutellariae*) 15g
Huanglian (*Rhizoma Coptidis*) 10g
Shengdihuang (*Radix Rehmanniae Recens*) 25g
Gancao (*Radix Glycyrrhizae*) 10g
Pugongying Gen (*Radix Taraxaci*) 60g
Machixian (*Herba Portulacae*) 60g
Wumei (*Fructus Mume*) 10g

The effect was highly improved after two doses were taken continuously, and the fever was brought down after five doses.

In this case, wind-cold attacked the patient first, and then it transformed into heat syndrome. Adding medicinals with sour flavor and cold nature into the previous prescription which contained pungent-cold and bitter-cold medicinals would enhance its effect.

In the autumn of 1947, Mr. Jin treated a 21-year-old male patient Mr. Jing. The patient had suffered from the disease for half a month. He had a little bit aversion to cold at the beginning, hiding fever, aching pain in joint, a rapid and soggy pulse. He had been diagnosed with common cold coupled with dampness and been treated in that way, but the treatment had no effect.

Afterwards, his symptoms turned into the following: slight aversion to cold, high temperature, aggravated pain in head and body, fullness sensation in stomach, poor appetite, unconsciousness at night, inhibited defecation, deep-colored and little urine, a dry and yellow tongue coating.

This case belonged to severe dampness-heat syndrome, in which pathogenic heat was more serious than pathogenic dampness. The turbid heat in the body covered seven orifices in the head. Therefore,

Mr. Jin prescribed *Sanren Tang* (*Three Kernels Decoction*) with *Huoxiang* (*Herba PogoStemonis*), *Peilan* (*Herba Eupatorii*), *Shichangpu* (*Rhizoma Acori Tatarinowii*), and *Yujin* (*Radix Curcumae*) to eliminate turbid dampness, to clear consciousness and to open orifices. *Huanglian* (*Rhizoma Coptidis*), *Huangqin* (*Radix Scutellariae*), and *Zhizi* (*Fructus Gardeniae*) with bitter flavor and cold nature were also added into the prescription to clear heat and dry dampness.

However, after the patient had taken several doses, the formula still had no effect on his disease and his condition even went worse. He got a higher temperature and coma sometimes with delirious speech and finger wriggling.

The patient was critically ill at that time, so Mr. Jin immediately replaced *Kuxingren* (*Semen Armeniacae Amarum*) and *Yiyiren* (*Semen Coicis*) in the previous prescription with 50g *Machixian* (*Herba Portulacae*), 10g *Wumei* (*Fructus Mume*), 15g *Baishao* (*Radix Paeoniae Alba*), 30g *Longgu* (*Os Draconis*) and 30g *Muli* (*Concha Ostreae*) (smashed and boiled first). He advised the patient to take the formula with fresh grape juice as water (it was the season for grape harvest).

After taking the formula for three days, the patient had his fever brought down and felt conscious. His stomach was not as full as before so that he could have half a bowl of porridge. Finally, his condition took a favorable turn.

Having taken six more doses of the formula, he had his temperature back to normal with a conscious mind. He could feel hungry. He gradually recovered after head and body ache was relieved.

The key to this effective formula was the addition of medicinals with sour flavor and cold nature but this is not a simple coincidence.

In the autumn of 1975, Mr. Jin treated a 38-year-old male patient, Mr. Ma, who had suffered hyperthermia for over 20 days. Once he had received transfusion treatment (with antibiotics and hormone), the fever would be brought down; however, his temperature would rise again the other day. Repeatedly, the transfusion had no effect on his disease. What was worse, he had alternating chills and fever every afternoon. It was not effective to take both Chinese medicinals and western medicines. The patient felt exhausted and had anorexia with a reddish tongue and a light yellow and dry coating. His pulse was wiry and moderate on both hands.

Symptoms were lighter in the morning, but at noon, he would suffer from alternating chills and fever.

Mr. Jin prescribed him with modified *Xiao Chaihu Tang* (*Minor Bupleurum Decoction*). The following was the prescription:

Chaihu (*Radix Bupleuri*) *15g*
Huangqin (*Radix Scutellariae*) *10g*
Qinghao (*Herba Artemisiae Annuae*) *15g*
Lianqiao (*Fructus Forsythiae*) *25g*
Zhimu (*Rhizoma Anemarrhenae*) *15g*
Pugongying Gen (*Radix Taraxaci*) *60g*
Gualou (*Fructus Trichosanthis*) *20g*
Machixian (*Herba Portulacae*) *50g*
Wumei (*Fructus Mume*) *10g*

After taking three doses, the patient felt relieved from alternating chills and fever.

Symptoms like alternating chills and fever, oppression in the chest, anorexia, a wiry and moderate pulse indicated that he suffered the syndrome of lesser yang, and should be treated by *Xiao Chaihu Tang* (*Minor Bupleurum Decoction*). Hereafter, the patient only had alternating chills and fever in the late afternoon, which revealed that the syndrome had transformed into overlap of diseases of lesser yang and yang brightness. Therefore, Mr. Jin combined *Xiao Chaihu Tang* (*Minor Bupleurum Decoction*) with *Baihu Tang* (*White Tiger Decoction*) to relieve pathogen from both lesser yang and yang brightness.

Qinghao (*Herba Artemisiae Annuae*) in this prescription was to improve the effect of *Xiao Chaihu Tang* (*Minor Bupleurum Decoction*) on harmonizing lesser yang.

Jinyinhua (*Flos Lonicerae*), *Lianqiao* (*Fructus Forsythiae*), and *Pugongying* (*Herba Taraxaci*) were used to improve the effect of *Baihu Tang* (*White Tiger Decoction*) on clearing heat from yang brightness.

Gualou (*Fructus Trichosanthis*) in the prescription was used to descend qi for smoothing the middle, to eliminate phlegm-heat and to relieve oppression in the chest.

Removing *Renshen* (*Radix Ginseng*) in the prescription of *Xiao Chaihu Tang* (*Minor Bupleurum Decoction*) was because the patient had no qi deficiency.

The dosage reduction of *Banxia* (*Rhizoma Pinelliae*) was due to the fact that the patient did not vomit.

The key of this prescription was to increase the dosage of *Machixian* (*Herba Portulacae*) and *Wumei* (*Fructus Mume*) for their sour flavor and cold nature in order to bring down the fever. This indeed had great effect on the disease.

Consequently, bringing down the fever by the medicinals with sour flavor and cold nature did have curative effect, but this method should not be applied to all syndromes.

TCM attaches importance to treatment based on syndrome differentiation. The mechanism of disease leading to high fever can generally be divided into two categories: one is internal damage fever which can be treated in the following methods: relieving fever with sweet and warm medicines, nourishing yin and clearing heat, and removing toxin and clearing heat; the other is external-contraction fever, including cold damage and warm disease.

The above cases cured by Mr. Jin and the case of infantile pneumonia treated by me all belong to external-contraction fever. As for internal damage fever, I dare not confirm that it can be cured by sour flavor and cold nature medicinals due to the lack of clinical experience.

Common medicinals with sour flavor and cold nature include *Machixian* (*Herba Portulacae*), *Wumei* (*Fructus Mume*) and *Shuiniujiao* (*rhinoceros horn*) (substituted by *Shuiniujiao* (*Cornu Bubali*) nowadays) and so on.

Wumei (*Fructus Mume*) with its sour flavor and moderate nature is the crucial medicinal to promote fluid production to quench thirst so that it is more suitable for warm disease.

A posthumous manuscript of Péng Zǐyì (彭子益) (edited by Zhàolán (赵兰)) was published in the first issue of Shanxi Medical Magazine released in 1966. The manuscript recorded cases of curing warm diseases with *Wumei* (*Fructus Mume*) and white sugar.

According to Mr. Peng's 50-year clinical experience, he used *Wumei* (*Fructus Mume*) and white sugar to effectively cure 13 patients suffering from warm disease.

The method of bringing down fever by sour flavor and cold nature medicinals sounds easy to imitate and master, but it was difficult for Mr. Jin to put it forward.

Mr. Jin was an authentic TCM doctor who strictly obeyed traditional principles of TCM. He had profound research of TCM classics and ideas of various famous doctors in different generations. Moreover, he was rigorous of research approaches and devoted his life to clinic. Such a veteran TCM doctor with a solid knowledge foundation as he was, he still felt helpless and could not figure out an effective prescription when facing patients suffering from persistent high fever. When dealing with the patient Mr. Niu who had persistent high fever, Mr. Jin was not able to find a suitable prescription until he was reminded of the words of 'treating fever without the medicinals with sour flavor and cold nature is like fire fighting without water'. Indeed, it was just like what Xīn Qìjí (辛弃疾) wrote, 'Having almost exhausted my energy searching for that person (vague), I suddenly turned my head, and there they were, standing at the far end of the street where the candlelight is the dimmest'.

I immediately mastered this method after Mr. Jin taught me using only few words. Therefore, how can people learn TCM without the support of teachers?

Nevertheless, he spent several years studying this method. In the early 1940s, he looked through a large number of medical cases recorded by predecessors and several ancient classics in order to look for effective medicinals that can bring down the fever. Having gathered as many cases as he could, he still acquired too little knowledge to confirm the success of the prescription. Afterwards, facing some patients suffering from persistent high fever, he had to try prescribing the medicinals with sour flavor and cold nature, and then unexpectedly received positive effect. This result that 'stands at the far end of the street where the candlelight is dimmest' was due to the fact that he 'had almost exhausted his energy searching for it'.

Madame Curie once said: "A great discovery does not issue from a scientist's brain ready-made, like Minerva springing fully armed from Jupiter's head; it is the fruit of an accumulation of preliminary work."

Indeed, this sour flavor and cold nature method to bring down fever was not discovered by Mr. Jin, but it did not groundlessly spring up from his mind. It is his effort of studying traditional medical cases and ideas that led to this result.

Ancient medical cases and ideas indicating the combination of TCM theories and practice reflect the wisdom of TCM. Studying ancient medical cases and ideas may not be immediately useful for current treatment, but it will enlighten doctors' minds in clinical medication, constantly enhance and improve the TCM idea so that doctors can instantly come up with different and creative methods when facing complex diseases. This is just as what Louis Pasteur, a French biologist, said: "fortune favors the prepared mind."

In 1930s, Yú Yúnxiù (余云岫) who was against TCM had a famous quote that it was 'coincidence' for TCM to cure patients. It seemed that he knew TCM could cure diseases, but he still thought hard to find out such a wording in order to be against TCM and the fact that TCM can cure diseases. It was just like the saying goes, 'A stick is quickly to find to beat a dog.'

Throughout the history of science, there are several 'coincident cases' that are delightful to talk about.

For example, Archimedes discovered the buoyancy law when taking a bath in the bathtub, after which he excitedly ran to the street naked to announce his significant discovery; Watt invented the steam engine after seeing the lid of the kettle getting lifted by steam during his vacation in his grandmother's house.

Isaac Newton discovered the law of universal gravitation when sitting under an apple tree for coolness and seeing the apple falling to the ground.

The above cases seem like coincidence, but are the results of having been studied by those scientists for a long time.

One should know that Newton had started his research of 'the law of universal gravitation' twenty years before seeing the apple falling to the ground.

These common and familiar phenomena that attracted no attention from ordinary people can become the opportunity to discover a scientific theory only when meeting with scientists and inventors with 'prepared minds'.

Similarly, all kinds of diseases, including complex problems in medical science such as cancers, can be 'accidentally' cured only when encountering conventional and authentic TCM doctors with 'prepared minds'. Not all people can meet with such a coincidence!

If a patient coughs, the doctor shall not relieve the cough first; if a patient has phlegm, the doctor shall not dispel phlegm first

— Discussing that the formula should be composed by the comprehensive analysis of pulse and symptoms by taking the example of curing intense nighttime cough by the therapeutic methods of 'taking away firewood from under the cauldron' and 'treating incontinent syndrome with dredging method'

On 20 December, 2011, I treated a nine-year-old boy, Lyu.

His parents told me that the patient child frequently had a severe cough in recent three days with white phlegm sometimes, causing him to be awake at night. Since they only told me the patient's symptoms without taking him to my clinic, I made a prescription with lung-diffusing, phlegm-reducing and cough-relieving medicinals. The prescription was as follows:

Ziwan (Radix Asteris) 10g
Baiqian (Rhizoma Cynanchi Stauntonii) 10g
Qianhu (Radix Peucedani) 10g
Fuling (Poria) 15g

Baibu (Radix Stemonae) 15g
Juhong (Exocarpium Citri Grandis) 6g
Zisu (Folium Perillae) 5g
Jiegeng (Radix Platycodonis) 10g
Gancao (Radix Glycyrrhizae) 6g

The parents took their child to my clinic the following day, saying the formula not only had no effect on their child but resulted in a more severe cough.

Having heard their words, I therefore carefully examined the patient child and knew that he only kept on coughing at night. Although he had white phlegm, the phlegm was too sticky to cough out. He had a dry throat, hoarse voice, feverish feeling in palms and soles, a reddish face.

His parents said that the boy had a very good appetite two days before he got sick and had diarrhea twice or third times per day with a swelling pain in abdomen.

I suddenly realized that his diarrhea was caused by heat retention with watery discharge when I felt his pulse condition as slippery and rapid. Therefore, the previous modified *Zhisou San* (*Cough-Stopping Powder*) I made was not suitable for this disease.

His disease was due to the syndrome of accumulation of excess heat in the large intestine. No wonder the prescription for ventilating lung, relieving cough, and resolving phlegm did not work well. Thus, I changed the prescription to modified *Da Chengqi Tang* (*Major Purgative Decoction*). The following was the prescription:

Dahuang (Radix et Rhizoma Rhei) 10g (later decocted)
Zhishi (Fructus Aurantii Immaturus) 10g
Houpo (Cortex Magnoliae Officinalis) 10g
Mangxiao (Natrii Sulfas) 10g (later decocted)
Yuanshen (Radix Scrophulariae) 10g
Maidong (Radix Ophiopogonis) 10g
Lianqiao (Fructus Forsythiae) 6g
Qingguo (Fructus Canarii) 6g
Gancao (Radix Glycyrrhizae) 6g

After taking one dose, he excreted faeces with feculence, and then the cough was relieved and the phlegm was eliminated.

This example indicates that although TCM holds the view that 'medicinals should be corresponding with symptoms', the 'symptoms' here must include 'pulse manifestations', that is, 'medicinals should be corresponding with both disease symptoms and pulse manifestations'.

This means the same disease may have different symptoms. Doctors must fully analyze symptoms instead of only treating the head when there are head aches or, in other words, taking stoppage measures.

Some may think that doctors should focus on the main symptoms in clinical treatment, which needs to be further discussed though this may be reasonable.

Symptoms should be divided based on its essence and appearance rather than main symptoms and minor ones. Some symptoms, apparent as they are, are only the appearance of the disease; others, despite their indistinctive nature, reflect the essence of the disease.

Doctors must make prescriptions by concentrating on the essence of the disease and can sometimes ignore its appearance. As long as the essential problem is solved, other surface problems can be readily dealt with. That is why TCM always stresses the importance of 'searching for the primary cause of disease in treatment'.

As for this child patient case, the reason why the former prescription for ventilating lung, relieving cough, and resolving phlegm had no effect on the patient is that it did not solve its essential problem.

In the old saying, it is not only the lung but also any other viscera that can cause a cough.

Severe the cough may be, it was only the appearance of the disease. The diarrhea (heat retention with watery discharge), swelling pain in abdomen, feverish feeling in palms and soles, red face, and slippery and rapid pulse manifestations, though not the main syndromes, indeed reflected the essence of the disease — yang brightness fu-organ excess syndrome.

Due to the fact that lung and the large intestine are interior-exterior related, excess heat from the large intestine was transferred into the lung, causing the malfunction of purification and descent function of the lung so that the patient had a more severe cough and phlegm. *Da Chengqi Tang*

(*Major Purgative Decoction*) could effectively and efficiently clear away the excess heat in the large intestine and excreted feculence. Afterwards, the lung regained its purification and descent function because it was no longer obstructed by the excess heat. That is why the cough was relieved and the phlegm was reduced without particular treatment.

This method, in the TCM field, is called as 'taking away firewood from under cauldron'. Water boiling in the cauldron is due to the firewood under the cauldron. If the firewood is taken away, the hot water will get cool. This is the principle of *Ḍa Chengqi Tang* (*Major Purgative Decoction*).

If doctors know nothing about this principle and only cool down the water by pumping it up, it will be as ineffectual as my former prescription.

Da Chengqi Tang (*Major Purgative Decoction*) was the prescription Zhāng Zhòngjǐng (张仲景) used most in his life. There are around 32 records of this prescription in *Treatise on Cold Damage Diseases* (*Shāng hán lùn*, 伤寒论) and *Synopsis of the Golden Chamber* (*Jīn kuì yào luè*, 金匮要略), such as 'There is no stool for five to six days, or even ten days, with tide-fever in the afternoon but no chill. The patient speaks to himself in an insane manner. In a serious case, the patient becomes unconscious to people around him and subconsciously touches his clothes and bed in terror; he also has a slight dyspnea and staring eyesight (the symptoms above indicate critical illness).'

'Delirious speech, tide-fever, sweating, sweating of palms and soles, constipation (two-yang overlap of diseases).'

'The patient has pain around the navel, restlessness and irritation appearing at certain times.'

'Dysuria, stool that is sometimes difficult to pass and sometimes easy, a light fever, dyspnea, and vertigo which makes the patient unable to lie in bed quietly.'

'Blurring of vision and low spirits, constipation, and a slight body fever.'

'Greater yang syndrome: fever and profuse perspiration.'

'After adoption of a diaphoretic, the syndrome is not gone. *Da Chengqi Tang* (*Major Purgative Decoction*) should be adopted urgently in a syndrome with abdominal distention and pain.'

'Lesser yin syndrome, the second or the third day: A drastic measure should be urgently adopted if the patient's mouth and throat feel parched. *Da Chengqi Tang* (*Major Purgative Decoction*) is curative.'

'Lesser yin syndrome: when watery stool of a bluish color, pain under the heart (at the epigastrium) and a parched mouth are diagnosed, a drastic, *Da Chengqi Tang* (*Major Purgative Decoction*), can be adopted.'

'Lesser yin syndrome, six to seven days: A drastic measure should be adopted urgently when there is no stool and there is abdominal distention. *Da Chengqi Tang* (*Major Purgative Decoction*) is curative.'

'Syndrome includes diarrhea with a moderate pulse at Cun, Guan, and Chi positions; when pressed, a hard mass is felt under the heart (at the epigastrium).'

'Syndrome includes diarrhea with a slow and slippery pulse.'

'Syndrome includes diarrhea with poor appetite.'

'After the diarrhea subsides, it will recur on the same day and same month of each year.'

'Patient who has diarrhea with a slippery pulse.'

'The pulse is floating and huge at Cun position, turning into an unsmooth pulse at Cun and Chi positions under pressure.'

'A rapid and slippery pulse.'

'After fever and restlessness are dispersed by the adoption of diaphoresis, the patient again has fever in the afternoon, like malaria.'

'Convulsive disease (Jing) can be manifested as follows: fullness sensation in the chest, trismus, serious opisthotonus that prevents the patient from lying flat on bed, with contraction of legs and grinding of teeth.'

'A tight pulse, like a rotating rope without a fixed form.'

'When abdominal distention is not reduced or only partially reduced, *Da Chengqi Tang* (*Major Purgative Decoction*) should be prescribed as a drastic measure.'

'A weak pulse ... If there is no stool for six or seven days with little urination and reduced food intake, a dose of purgative will cause watery stool, as there are hard feces only at the beginning, followed by watery stool. When urination returns to normal there will be constipation and a purgative can then be used. *Da Chengqi Tang* (*Major Purgative Decoction*) is the remedy.'

'(Postpartum) after the syndrome subsides, the patient has a good appetite. Seven or eight days later, fever recurs.'

'On the seventh or eighth day after delivery, the patient does not suffer greater yang syndrome but suffers abdominal aisteneion and pain. This is a case of profuse lochia. *Da Chengqi Tang* (*Major Purgative Decoction*) can be adopted when the following symptoms and signs are observed: constipation; fever with restlessness and irritability; and slightly excessive pulse; fever aggravated in the afternoon; poor appetite. If food is taken, delirium will occur but the patient will quiet down at night. This is a case with accumulated pathogenetic heat in the urinary bladder.'

'A huge and tight pulse indicates that yang contains yin.'

As for the applications of *Da Chengqi Tang* (*Major Purgative Decoction*) based on varied pulse conditions, some think the pulse condition should be wiry, some think the pulse should be moderate at Cun, Guan, and Chi positions, some think the pulse should be slow and slippery, some think the pulse should be slippery, some hold the view that the pulse should be rapid and slippery, some have another view that the pulse should be tight, like a rotating rope without a fixed form, some also have a different opinion that the pulse should be sufficient while some stand for a little bit sufficient pulse, and others think that the pulse should be huge and tight.

Based on some studies, the slippery and rapid pulse is the main pulse condition while others are all modified ones.

In Zhāng Zhòngjǐng (张仲景)'s opinion, dry feces, retained food or hard stool from the above cases, are the basic clinical applications of *Da Chengqi Tang* (*Major Purgative Decoction*). In his book, he described the solutions to these situations as 'purgative method must be used instantly', 'purgative method could be the remedy', 'purgative method is the better choice for curing disease', or 'purgative method should be used', which depends on disease severity.

In *Treatise on Cold Damage Diseases* (*Shāng hán lùn,* 伤寒论), Zhāng Zhòngjǐng (张仲景) described this prescription in the most detailed way and regarded it as the formula of drastic purgation. Although it is not as widely used as *Guizhi Tang* (*Cinnamon Twig Decoction*) and *Chaihu Tang* (*Bupleurum Decoction*), it indeed has more important meaning.

Excess heat stagnated in the stomach and intestines may cause death. In this crucial situation, *Da Chengqi Tang* (*Major Purgative Decoction*) is the only formula that can have effect on the disease; however, if this prescription is not utilized correctly, it may undermine a patient's condition in a very short time. Just as the saying goes, a miss is as good as a mile. That is the reason why Zhāng Zhòngjǐng (张仲景) spent plenty of time in analyzing and describing this prescription, and in stressing its importance to younger generations. How considerate and precise he is!

My respected teacher Huáng Jiéxī (黄杰熙) once noted, "If TCM learners can master the application of this decoction, they will be the master of harmful hyperactivity and responding inhibition, which is the mainstay of therapeutic methods in TCM!"

Some may ask: Zhāng Zhòngjǐng (张仲景) had used most detailed description on *Da Chengqi Tang* (*Major Purgative Decoction*) without any words related to coughing. Then why did I apply this prescription to my patient?

As far as I am concerned, one reading books written by Zhāng Zhòngjǐng (张仲景) should certainly keep his words in mind, but what is more important is to understand his principle of prescription making, instead of blindly copying his prescription in clinical treatment.

We should creatively study and apply his knowledge to practice when reading Zhāng Zhòngjǐng (张仲景)'s classics rather than sticking to theories.

Masters endow people with rules and theories; it is we that apply them creatively to the practice.

Taking this patient child as an example, he was taken to my clinic because of severe cough. After knowing his cough was more serious at night instead of daytime, seeing his red face, feeling his pulse slippery and rapid, and being told by his mother that he had a very good appetite with diarrhea, I diagnosed him with excess heat (caused by food accumulation) in the intestines and stomach. Therefore, I changed the prescription into *Da Chengqi Tang* (*Major Purgative Decoction*) and cured him with one dose.

If I only focused on main symptoms, I might have regarded severe cough with vital importance. We should see through the appearance to perceive the essence.

This reflects what TCM stresses: 'Diseases should be treated by searching for the primary cause.' 'Primary cause' here means the pathogenesis and etiology. Although every kind of cough is related to the lung, the lung is not the only viscera that should be focused on in treatment. A cough maybe caused by six excesses of external contraction, seven emotions of internal damage, eating and overstrain, all of which should be treated by 'understanding its primary cause through main symptoms'.

Making prescriptions based on causes can help to cure diseases in a few doses.

The wording 'It is all viscera not only the lung that cause a cough' recorded in *Plain Questions · Treatise of Cough* (*Sù wèn·Kélùn*, 素问·咳论) is the principle of TCM. How can modern medicine studies know about it?

Overall, if this method had not been applied, not only was the cough hard to be cured, the disease might have also threatened the child's life.

The child patient had watery stool, which is called diarrhea in *Treatise on Cold Damage Diseases* (*Shāng hán lùn*, 伤寒论). In this case, diarrhea should be treated with drastic purgation medicinals with bitter flavor and cold nature, and the therapeutic method should be treating incontinent syndrome with dredging method, which is the 'reverse treatment' in TCM.

Toxic or not toxic

— The discussion on the toxic
side effects of Chinese medicinals

In the early 1990s, *Xiao Chaihu Tang Keli* (*Minor Bupleurum Decoction Granule*) caused death in Japan; recently, similar accidents happened due to *Longdan Xiegan Wan* (*Gentian Liver-Draining Pills*) and *Houttuynia Cordata Injection*. Therefore, the problem of the toxic side effect of the Chinese medicinals has been widely noted in public as well as in the TCM field.

Some experts and scholars seem to find the New World, warning people to thoroughly eliminate their false opinion that traditional Chinese medicinals have no toxic side effect. Some 'wise men' even put forward that the toxic side effects should be clearly highlighted in the usage instructions just as in western medicines. There are numerous similar opinions towards this event, making people confused and perplexed.

All in all, the study of the safety of Chinese medicinals is not comprehensive and deep enough.

Medication safety, whatever in Western Medicine or TCM, is a matter of vital importance — because it relates to people's lives.

The scientification and modernization of TCM have been going on for decades, among which medication safety should have been included. Why has it not been given enough attention?

Just as what experts have pointed out, "Natural *Houttuynia cordata* for example has at least 48 components, but it is unclear which components are antibacterial and which are for immune-regulation. It is actually a general problem in Chinese medicinals that the quantity and quality of every medicinal are not clearly defined." Science is rigorous, so are experts' opinions.

So far, since the quality and quantity of Chinese medicinals are not clearly defined, we clinical TCM doctors can only make prescriptions everyday as 'a blind man on a blind horse'.

However, please calm down, because scientists will figure out this problem for us.

One day I was reading the newspaper, a highlighted headline just came into my sight: 'Rewriting *Compendium of Materia Medica* (*Běn cǎo gāng mù*, 本草纲目)'! with the subheading as 'revealing the essence of traditional Chinese medicinals and achieving the modernization and inter-nationalization of traditional Chinese medicinals', which was undoubtedly a piece of very good news.

After reading the content carefully, I found it a news special of Shanghai from China News:

> *Compendium of Materia Medica* (*Běn cǎo gāng mù*, 本草纲目), the pre-cious heritage in China's medical treasure-house and 'the great classic of oriental medicinals' is looking forward to a reborn after over 400 years.
>
> Recently, scientists in China proposed a scheme, 'Herbalome Project', planning to rewrite *Compendium of Materia Medica* (*Běn cǎo gāng mù*, 本草纲目) in vernacular Chinese [...]. At present, the 'Herbalome Project' has passed the first round of verification and will start the second round this May [...]. The project is not to literally rewrite *Compendium of Materia Medica* (*Běn cǎo gāng mù*, 本草纲目) but comprehensively ana-lyze the components, structures and functions of Chinese medicinals, establish a resource library of Chinese materia medica and explain the synergistic and complementary mechanisms of multi-components on multi-targets all by utilizing modern science and technology [...]. A researcher from a research institution of Chinese Academy of Sciences noted that Chinese medicinals are effective, but they are difficult to be accepted by international medical field due to the fact that they have com-plex ingredients and undefined material basis and mechanism of action. For example, *safflower oil* contains at least 310 thousand compounds, among which only one hundred have been discovered by us.

He said: "The above problem will not be solved until both effective and toxic ingredients in Chinese medicinals are clearly defined."

"The 'Herbalome Project' is put forward to deal with this problem," he added, "After finishing this project, people will know whether there are toxic compounds in Chinese medicinals and what exact compounds they are [...]. It will fundamentally guarantee the stability and controllability of medical quality as well as the safety and effectiveness of medical property, and achieve the modernization and internationalization of Chinese medicinals [...]. This will be quite a complex project."

The doctoral researcher mentioned that the overall five-year plan of this project is to select and study 30 prescriptions and 300 medicinal materials under the guidance of TCM theory and to establish a resource library containing 120 thousand standard components and 30 thousand compounds with relevant information and data to clearly catalog toxic components of Chinese medicinals.

I have no idea whether such a huge and complex project can successfully go through the approval or when it will start and finish. I am afraid, however, that even an enormous amount of scientific research fund is still not enough to support this project.

Although I understand that this project is a significant measure taken by Chinese scientists to achieve the scientification, modernization and internationalization of Chinese medicine, as a TCM doctor making prescriptions for treatment every day, I am unlikely to look forward to it.

If we only discover 100 compounds contained in *safflower oil* after studying for decades, how many years on earth do we need to figure out the other 310 thousand compounds, not to mention the study of hundreds of Chinese medicinal materials? Maybe this would not be achieved by the end of the world.

Even if the study is indeed achieved, I doubt that not only conventional TCM doctors, but also modern TCM doctors and even trans-modern TCM doctors, will not know how to make prescriptions when facing 310 thousand compounds in *safflower oil*.

TCM doctors will have nothing to prescribe if we over-rely on the modern scientific study of toxicity of Chinese medicinals.

Certainly, there are very few Chinese medicinals that are deadly toxic, such as *hydragyrum*, *cantharides* and *arsenic*, which require processing and use in a special way. However, most of Chinese medicinals are made of natural bark and roots; they as plants are totally different from synthetic drugs.

TCM has held the view since ancient times that medicine does have some toxicity.

The old saying that 'Shénnóng (神农) encountered 70 toxic herbs on one day of tasting materia medica' is not fully exaggerated.

Even *Internal Classic* (*Nèi jīng, 内经*) also records, If 'medicinals with extreme toxicity can only cure the disease for 60%, then the medicinals shall not be taken. Similar case is made for normal toxicity for 70%, little toxicity for 80%, and toxicity free for 90%. After that, grain, meat, fruits, and vegetables, as dietary treatment, shall be taken for complete recovery. Medicinals with toxicity cannot be taken in overdose, otherwise they will harm health.'

This is a very common theory among TCM doctors.

Although both TCM and Western Medicine have pointed out the 'toxicity', they consider it as totally different meanings in practice. The thinking pattern on toxicity of Western Medicine should not be applied to TCM opinion of 'medicine does have some toxicity'.

In 2007, my daughter got pregnant. She had edema legs and constipation. Her pulse was slippery and weak on both hands. Her symptoms indicated that she had a puffiness habitus. Therefore, I advised her to decoct and take 60g of *Dangshen* (*Radix Codonopsis*) per day. Except for taking several doses of other decoctions when suffering from severe urticaria in the sixth month, she took *Dangshen* (*Radix Codonopsis*) once a day or every two days almost during her whole pregnancy; otherwise her legs would have edema and she would have constipation.

My wife was very concerned, saying, "It will be so terrible if she gives birth to a baby with dark skin since she takes this disgusting decoction every day!"

I comforted her, "Please be at ease! Our grandchild will be definitely smart!"

Although I really meant it, my wife still felt worried (she was a professionally trained TCM doctor and had been in charge of wards in a major hospital for years).

On the parturient day, all our relatives, such as my daughter's aunt and uncle were anxiously waiting outside the delivery room with my wife and son-in-law, worrying that she would give birth to a child with dark skin or any other problem because they had known she took many decoctions.

However, when twenty newborns were brought out from the delivery room, my granddaughter was the one with the fairest skin.

Finally, they all got relieved.

My granddaughter is four years old now. She has a very healthy body and is very smart like I have said before.

Some may wonder that a woman's body is very sensitive during pregnancy and she needs to be particularly careful when taking medicines, otherwise it will have influence on the fetal development. According to some reports, the disability rate of newborns in China has already surpassed the world average level, which is directly correlated with the abuse of antibiotics and chemical synthetic medicines as well as environmental pollution.

My daughter absolutely refused to take western medicines when she got pregnant (she believes in TCM), and she only took Chinese medicinals when feeling uncomfortable.

TCM has a very famous saying that, 'Prescribing drastic and toxic medicinals strictly according to the pathogen will do no harm to the pregnant woman and the fetus', which is often applied to guiding the TCM doctor to treat diseases of pregnant women. That I advised my daughter to take *Dangshen* (*Radix Codonopsis*) decoction every day was to treat her qi deficiency, spleen deficiency, and low-grade fever during pregnancy.

Dangshen (*Radix Codonopsis*) as a 100% Chinese medicinal was taken by my daughter and approximately 15 kilograms were taken during her pregnant period. If 'medicine does have some toxicity', to what extent would my daughter have been poisoned, and how could she have given birth to such a healthy baby?

The reason why I insisted that my daughter should take *Dangshen* (*Radix Codonopsis*) in her pregnancy is that, according to the first medicinal record in the first section of *Shennong's Classic of Materia Medica* (*Shén nóng běn cǎo jīng,* 神农本草经), '*Renshen*, with its sweet flavor, slight cold nature and toxic-free compounds, can mainly be used to tonify five zang-organs, tranquilize mind, relieve anxiety, calm fright, and eliminate pathogen, as well as to open heart orifice, improve vision and develop wisdom; long-term use is beneficial for life prolonging.'

However, this *Renshen* recorded in *Shennong's Classic of Materia Medica* (*Shén nóng běn cǎo jīng,* 神农本草经) does not refer to the *Renshen* (*Radix Ginseng*) we see nowadays but *Dangshen* (*Radix Codonopsis*).

According to *Explaining and Analyzing Characters* (*Shuō wén jiě zì,* 说文解字), '*Shen* refers to *Renshen,* a kind of Chinese materia medica originally from Shangdang, Shanxi Province.'

Later generations however misunderstood the nature, flavor and function of *Dangshen* (*Radix Codonopsis*) as *Renshen* (*Radix Ginseng*) and recorded it into the TCM textbooks, leading to a historical mistake.

The 'slight cold nature' of *Dangshen* (*Radix Codonopsis*) is similar to the 'slight cold nature' of rice we eat. Is anyone poisoned by eating rice? Therefore, *Dangshen* (*Radix Codonopsis*) has not done harm to human's health so far. The main function of *Dangshen* (*Radix Codonopsis*) is to tonify five zang-organs due to the fact that they will help to build a healthy body and then bring benefit to tranquilizing mind, relieving anxiety, calming fright, and eliminating pathogen as well as opening heart orifice, improving vision and developing wisdom. How can such a life-prolonging treasure be toxic?

Nourishing the five zang-organs is better than only concentrating on one organ for the reason that the five zang-organs are interrelated and closely connected. They reinforce each other.

Pregnant women will be very healthy if five zang-organs are well tonified, and they will of course give birth to healthy infants. More importantly, *Dangshen* (*Radix Codonopsis*) can develop intellectual capacity, so I am pretty sure my granddaughter is definitely smart.

My mother-in-law is 94 years old with a vulnerable physique. She has had fracture five times: femur fracture for twice, one leg with implant of stainless steel caput femoris and the other with stent; and clavicle fracture, humerus comminuted fracture and left-hand middle finger fracture once eadn.

Except for the first fracture having happened in 1985, the other four times all took place in recent years, resulting in her not being able to do exercise in the park nearby.

She had a bad appetite and little sleep. She often felt uncomfortable, and I have approximately prescribed her medicinals four to five times every month especially in recent years.

My mother-in-law is particularly serious in taking medicines; she is totally a valetudinarian since she almost takes medicine every day.

Actually, the prescriptions I made for her were quite simple, which are either good for strengthening the spleen and stomach or for tonifying qi and nourishing blood. However, I added 30g to 60g of *Dangshen* (*Radix Codonopsis*) in every prescription or even advised her to decoct only this medicinal to drink.

In August, 2010, she was able to climb six floors of stairs (I was on the sixth floor) alone when she came to my apartment in Weihai, Shandong Province from Beijing.

Most unexpectedly, when she had CT examination in the hospital, the doctor said surprisingly: "Wow, in such an age, you have a clearer brain pattern than young people."

In fact, despite a little bit deaf, my mother-in-law has very clear thoughts so that she could remember everything in the past and has quite quick reaction. She often transcribes font size five characters page by page with pretty clear handwriting.

There are of course other reasons that keep her as a feeble person in such a good condition, but taking *Dangshen* (*Radix Codonopsis*) also definitely helps her to a large extent.

I got presbyopia and blurred vision five years ago, and then I started to decoct *Dangshen* (*Radix Codonopsis*) from 60g to 100g for drinking frequently or to take *Dangshen* (*Radix Codonopsis*) powder for around 10g once or twice a day.

Thanks to taking *Dangshen* (*Radix Codonopsis*), although I am in my seventies now, I can still read small characters in Ci Hai (a comprehensive dictionary) without wearing glasses.

One's eyes can reflect a people's condition of five zang-organs, so healthy organs will lead to bright eyes. That is the reason why *Dangshen* (*Radix Codonopsis*) has the function of improving vision.

Zhāng Yǐn'ān (张隐庵) had the most proper explanation of *Dangshen* (*Radix Codonopsis*) recorded in *Shennong's Classic of Materia Medica* (*Shén nóng běn cǎo jīng, 神农本草经*): 'It has sweet flavor with slight bitterness, and slight cold nature. *Ginseng,* which belongs to the first class of medicines, is toxic-free [...] so that it is mainly used to tonify five zang-organs. Substance stored in five zang-organs: kidney stores essence, heart stores spirit, liver stores corporeal soul and spleen stores wisdom.

To keep essence, spirit, corporeal soul, and wisdom at normal state is to tonify primordial qi in the heart, kidney, lung and liver. As long as primordial qi is sufficient, people will be in a balanced condition of both internal and external states. Essential qi from five zang-organs upward transfuses into the eye. *Ginseng* can open heart orifice which is the commander of five zang-organs. It can also dominate spleen due to the fact of improving wisdom. *Ginseng,* which belongs to the first class of medicines, can be taken for long periods to both cure diseases and tonify qi. Therefore, taking *Ginseng* can prolong one's life (*editor's note: the word Ginseng in this section is actually Dangshen nowadays*)."

Yè Tiānshì (叶天士) also delivered an appropriate explanation of the former section by Zhāng Yǐn'ān (张隐庵): '[...] qi deficiency will easily cause fright while blood deficiency will easily result in palpitation. *Ginseng* can tonify qi and with sweet flavor can nourish blood so that the fright and palpitation will be relieved. According to the old saying, 'Invasion of pathogen must be due to deficiency of essential qi', therefore *Ginseng* can tonify qi so that the pathogen will be eliminated after qi is sufficient. [...]. Heart is where spirit is stored. Comforting one's spirit (open heart orifice) will help to relieve palpitation; kidney is where essence is stored. One's wisdom will be developed when essence is sufficient. Taking it for a long period will help to tonify qi so that one can feel comfortable and prolong life (*editor's note: the word Ginseng in this section is actually Dangshen nowadays*).'

I often request medicinal herb growers to pick up *Dangshen* (*Radix Codonopsis*) in the mountain for me, and I notice they always add one or two servings of it into their porridge.

Why do they do that?

They told me adding *Dangshen* (*Radix Codonopsis*) into porridge can enrich the sweetness; besides, they feel energetic after having such porridge; it makes them not easy to be thirsty when doing work and get rid of bad cold.

My mother-in-law was prone to getting a bad cold before she took *Dangshen* (*Radix Codonopsis*). After she kept taking it, she seldom got a cold or recovered easily even if she accidentally got a bad cold due to wind cold. This is what is called sufficient qi will help to eliminate the pathogen. Therefore, *Dangshen* (*Radix Codonopsis*) is beneficial to 'eliminate pathogen'.

Once I saw a thick *Dangshen* (*Radix Codonopsis*) when climbing the mountain with two friends. We shared it raw immediately due to its sweet flavor. Afterwards, we climbed up and down full of energy and without any feeling of thirsty. When I came home that day, I had a mild diarrhea and then felt very comfortable. Wasn't it contributed by its properties, like, 'slight cold nature', 'opening heart orifice' and 'tonifying five zang-organs'?

Based on my understanding of '*Ginseng*(*Dangshen*)', the first medicinal recorded in *Shennong's Classic of Materia Medica* (*Shén nóng běn cǎo jīng*, 神农本草经), and tasting in person as well as site observation, I knew that the key function of *Dangshen* (*Radix Codonopsis*) is to tonify five zang-organs, making it a good remedy to cure diseases and to prolong lives.

If that 'medicine does have some toxicity' is true, to what extent have my family members been poisoned since I advised them to keep taking large amounts of *Dangshen* (*Radix Codonopsis*). How dare I play jokes on my families' lives!

Nevertheless, I only use *Dangshen* (*Radix Codonopsis*) picked up in person because of my favorable location.

By contrast, most of *Dangshen* (*Radix Codonopsis*) sold in the market is grown in large areas so that it has very different flavor and nature compared with the wild one. I am unable to define its function since I seldom use it.

Although *Dangshen* (*Radix Codonopsis*) is a tonic, it is not suitable for everyone. I dare not prescribe it if I treat patients who have dampness-heat habitus or suffer from aphtha and inflammation. Otherwise, their condition will be more severe, which shows 'medicine does have some toxicity'.

Sūn Sīmiǎo (孙思邈) started to learn TCM because he was easy to get ill in his childhood. There are of course many reasons leading to him living over a hundred years, among which 'keep taking tonics' definitely plays an important role.

There is no doubt that Péng Zǔ (彭祖) is the person who lived the longest life in China so far. He thought a person must obey the following rules in order to prolong life:

- The first one is to be optimistic.
- The second is to do exercise regularly.
- The third is to take tonics.

These are also the reasons why many TCM doctors can live a long life since the ancient time.

It is well-known that life lives in exercise. As a TCM doctor, especially a veteran doctor, however, I often have to treat more than ten or even dozens of patients a day, besides that, I also need to do some reading. That is how I make a living by treatment in the daytime and by reading in the evening. In this situation, how can I have time to do Tai Chi as most of the elderly do? All I can rely on is to preserve my health by taking tonics.

Taking tonics, as one of the eight therapeutic methods for life prolonging, contributes to both treatment and health keeping. Considering current opinions on toxic and side effects of Chinese medicinals, however, this method should be abandoned.

Actually, as long as the prescription is made correctly, the toxic medicinals can be toxic-free as well, so it is unnecessary to fear toxic medicinals as evil such as snakes and scorpions. The first medicinal recorded in the third section from *Shennong's Classic of Materia Medica* (*Shén nóng běn cǎo jīng,* 神农本草经) is pungent-warm *Fuzi* (*Radix Aconiti Lateralis*) with high toxicity. Its clinical indications include: 'wind-cold cough with dyspnea, cold-dampness arthralgia, limb spasm and gonatalgia, walking difficulty, accumulation-gathering, movable mass, and incised wound.'

Chén Xiūyuán (陈修园) had a very precise explanation of this record: 'wind-cold cough with dyspnea' refers to the fact that pathogen cold ascends via counterflow to the upper energizer; 'cold-dampness arthralgia, limb spasm and gonatalgia, walking difficulty' means the pathogen mainly accumulates in the sinew and bones of lower energizer; 'accumulation-gathering, movable mass, and incised wound' relates to congealing cold and blood stagnation.

According to *Collected Classified Meteria Medica* (*Dà guān běn cǎo,* 大观本草), 'pathogen causing cough with dyspnea' is followed by 'healing incised wound by warming the middle'; 'pathogenic cold can be eliminated by warm nature, and wound can be healed by warm nature [...]. The warm nature of the medicinal could spread over the whole body. Therefore, diseases caused by cold-dampness can always be treated by warm natured medicinals. For the reason that yang deficiency can cause cold inside the body, resulting in sweating, diarrhea, asthma, stroke, and coma, the treatment of which should rely on the medicinal with strong efficacy like *Fuzi* (*Radix Aconiti Lateralis*).' Chén Xiūyuán (陈修园) also mentioned: 'Medicinal with a strong nature in only one aspect will produce toxicity, and the stronger the nature is, the more toxic the medicinal is; therefore, *Fuzi* (*Radix Aconiti Lateralis*), as highly toxic as it is, has extreme warm nature and pungent flavor.'

Extreme warm nature tends to be strong hot nature; extreme pungent flavor quickly leads to fire which circulates through twelve meridians, sinews, bones, skins and muscles. Thus, *Fuzi* (*Radix Aconiti Lateralis*) is the key medicinal to restore yang and expel cold. The high toxicity of this medicinal here actually refers to the strong hot nature.

Zhāng Yǐn'ān (张隐庵) once said: "*Fuzi* (*Radix Aconiti Lateralis*) has the warm-hot nature which is full of power. Therefore, it is highly toxic […]. This is what is called medicinal with extreme toxicity can eliminate pathogen in one's body. In other words, the elimination of the pathogen will lead to the recovery of healthy qi, i.e. eliminating is equal to tonifying."

Therefore, in the situation where the patient has deficiency of yang with exuberance of yin, *Fuzi* (*Radix Aconiti Lateralis*) with its strong pungent flavor and strong hot nature can immediately restore yang to rescue one's life, under which circumstance, this medicinal has become toxic-free elixir of life.

On the contrary, if it is prescribed to deal with yin deficiency and internal heat or yin deficiency with yang hyperactivity, the toxicity will be highly enhanced and may cause a severe consequence.

In 1960s, my respected teacher Lǐ Kě (李可), with his talent and intelligence, created *Poge Jiuxin Tang* (*Breaking the rule and heart-saving decoction*), which contains *Fuzi* (*Radix Aconiti Lateralis*) for 30g, 100g or even 200g, in order to rescue lives by tonifying yang and relieving excessive yin.

Some may think that based on chemical analysis, the toxicity of *Fuzi* (*Radix Aconiti Lateralis*) comes from 'aconitine', and decocting *Fuzi* (*Radix Aconiti Lateralis*) for a long time can destroy the compounds of 'aconitine' so that the toxicity will be eliminated.

However, when treating critically ill patients with cold limbs, faint blood pressure and pulse, slightly warm chest, faint breath and heart beat, doctors have no enough time to long boil *Fuzi* (*Radix Aconiti Lateralis*) but to decoct it in a short time with strong fire as well as to feed the patients the decoction in the meantime. One hour later, the dying patient can be brought back to life.

In accordance with modern research of pharmacology, decocting *Fuzi* with strong fire for one hour will stimulate the decomposition of its toxicity. The moment when the 'aconitine' is not damaged yet is exactly the time that the toxicity of *Fuzi* becomes elixir. In this situation, feeding the patient with any toxic-free food, even pure water, may cause his or her death, not to mention the medicinal with slight toxicity or *Fuzi* with high toxicity.

On the contrary, it is the toxic *Fuzi* that becomes the last elixir which rescues patients' lives.

Only with the support of experienced, authentic and superb TCM thoughts, can *Fuzi* become elixir from a poison!

I would like to share more about *Fuzi*.

In 1870s, Zhāng Zǐlín (张子琳), one of the four famous doctors in Shanxi Province, noted in his collection of medical expertise that his father usually treated patients with *Fuzi* with a dosage from 30g to 60g, which often had great effects. He once said: "*Fuzi* should either be removed from prescriptions or be added to in large amounts; otherwise, small amounts of it may have the opposite effect on patients." In other words, *Fuzi* is a medicinal which targets the lower energizer, small amounts of which are not able to go to the downside of the body, causing inflammation in the upper energizer of the body.

Moreover, the decoction of *Fuzi* should be taken in cold temperature due to treating cold with cold which is called the reverse treatment; if taken in hot temperature, the medicinal will remain in the upper energizer and cause side effects, such as numb lips, numb tongue and body paralysis. However, it is unnecessary to panic when encountering such a situation because drinking plenty of water or taking a rest for half a day can relieve this symptom.

The clinical indications of *Fuzi* include: a deep and slow pulse, blue-black lips and nails. As long as patients have such symptoms and pulse manifestations, *Fuzi* can be certainly used and will bring positive effect.

Zhāng Zǐlín (张子琳) also said: "*Fuzi* grows in Sichuan Province where local people get used to taking it. A friend of mine is a monk from

Mount Wutai in Sichuan who often stores more than ten kilograms of *Fuzi* and takes 250g every time. Although there is no side effect of constantly taking it, it is better not to imitate him."

That I quote the above sentences from Zhāng Zǐlín (张子琳) is on the one hand to help people new to learning TCM to deepen the understanding of *Fuzi*, and on the other hand to explain that TCM has a very different medicine system compared with Western Medicine. Their ideas toward the toxic and side effects of medicinals are also opposite, so it is not appropriate to generalize them; otherwise, in Western Medicine's opinion, they may misunderstand the toxic side effect of Chinese medicinals based on their modern science. Despite their reasonable evidence, their words may push TCM into a terrible situation where people think TCM doctors do not know how to cure patients. TCM, however, treats patients with the thinking pattern of *Tao-like medicinal knowledge* rather then relying on those chemical compounds in Chinese medicinals. The monk from Sichuan who took large amounts of *Fuzi* must have had yang deficiency and the place he lived, Mount Wutai was the coldest place in winter. With decocting the medicinals in a correct method in the guidance of some masters, he took the decoction to prevent cold by extreme warm. This method however should not be imitated by other people.

TCM is able to cure patients that Western Medicine fails to cure mainly by the scientific principle of treatment and prescription that are totally different from Western Medicine.

The principle has been clearly illustrated in the first prescription, *Guizhi Tang* (*Cinnamon Twig Decoction*), recorded in *Treatise on Cold Damage Diseases*(*Shāng hán lùn, 伤寒论*) by Zhāng Zhòngjǐng (张仲景).

What kind of diseases can *Guizhi Tang* cure? Symptoms such as 'headache, fever, sweating and fearing wind', 'prescribe *Guizhi Tang* when the patient feels averse to wind, uneasy because of a fever, nauseous and with a tendency to snore', 'a floating and weak pulse, or a floating and rapid pulse', 'if a patient is not suffering from other diseases but has a fever and perspires now and then, it shows the abnormal condition of the vital resistance', 'patient who has a slow pulse with profuse perspiration and is slightly averse to cold should be treated with *Guizhi Tang*', 'vexing heat in chest, fever in the afternoon, like malaria, [...], a floating and weak pulse', 'a constant body pain', 'epigastric stuffiness, unresolved aversion to cold and exterior syndrome', 'after a dose of purgative, the patient feels an ascending air from the chest', are all included. These are the criteria for TCM doctors to prescribe *Guizhi Tang*.

No matter what the disease is defined in modern medicine, this decoction can be prescribed as long as the patient has these symptoms, even before or after the pregnant period.

However, it is noted that, 'after taking one Sheng of the decoction, if the symptoms have gone, stop taking the rest of the decoction.' In another word, stop taking the medicines when the illness is cured.

This is not only the principle of taking *Guizhi Tang*, but also the principle of all treatments and prescriptions made by TCM doctors.

The medicines are only taken when patients have relevant symptoms, otherwise patients should stop taking them.

Occasionally, symptoms are relieved just after one dose, after which the second dose is unnecessary to be taken. This happens frequently in TCM clinic treatment.

The elimination of symptoms indicates 'the balance of yin and yang' which refers to the cure of all diseases. This is the secret of Chinese medicinals which produce toxic-free prescriptions by toxic medicinals.

Poison or not poison

— The second discussion on the toxic side effects of Chinese medicinals

Toxicity or not is a relative concept. People should neither be too worried about it nor have something too much considering it non-toxic.

What is toxicity? It simply means something that may do harm to one's body or organs in the body, causing diseases or death! This is where toxicity comes from.

Does it mean things without toxicity will not damage one's body? Of course not! Things without toxicity may produce harmful things as well!

Meat products we have every day should not be toxic, shouldn't it? In modern society, however, the annoying obesity just originates from having too much meat.

According to the Health Bureau of Beijing, there are 9% of children under 15 in Beijing having dyslipidemia, 8.5% having abnormal heart rate. There are more and more people suffering from cardiac and cerebral diseases at a younger age, causing unbearable burden for both individuals and the country. All of these resulted from non-toxic food.

Internal Classic (*Nèi jīng,* 内经) has noted this more than two thousand years ago: 'Fat meat and fine grain with favorable taste cause severe diseases.' The more 'feasts' we have, the higher the risk of suffering from diseases.

The saying that, 'Fat-rich food causes people to die young while simple food protects our lives', also refers to the same principle.

Zuǒ Zōngtáng (左宗棠) in late Qing Dynasty was a great general good at fighting battles. He used to be the first rank among other officials.

However, since he was addicted to eating meat and refused to have any rice, he suffered hemiplegia before 70 years old and then got general paralysis. It is said that every time he had meals, his servant fed him with slices of meat, and he could have more than ten slices of meat without any rice and vegetables for one meal. He died in dreariness when he was 73. White rice and fine milled flour are definitely non-toxic, but they are the criminal causing diabetes.

Complication appearing in the advanced stage of diabetes makes patients even more painful. The non-toxic white rice and flour are so-called the 'drug trafficker'.

Every time I treat patients with diabetes, I always advise them to add at least two small cups (the more, the better) of bran to their meal per day besides prescribing them some relevant medicinals. Those who keep taking bran according to my advice mostly get complete recovery.

Some may think how I as a person without any knowledge of modern science can possibly know bran is able to cure diabetes.

Actually, in the 1960s, I suffered from starvation for over ten years. Most of people at that time only ate bran and other simple food. Hardly could we have chance to enjoy a white flour steamed bun, during which period of time however I never saw a person with diabetes. Therefore, I assume that it is too much fine food we have nowadays that causes so many patients suffering from diabetes. In a more modern expression, it is caused by imbalanced diet. In this situation, to keep a balanced diet is the way to deal with this disease, which is similar to the principle of TCM that 'treating heat with cold and treating cold with heat'.

It is not those white rice and fine flour that have toxicity but people are not able to keep a diet. The more we eat, the more toxic they are, and finally severe diseases would be formed. Trepang, as one of the eight delicacies in the ocean, is a precious cuisine with its delicious taste and rich nutrition. It can tonify kidney and supplement essence, nourish yin and blood, moisten dryness and regulate menstruation. As a tonic product with great quality, it is called 'the ginseng from the ocean'.

According to modern research, trepang is rich in protein, minerals and vitamins. Every 100g of dried trepang has 557mg of protein, 114mg of iron and even 1109mg of magnesium, making it ranked first among all other marine food products. Magnesium is the essential element in human body and the component of bones and teeth. Magnesium deficiency may cause myocardial necrosis. Moreover, the chondroitin sulfate contained in trepang even has the special function of improving skin condition and anti-aging effects.

I experimented with myself by eating one trepang every day. Having it for one to two months, my frequent urination symptom was relieved and I was not easy to have bad cold.

Mr. Dong (over 70 years old) was one of my classmates. He used to have cold feet and hands, but the symptoms were relieved after taking trepang for a while and his feet even started to sweat (the old normally have dry feet without sweat due to aging, so sweating feet refers to vigorous metabolism). He felt much healthier than before.

A teacher is said to suffer from neurasthenia and chronic tracheitis with feeble habitus. Once he heard that trepang is a great tonic, he started to have it and then his habitus got better. He started to feel energetic and was full of physical strength, making him quite a different person than before.

However, does this mean that trepang is suitable for every person? Of course not.

Another classmate of mine, Mr. Ren, was also over 70 years old, with heart disease. He was in a good economic condition, so he purchased stichopus japonicus with the best quality at a quite high price. However, every time he had it, he would have nosebleed and toothache. After several times, he gave up eating it.

Why did it happen? The reason is quite simple. He is the person with yang exuberance habitus though in such an age.

After all, trepang is warm in nature, so having trepang was like pouring oil on the flames.

If he only blindly believed in the high content of magnesium in trepang, continuously eating trepang might have killed him!

Therefore, the trepang honored as the ginseng from ocean suitable for most people may become toxic for people with yang exuberance habitus, not to mention the real ginseng.

According to the modern research by scholars, *Renshen* (*Radix Ginseng*) is mainly composed of carbohydrate (accounting for approximately 70%, which produces the sweet taste of ginseng), so is carrot. The ginseng alkynol extracted from *Renshen* is totally the same as the alkynol from carrot. In this situation, having carrot will have the same effect as having *Renshen*, but who has ever seen people get poisoned or cured by carrot?

Hence, those who criticize TCM seem to finally have something on TCM, claiming that *Renshen* is very unlikely to cure any kind of disease and that the worship of *Renshen* in China is to a large extent caused by historical and cultural factors.

In fact, as long as they taste *Renshen* in person, those people will realize whether *Renshen* is the same as carrot or not. Unfortunately, although they keep on discussing science, they have no 'hands-on' scientific spirit but to make irresponsible remarks.

There are other scholars claiming that *Renshen* has various kinds of pharmacologic actions that 'have positive influence on central nervous system, cardiovascular system, immune system and endocrine system, and that can improve the capacity of both physical and mental work, relieve fatigue, and prevent and cure number one killer diseases in modern world, such as high blood pressure, coronary disease, angina and diabetes'. In their opinion, *Renshen* seems to become the tonic without any side effects or toxic harm.

Nevertheless, it is reported that 'an American medical institution has warned several years ago that *Renshen* (*Radix Ginseng*) and *Xiyangshen* (*Radix Panacis Quinquefolii*) should not be taken to tonify qi during intra-operative period, otherwise it may result in hemorrhoea.'

It is also said that *Renshen* was once recorded in the United States Pharmacopeia-National Formulary but was deleted in 1880 and 1937 respectively. In 2005, however, it was again included in that book.

Moreover, some people say that the argument of the effectiveness of *Renshen* (*Radix Ginseng*) and *Xiyangshen* (*Radix Panacis Quinquefolii*) has lasted for over one century in the modern medical field.

Some other scholars report that taking *Renshen* for anti-aging effects has caused 35.5% of people have diarrhea, 24.5% rash, 19.5% insomnia, 15.5% nervousness, 16.5% high blood pressure and 10.5% edema and so on. Therefore, the academia defines the symptoms of the excitation of corticosteroids nervous centralis after taking *Renshen*, such as excitement, agitation, epistaxis, anxiety, insomnia, chest suppression, asthma, even personality lost and insanity, as '*Renshen* syndrome'.

Actually, all the above information results from taking *Renshen* blindly without enough understanding of Chinese Medicine. In other words, it is people's fault instead of the fault caused by *Renshen*!

Studying components of *Renshen* without the support of TCM theory is actually the research of botanical medicine through modern scientific and technological approach. If *Renshen* has so many side effects, how come it is called an anti-aging medicine?

As a TCM doctor, how dare I prescribe patients with *Renshen*?

If the study of toxic and side effects of Chinese medicinals by Western Medicine is taken into consideration, there are almost no medicinals TCM doctors can prescribe. Once *Renshen*, as one Chinese medicinal, has been studied by modern science, it will make people confused and misunderstand TCM, not to mention the entire TCM theories.

The so-called scientific TCM will be too aimless to know what to do! Under this circumstance, it will be too difficult to cure diseases by Chinese medicinals. Moreover, there will be more reports claiming the side and toxic effects of Chinese medicinals, causing the argument of *Renshen* lasting for at least ten thousand years!

However, if people can abandon the study result of *Renshen* by so-called modern science and go back to TCM thoughts, they will have a rather clear understanding of TCM.

Renshen (*Radix Ginseng*) is pungent-bitterness in flavor and warm-hot in nature, and can greatly tonify primordial qi.

People with deficiency-cold habitus can gain energy and prolong life by frequently taking it in small amount.

By contrast, patients suffering from severe diseases can instantly survive by taking it in a large amount even though they are not able to be cured by Western Medicine and are dying.

The strong evidence is *Poge Jiuxin Tang* (*Breaking the Rule and Heart Saving Decoction*) created by my teacher Lǐ Kě (李可).

Renshen (*Radix Ginseng*) has been one of the four medicinals for life saving (*Renshen* (*Radix Ginseng*), *Fuzi* (*Radix Aconiti Lateralis*), *Shigao* (*Gypsum Fibrosum*), and *Dahuang* (*Radix et Rhizoma Rhei*)) since ancient times.

Therefore, people sometimes can see a sere mountain ginseng in pharmacy being priced from ten thousand yuan to over one hundred thousand yuan. The reason of its high price is that it can save one's life. Thus, it is so stupid to assimilate ginseng as carrot.

In China, there are plenty of people who know about TCM or follow the guidance of authentic TCM doctors by taking small amounts of *Renshen* every day, especially the old that still have sufficient energy though in their nineties. They are all people who do well in preserving their health.

It is said that Emperor Qiánlóng (乾隆) in Qing Dynasty used to be fond of eating *Renshen*. In one year, he even took 3g *Renshen* every day. He must have been too aged to have sufficient primordial qi that year so that he had to rely on taking *Renshen* to reinforce vital energy. If he had taken *Renshen* in the same way in his youth, he must have had severe problems in his health and his imperial physician would definitely have not prescribed him with such a large amount of *Renshen*.

A friend of mine used to blindly take *Renshen* to build up his health when he was young, causing him to lose all his hair. This was due to the fact that taking *Renshen* made him suffer blood-heat.

When I was in my forties, I tried to take *Renshen* for several times with 3g to 5g per time; however, I would have my hair fallen every time after I took it. Afterwards, I dared not taste it any more. Last winter however I fell ill and kept sweating, so I started to decoct and take one *Renshen* (around 10g) every day for over ten days before I stopped sweating.

Why does *Renshen* have opposite effects on the same person in different times?

The reason is that when I was 40, I still had sufficient energy so that taking *Renshen* in a healthy condition caused me blood-heat and my hair fall.

By contrast, when I was 69 and had primordial qi deficiency after a severe disease, taking *Renshen* could nourish my vital energy and stop me from sweating so that I did not have alopecia. Moreover, I immediately stopped having it after I recovered; otherwise I was afraid *Renshen* would 'have toxic and side effects' on me again.

A 50-year-old female patient suffered from uterus hemorrhoea with short and faint breath and a hollow pulse, so I immediately asked her to decoct and take *Renshen* (around 15g), after which she stopped bleeding and gradually recovered. Just as the old saying goes, 'When facing hemorrhoea, invisible qi should be used to consolidate bleeding due to the fact that visible blood can not be produced immediately', or 'qi is the commander of blood'.

Nevertheless, it is reported that people who had no primordial qi deficiency suffered uterus hemorrhoea after taking *Renshen*.

A 90-year-old person from Hong Kong says that he takes a small amount of *Renshen* every day so that he still has sufficient energy in such an advanced age. He is really a person good at preserving his health.

There are instances of people with yang exuberance habitus, becoming insane or even dead after taking several grams of *Renshen*. In this situation, it is the people who take *Renshen* without understanding of TCM rather than *Renshen* itself that should be blamed.

It is not only *Renshen* but also other Chinese medicinals that become toxic because people blindly take tonic for anti-aging properties without any knowledge of human habitus and TCM thoughts.

The most typical example is the case of *Xiao Chaihu Tang* (*Minor Bupleurum Decoction*) which is well-known around the world.

Zhāng Zhòngjǐng (张仲景) would have created *Xiao Chaihu Tang* (*Minor Bupleurum Decoction*) specially for lesser yang disease.

The precondition of taking *Xiao Chaihu Tang* (*Minor Bupleurum Decoction*) is that 'people suffering from lesser yang disease with bitter taste, dry throat and dizziness'. Specific symptoms include 'intermittent chills and fevers, feels distention and a sensation of oppression in the chest and costal region, reluctant to speak and eat, restless and nauseous, or to be restless but not nauseous, with thirst for water, with abdominal pain, with mass below the costal margin, with palpitation and dysuria, no thirst of water but with a slight fever, with cough', all of which are the evidence to prescribe *Xiao Chaihu Tang* (*Minor Bupleurum Decoction*).

Zhāng Zhòngjǐng (张仲景) especially noted that when one of the symptoms of *Xiao Chaihu Tang* syndrome is observed, a diagnosis of *Xiao Chaihu Tang* can be established.

Above is the criterion of taking *Xiao Chaihu Tang* (*Minor Bupleurum Decoction*), following which the disease will be cured in time. How possibly can this do harm to one's health?

Once after the symptoms are relieved and people get recovery, patients should stop taking the decoction.

Why? Because yin and yang as well as qi and blood have been kept in balance and no longer need to be adjusted by the decoction; otherwise, another imbalance would occur and may cause more severe diseases to threaten one's life.

Keeping balance as the eternal principle for TCM to make prescriptions needs great wisdom. In other words, adjusting imbalanced conditions back to balance makes the medicinals remain toxic-free while changing a balanced condition to an imbalanced one causes the medicinals to become toxic. Doctors should carefully apply this principle to prescriptions rather than impulsively doing it.

However, once TCM is westernized, it would be impetuous.

In 1970s, *Xiao Chaihu Tang* (*Minor Bupleurum Decoction*) was produced into granula in Japan, making it a bestselling medicine for chronic hepatitis treatment for a time. A Japanese professor, Arichi Shigeru, who studied Chinese prescription once wrote in his article, '*Xiao Chaihu Tang* (*Minor Bupleurum Decoction*) is very safe in treating hepatitis and liver cirrhosis even for long-term use.'

This totally deviated from the TCM principle of adjusting imbalance into balance, causing serious problems.

Till 1990s, within five years there were 188 people suffering from interstitial pneumonia due to long term use of *Xiao Chaihu Tang* (*Minor Bupleurum Decoction*), 22 among whom even died.

The toxic and side effects of *Xiao Chaihu Tang* (*Minor Bupleurum Decoction*) then caused a significant disturbance among the world overnight.

It is not *Xiao Chaihu Tang* (*Minor Bupleurum Decoction*) itself that has toxic side effects but the incomprehension of TCM and the misuse of the decoction that cause the consequence. However, *Xiao Chaihu Tang* (*Minor Bupleurum Decoction*) has to bear all blames. What an injustice!

Similarly, *Longdan Xiegan Wan* (*Gentian Liver-Draining Pill*) is supposed to mainly treat symptoms caused by excess heat in liver-gallbladder meridians, or dampness-heat pouring down and upward reversal, such as hypochondriac pain, deafness, ear swelling, bitter taste, sinew flaccidity, genital sweating, swelling of vulva, vaginal pain, gonorrhea, haematuria and so on, all of which are the criteria of prescribing *Longdan Xiegan Wan*.

After the excess heat or dampness-heat in liver-gallbladder meridians are relieved and all of the above symptoms are eliminated, patients should not take the pill any more. This is quite a simple TCM common sense. Nevertheless, some people regard this pill as an anti-inflammation medicine that should be taken as long as they get inflamed, so they take large amounts of it, causing their kidneys to be damaged. Under this circumstance, the toxic and side effects of *Longdan Xiegan Wan* attract people's attention as well. Chinese medicinal once again suffers the fault of humans!

Lately, that the houttuynia cordata injection caused 35 deaths aroused people's attention to the toxic and side effects of Chinese medicinals for a third time.

Experts once again said that there were no comprehensive studies of the safety of Chinese medicinals and appealed to produce a standardization of those medicinals. In fact, those incidents had no relation to Chinese medicinals; instead, they were caused by the problem of the westernization of Chinese medicinals. More precisely, it is the problem of using botanic medicine injection by Western medicine doctors.

Houttuynia cordata has pungent flavor and slight cold nature. It is supposed to be the medicinal for clearing heat and removing toxin, as well as promoting diuresis and relieving stranguria. People in Sichuan Province even regard it as an eatable vegetable. How does it have toxicity? Chinese medicinal was treated as a scapegoat again!

The idea of criticizing Chinese medicinals in the thought of Western Medicine research and botanic medicine application in the name of science can only confuse the public. Similar situations may happen endlessly.

I have no idea how current TCM can be double cautious in order to avoid the toxic and side effects of Chinese medicinals. If so, in what approaches can TCM doctors treat their patients? In terms of TCM, what is the meaning of treatment if doctors are only aware of the toxic and side effects of Chinese medicinals but ignore curative effects when making prescriptions.

If they face patients in danger and only choose to prescribe so-called safe medicinals with little curative effects, aren't those safe medicinals the same as poisons?

When Guāngxù (光绪) Emperor in Qing Dynasty was crucially ill with reversal cold of limbs and a faint pulse, he badly needed large amounts of *Fuzi* (*Radix Aconiti Lateralis*) to restore yang to save him from collapse. However, his imperial physicians prescribed him the following three mild medicinals: *Renshen* (*Radix Ginseng*), *Maidong* (*Radix Ophiopogonis*), and *Wuweizi* (*Fructus Schisandrae Chinensis*) for 3g each. The emperor then passed away without any favorable turn after taking those medicinals.

Didn't those doctors know how to restore yang to save from collapse? Was there anyone of them who never read *Treatise on Cold Damage Diseases* (*Shāng hán lùn*, 伤寒论)? How could they make such a mild prescription only to tonify qi and nourish yin when treating the emperor who had severe deficiency of yang?

Although Guāngxù (光绪) was an emperor, he was not a family member of those doctors. After all, his life and death had no relation to them. Making such a mild prescription without any toxicity would protect them from being blamed for the death of the emperor. They did not need to take any responsibility of 'poisoning' their emperor.

If they had prescribed toxic *Fuzi* (*Radix Aconiti Lateralis*), they would have inevitably been blamed for prescribing poison for the emperor no matter Guāngxù (光绪) took it or not. How could they bear such a serious charge? Therefore, a mild prescription having neither toxicity nor curative effects would help them get rid of responsibility even if Guāngxù (光绪) Emperor died after taking it.

Maybe those doctors had no choice but to save their lives in a wise way. It is quite reasonable that all famous doctors were unwilling to be imperial physicians in ancient times.

On the contrary, if TCM doctors nowadays only persist in prescribing medicinals without toxic side effects, they will have significant negative effects on revitalizing TCM and curing sickness though they themselves may make no mistakes.

TCM is deeply rooted among the people

— The discussion on folk TCM by taking the example of 'Wu Gen Tang'

In 2008, my elder sister came to visit me from Inner Mongolia, and talked about one thing when chatting with me.

It was in the late 1970s when my nephew Fu was six years old and his tonsil festered and he got a high fever of 39°C. My sister was very worried and took his son to a major hospital of Inner Mongolia immediately. The boy had to be hospitalized and received tonsillectomy after the diagnosis.

Since my sister was so anxious that she did not bring enough money with her, she went back home to get money in a hurry. Unexpectedly, she met Lǐ Fènglín (李凤林), the director of the TCM department of that hospital before she left there.

After knowing the situation, Doctor Li said: "He has no need to be hospitalized. Taking *Wugen Tang* (*Five Kinds of Radixes Decoction*) is enough!"

Afterwards, he prescribed two bags of *Wugen Tang* that only cost less than ten cents at that time. After taking those decoctions, my nephew's fever was brought down and got relieved from tonsil fester.

My sister still appreciated Lǐ Fènglín (李凤林) a lot when mentioning this matter, saying: "If I had not met such a great TCM doctor, my son's tonsil would have been excised."

As a TCM doctor, I occasionally treat child patients suffering acute or chronic tonsillitis though I do not specialize in pediatrics.

This disease often happens in spring and summer time. Child patients usually have symptoms such as fever, red and swollen throat with pain in one side or both sides, and purulent secretion on the surface of the throat. Due to the moth-shaped red and swollen throat and nipple-shaped pick, TCM calls it as *Ru'e* (*nipple-moth*).

It is also called as *Hou'e* (*throat-moth*) because it appears in throat: single moth for swelling on one side and double moths for swelling on both sides.

TCM doctors also call it as *Houbi* (*pharyngitis*) because the swollen throat may cause patients having difficulty in eating.

If patients do not have their fever brought down and swelling reduced immediately, they may die due to the pathogen doing harm to heart and stomach. Therefore, this disease is one of the most acute syndromes in pediatrics.

The disease is usually caused by a bad cold. If the patient suffers external-contraction of pathogenic wind-heat with severe symptoms caused by exterior pathogen, he would tend to have a fever, slight aversion to wind-cold, adiapneustia, slight cough, a sore throat, a red and swelling nipple-moth, a thin and white tongue coating, and a floating and rapid pulse.

If the patient suffers severe symptoms caused by heat accumulation in lung and stomach meridians, he would tend to have a high fever with no aversion to cold, a reddish face, thirst, a red and swelling nipple-moth sometimes with whitish yellow pus patches, difficulty in swallowing, constipation, a yellow tongue coating, and red lips.

The former patients need to relieve pathogenic wind-heat, so I often prescribe them with *Yin Qiao San* (*Lonicera and Forsythia Powder*) (ingredients: *Lianqiao* (*Fructus Forsythiae*), *Jinyinhua* (*Flos Lonicerae*), *Jingjie* (*Herba Schizonepetae*), *Zhuye* (*Herba Lophatheri*), *Niubangzi* (*Fructus Arctii*), *Bohe* (*Herba Menthae*), *Douchi* (*Semen Sojae Preparatum*)), or *Niubang Ganjie Tang* (*Great Burdock Achene, Liquorice Root, and Platycodon Root Decoction*) (ingredients: *Niubangzi* (*Fructus Arctii*), *Gancao* (*Radix Glycyrrhizae*), *Jiegeng* (*Radix Platycodonis*), *Chenpi* (*Pericarpium Citri Reticulatae*), *Huanglian* (*Rhizoma Coptidis*), *Tianhuafen* (*Radix Trichosanthis*), *Chishao* (*Radix Paeoniae Rubra*), *Chuanxiong* (*Rhizoma Ligustici Chuanxiong*), *Sumu* (*Lignum Sappan*)) based on their conditions.

For latter ones, I usually prescribe *Puji Xiaodu Yinzi* (*Universal Relief Decoction for Eliminating Toxin*) (ingredients: *Niubangzi* (*Fructus Arctii*), *Huangqin* (*Radix Scutellariae*), *Huanglian* (*Rhizoma Coptidis*), *Jiegeng* (*Radix Platycodonis*), *Banlangen* (*Radix Isatidis*), *Mabo* (*Lasiosphaera seu Calvatia*), *Lianqiao* (*Fructus Forsythiae*), *Xuanshen* (*Radix Scrophulariae*), *Shengma* (*Rhizoma Cimicifugae*), *Chaihu* (*Radix Bupleuri*), *Bohe* (*Herba Menthae*), *Jiangcan* (*Bombyx Batryticatus*)) for treatment.

If the patient who has the above symptoms suffers pathogenic phlegm-heat, he would be treated as follows. Patients should first be treated by collateral pricking for letting toxic blood out and then take *Gan Jie Tang* (*Licorice and Platycodon Decoction*) (ingredients: *Gancao* (*Radix Glycyrrhizae*), *Jiegeng* (*Radix Platycodonis*), *Yuanshen* (*Radix Scrophulariae*), *Lianqiao* (*Fructus Forsythiae*), *Fangfeng* (*Radix Saposhnikoviae*), *Jingjie* (*Herba Schizonepetae*)).

If the constipation has continued for 3 to 5 days and the tongue coating is yellow and rough, *Huangqin* (*Radix Scutellariae*), *Huanglian* (*Rhizoma Coptidis*), *Dahuang* (*Radix et Rhizoma Rhei*), and *Mangxiao* (*Natrii Sulfas*) should be added; if the symptoms caused by pathogenic heat are severe, a large dose of *Shigao* (*Gypsum Fibrosum*) should be added. Based on the above therapies, I have cured all my patients suffering from this disease.

However, compared with *Wugen Tang* prescribed by Lǐ Fènglín (李凤林), mine seems a little bit complicated and disordered.

What on earth does *Wugen Tang* refer to? I was still not sure after thinking of all drugs in Chinese medicinals related to 'radix'.

Therefore, I asked my sister: "Do you know the composition of *Wugen Tang*?"

My sister answered: "I only asked my son to take the medicine. How can I possibly know what specific medicinals it contains? Doctor Li also has various prescriptions, such as *Qing Fei San* (*Lung Clearing Powder*) to cure children cough and *Zhi Xie San* (*Diarrhea Relieving Powder*) to cure child diarrhea, with great curative effects and they only cost several cents!"

After I heard what my sister said, an idea came into my mind that I would like to acknowledge this veteran TCM doctor, Lǐ Fènglín (李凤林), as my teacher.

Several years ago, my sister introduced me to a veteran TCM doctor, Méi Qīngtián (梅青田), who worked at the infirmary of Inner Mongolia Normal University. After meeting with him, I knew that he graduated from the department of foreign languages in Shanxi University. Due to the love of acupuncture and moxibustion, he changed his occupation to a TCM doctor as well. Despite being a school doctor, he was often invited to treat shepherds in pasture. I regarded him as my senior fellow apprentice because he was more than ten years my senior. We saw each other as friends immediately after we met due to the same hobby.

Having heard that I suffered from scapulohumeral periarthritis, he gave me some powder, which he said was an ancestral secret prescription from his apprentice to set broken bones.

He unintentionally used this powder to cure his scapulohumeral periarthritis. After taking it, I really recovered.

Afterwards, I added some other medicinals based on this prescription and successfully cured my severe lumbar disc herniation. More surprisingly, the disease has not relapsed for 20 years so far.

At this time my sister introduced me to another veteran TCM doctor, Lǐ Fènglín (李凤林). As far as I am concerned, it might be a destiny between me and Inner Mongolia, so I said I would like to go there to visit him.

My sister said however: "I am afraid you can't because he is no longer in that hospital."

"At one year the hospital he used to work at conducted a professional review of the doctors to confer them with titles. Although he was the director in the TCM department and effectively cured many patients and received high reputation, the hospital failed to assess his professional title because he did not have a relevant diploma or degree. Other doctors all had been reviewed except for him. He could not work there any longer, so he resigned and left the hospital. I was not able to find him since then, and later I heard that the TCM department of that hospital was closed!" My sister added.

I got totally shocked after hearing that! It seemed that I would never know about *Wugen Tang*. However, I could not stop thinking of it.

Three years later, when I read *The Collection of Curative Prescriptions and Skills for Pain Treatment* (*Téng tòng miào fāng jué jì jīng cuì,*

疼痛妙方绝技精粹) by Liú Yǒuyuán (刘有缘), I suddenly noticed the words of *Wugen Tang* in the appendix at the end of the book. I was so excited that I instantly read it. It was indeed the *Wugen Tang* by Lǐ Fènglín (李凤林) from Inner Mongolia. The prescription is as follows:

Gegen (*Radix Puerariae*) 6g
Banlangen (*Radix Isatidis*) 6g
Shandougen (*Radix Sophorae Tonkinensis*) 6g
Baimaogen (*Rhizoma Imperatae*) 6g
Lugen (*Rhizoma Phragmitis*) 6g
Huoxiang (*Herba PogoStemonis*) 6g
Honghua (*Flos Carthami*) 3g
Dahuang (*Radix et Rhizoma Rhei*) 2g

All the ingredients should be decocted with water twice and reduced to 70 ml decoction each time. Take the decoction two to three times a day.

The editor said that in the late 1950s, Lǐ Fènglín (李凤林) had already started to create and produce a prescription that not only could cure pediatric fever caused by infection but also balance deficiency and excess, cold and heat according to different symptoms of varied patients. Although it was against the common sense in TCM, he finally made it come true after persistent endeavor — he created and developed the famous prescription *Wugen Tang*.

The clinical application to more than 100 thousand child patients within three decades has successfully proved that this decoction not only has the effect on diminishing inflammation and antivirus effect, but also can work in any season no matter it is fever or aversion to cold and wind. It is particularly suitable for the fever caused by a bad cold, amygdalitis and scarlatina, as well as bringing down the fever caused by unknown pathogen.

Wugen Tang indeed has extraordinary clinical effects! Having considered the prescription for many years, I was so pleased that I could finally find it. It is really convenient to be applied to clinical treatment; besides, due to its mild property, people having no knowledge of TCM can also utilize it for treatment without any hesitation. Common people can store several doses of this prescription at home for possible periods of need.

Based on my clinical application, I think the followings are the reasons why this prescription is so effective:

Gegen (*Radix Puerariae*), which is pungent in flavor and cold in nature, is suitable for releasing flesh heat and bringing down fever, making it the key medicinal to treat dampness-heat seasonal epidemic.

Bringing down the fever is the crucial task when encountering any diseases related to pyrexia, otherwise how can other symptoms be relieved? The swollen sore throat caused by fever indicates the formation of severe internal heat and toxicity. *Shandougen* (*Radix Sophorae Tonkinensis*) with its bitter flavor and cold nature could clear away heat and relieve toxicity, so it is the preferred medicinal for relieving swollen sore throat through direct treatment; *Banlangen* (*Radix Isatidis*), with the function of clearing away heat and removing toxicity due to its sweet flavor and cold nature can be added into the prescription as an auxiliary medicinal which plays a very important role in cooling blood, relieving sore throat and swelling. How can swelling be relieved without cooling blood? The three radixes above are the main curative medicinals, supplementing the other two radixes to protect fluid from over heat. *Lugen* (*Rhizoma Phragmitis*) with its sweet flavor and cold nature can clear heat and promote fluid production; besides, since it grows from water to air, it has cold nature and has the priority action of ascending, so ancient formulas often use it as a guiding drug to cure swollen-head infection. *Lugen* (*Rhizoma Phragmitis*) to the prescription is what the guide is to army in battle. *Baimaogen* (*Rhizoma Imperatae*) with its sweet flavor and cold nature not only can remove heat and promote fluid production but also can cool blood and improve diuresis, from which the heat can be removed. All of the above compose *Wugen Tang*!

Recognizing that this syndrome mostly happens during the influenza eruption in spring and summer time, Li added *Huoxiang* (*Herba PogoStemonis*) to eliminate dampness with aromatics and to expel external pathogen from skin; *Dahuang* (*Radix et Rhizoma Rhei*) is added to relieve the stagnation of intestines and stomach in order to remove internal pathogen through excrement.

All kinds of swelling pain are related to blood stasis, so a small dosage of *Honghua* (*Flos Carthami*) can help to promote blood circulation to remove blood stasis, which is like damaging the enemy from inside in order to attack them as fast as it can be. Although there are only eight medicinals included in *Wugen Tang*, they treat the patient from both internal and external factors and closely follow the TCM principles of amygdalitis treatment. Therefore, this prescription had very good effect on my nephew. It is really a prescription with significance, which not only can cure fever in children but also can treat fever in adults with a few alternations.

Just like people should never forget where the happiness comes from, I really appreciate what Lǐ Fènglín (李凤林) has done though I never meet him while I also feel deeply sorry that he had to leave the hospital. 'One curative prescription is much harder to get than a thousand of other ones.' Didn't Zhāng Zhòngjǐng (张仲景) only aim to get one useful prescription by 'looking through numerous medical formulas'?

The sentence 'keep children away from antibiotics' is not only an appeal from people of vision but also a serious problem faced by human being's health. In this situation, how to treat diseases caused by inflammations, such as bad cold and fever, without antibiotics? Certainly, it is then TCM doctors' duty. The society should promote all convenient, curative and cheap methods, such as *Wugen Tang*, infantile massage, and incision therapy of Sifeng (EX-UE 10). Otherwise, 'keep children away from antibiotics' will be a meaningless slogan having no practical significance no matter how popular it is.

In 2009, I met a private TCM doctor Mr. An who told me that two western persons from a Sino-US cultural exchange organization in America just came and invited him to participate in a traditional medical academic exchange and make several treatments in the US. He refused them because he had other plans and recommended them several other TCM doctors graduated from the college of TCM. However, the two westerners said: "No! No! We only want TCM doctors without any professional title, because we think they are the real and authentic TCM doctors!"

I still remember that in the autumn of 2009, my patient Mr. Bi's daughter came to visit me because I cured her parent's prosopalgia. She said she was admitted to a university of TCM. On the first day of school, her teacher told all freshmen during the induction ceremony: "More than 80% of present students will change career after graduation!"

On the one hand, taxpayers complain about the difficulties and high cost of getting medical treatment, eagerly expecting they could find TCM doctors with simple treatment procedures, low cost and curative effects; on the other hand, those universities of TCM spend money from taxpayers in cultivating talents good at the combination of TCM and Western Medicine without any guilt, causing most of outstanding students to change their possession. How can those teachers face such a disappointing situation?

It is quite reasonable for universities of Western Medicine to train authentic Western Medicine doctors; why can't universities of TCM cultivate authentic TCM doctors?

Students applying for TCM universities are supposed to learn TCM skills, but those universities arrange most of their time to learn about Western Medicine (courses of Western Medicine account for over half of course time in TCM universities, some of which even set the Classics of TCM as an optional course). Universities train students to talents with knowledge of the combination of TCM and Western Medicine and claim that only by doing so can them adapt to the modern society.

According to their logic, TCM universities themselves do not adapt to the modern society and should be changed into 'universities of the combination of TCM and Western Medicine' or 'universities of new medicine', which follows their essence. Why do they still keep such an 'obscure' university name?

In 2010, a friend of mine suddenly came to me, saying that a veteran TCM doctor in Hangu Pass could make the tumor subside gradually only by sprinkling some white powder on it. This reminded me that Liáng Xiùqīng (梁秀清) could also do the same by plastering some red powder. However, since he passed away many years ago, this special skill has vanished.

Therefore, I rushed to the house of that veteran TCM doctor by car. The doctor, Mr. Gao was 75 years old then. He was a little bit deaf and could not clearly hear my words, while I could not understand his dialect except for several words I used to learn from ancient books, such as, *'Da Jin Dan'*, *'Xiao Jin Dan'*, *'Bai Jiang Dan'*, and *'Jiuzhuan Lingdan'*. I had to ask the local guide to interpret for me.

Mr. Gao took out a toad with three legs having been preserved in cinnabar for over 100 years, saying that no matter what severe or big ulcers his father had met with, they would be cured very soon by inserting the tail of this toad into the ulcer. His father said it was the real toad!.

Mr. Gao also said that one of his patients told him he used to see such kind of toad with three legs in a valley in Shanxi Province, but he could not remember clearly which valley it was. However, he told me that there is record about the toad in *Compendium of Materia Medica* (*Běn cǎo gāng mù,* 本草纲目), from which I indeed found out the discussion of this three-leg toad in Volume 42, Toad.

Kòu Zōngshì (寇宗奭) said: "The rumor that only three-leg toad is the real toad is so popular that someone deceives people with dried three-leg toads. However, it is easy to expose the lie after soaking the dried toad in water for half a day. In other words, there is no inborn three-leg toad."

On the contrary, Lǐ Shízhēn (李时珍) held another view: "Mr. Xu said only three-leg toads are real toads while Mr. Kou put forward an opposite opinion; as far as I am concerned, it can make sense to admit there are three-leg toads because people have seen three-leg turtles, but the real mistake is to claim that only three-leg toads can be used as a medicine."

Certainly, no evidence can be found now to prove whether there were three-leg toads at that time. The problem is that *Explaining and Analyzing Characters* (*Shuō wén jiě zì,* 说文解字), as the first book to analyze the shapes and study the origins of characters in China, was composed by Xǔshèn (许慎) in the Eastern Han Dynasty and was completed in the twelfth year of Emperor He period in the Eastern Han Dynasty, while Kòu Zōngshì (寇宗奭) who wrote *Amplification on Materia Medica* (*Běn cǎo yǎn yì,* 本草衍义) was the medical official in Song Dynasty, a thousand year after Han. How many species might be extinct or become rare during such a long period? Nevertheless, surprisingly, Mr. Gao could still keep one three-leg toad which according to his father cost three silver dollars at that time. Once a friend from Xiamen, Fujian Province came to me, saying there were tea sets in Fujian with weird 'three-leg toads' paintings. He felt strange why there were toads like that? Who is able to know how many secrets of the nature have been lost to history, the secret of TCM included?

This reminds me of my teacher Huáng Jiéxī (黄杰熙). When I acknowledged him as my teacher in 1980s, he told me that the key of learning Chinese medicinals is to master *Shennong's Classic of Materia Medica* (*Shén nóng běn cǎo jīng, 神农本草经*) which he thought was compiled together by famous doctors at that time and named after Shénnóng (神农). Most prescriptions mentioned in this book are very curative in clinical treatment; other books about medicinals in later times however mostly have individual conjectures, making those prescriptions less effective, so I could only observe those useful principles instead of spending too much effort on them. I benefit a lot from what Mr. Huang said, understanding what kind of books I should devote to when acquiring knowledge of Chinese medicinals. Accordingly, the reason of acknowledging a good teacher when leanring TCM is that a great teacher will help us avoid many mistakes and obstacles so that we can get more effects with less effort.

At that time, I was always carefully reading up *Notes about Materia Medica by Three Doctors* (*Běn cǎo sān jiā hé zhù, 本草三家合注*), thinking about those notes by Zhāng Yǐn'ān (张隐庵), Yè Tiānshì (叶天士) and Chén Xiūyuán (陈修园) and consulting Mr. Huang for the details of every medicinal.

When getting up to the medicinal, *Kongqing (Azurite)*, in the book, I noticed there was only one sentence from the original text, '*Kongqing (Azurite)* which is sweet and sour in flavor, cold in nature and has non-toxic components, is mainly used to treat bluish blindness and deafness, to improve vision, to relive nine orifices, to promote blood circulation, to nourish essence and spirit, to tonify liver qi, as well as to prolong life after taking it.' I wondered why there was no note for this sentence and turned to Mr. Huang for answers.

He said: "*Kongqing (Azurite)* is a rare treasure with its price ten times higher than gold. *Kongqing (Azurite)* from gold mines are with the highest price, followed by those from copper mines. Certainly, these three famous doctors never saw it or use it before so they were not able to make any comments."

Mr. Huang also mentioned that his father used to receive one *Kongqing (Azurite)* as bright as a black bean with light weight. And he remembered Yuán Lǐwén (袁礼文), a friend of his grandfather had had bluish blindness for thirty years.

Bluish blindness here refers to the condition that there are no abnormalities of the white of the eyes or the eyeballs, but the patient still cannot see anything, symptoms of which are equal to the optic atrophy in modern medicine. Yuán Lǐwén (袁礼文) had already lost confidence after facing so many treatment failures, but Huang's grandfather still decided to try for the last time. He cracked *Kongqing* (*Azurite*) in a porcelain bowl and some oil juice came outside; he then dissolved the oil juice into 2 ml distilled water. Mr. Huang tasted the water by dipping a thin glass rod in it and found it with the same taste as described in *Shennong's Classic of Materia Medica* (*Shén nóng běn cǎo jīng,* 神农本草经).

Yuán Lǐwén (袁礼文) was then asked to take off his clothes and go to sleep at 9pm that night. The grandfather instilled three drops of the medicinal juice into each eye and moistened two eyebrows by gauze with it. He also fed him the rest of the medicinal juice brew with half cup of hot water.

At seven the next morning, they heard Yuan shouted: "I can see everything!"

Hearing that, everyone rushed to his room to make sure Yuán Lǐwén (袁礼文) was not dreaming.

After being blind for 30 years, he was cured by *Kongqing* (*Azurite*). How magic it is!

Mr. Huang would not have believed what the book recorded if he had never witnessed it.

Therefore, although three famous doctors had no comments on *Kongqing* (*Azurite*), my teacher Mr. Huang could explain himself: "*Kongqing* (*Azurite*) is sometimes as big as an egg or as small as a soya bean both with oily juice inside. For its metal property in terms of five elements, it belongs to lung meridian of hand greater yin. For its cold nature, it belongs to kidney meridian of foot lesser yin. For its sweet flavor, it belongs to spleen meridian of foot greater yin. For its sour flavor, it belongs to liver meridian of foot reverting yin."

"It is mainly used to treat patients with bluish blindness and deafness. Eyes are the orifices of liver and ears are the orifices of kidney. Its cold nature can produce water and nourish orifices through kidney and its sour flavor can relieve orifices through liver. Things with metal property can make sounds and improve vision, so *Kongqing* (*Azurite*) has the functions of curing deafness and blindness."

"Vision can be improved by nourishing kidney essence. Nine orifices include seven apertures in the head and two in the external genitalia and anus, all of which are places where spirit qi of five zang-organs will go through. *Kongqing* (*Azurite*) with its black cyan color and sour flavor can tonify liver and produce heart fire; its cold nature can tonify kidney; its sweet flavor can tonify spleen; its metal property can tonify lungs. All five zang-organs are tonified and the spirit qi is at full, so it is beneficial to relieve nine orifices, leading to the promotion of blood circulation, the nourishment of essence and spirit, and the improvement of liver qi."

Having heard what Mr. Huang said, I knew that there definitely existed *Kongqing* (*Azurite*) in the nature.

Afterwards, when I looked through *Compendium of Materia Medica* (*Běn cǎo gāng mù*, 本草纲目), I found it also recorded *Kongqing* (*Azurite*) in Volume Ten of Rock Section. Other books of medicinals recorded this medicinal as well, saying it is 'the elixir for eyesight treatment' that can cure 'all eye diseases (sparrow vision (night blindness), pinkeye (infectious conjunctivitis), bluish blindness (optic atrophy), acute nebula (epidemic keratoconjunctivitis), and trachoma).' Some books, such as *Golden Prescriptions for Emergencies* (*Qiān jīn fāng*, 千金方) and *General Records of Holy Universal Relief* (*Shèng jì zǒng lù*, 圣济总录), introduce the 'instilling' methods and says 'the eyesight will recover the next day'. *Records of Meteria Medica in Ming Dynasty* (*Dà míng běn cǎo*, 大明本草) even says that 'it is very curative to cure facial palsy of wind stroke by keeping *Kongqing* (*Azurite*) in mouth'.

Kòu Zōngshì (寇宗奭) also noted, 'Emperor Zhenzong of Song used to ask people to look for *Kongqing* (*Azurite*) with juice inside, and he finally received one after a long time.'

I was so curious that I tried to look for *Kongqing* (*Azurite*) from mineral heaps in Sijiawan Copper Mine a hundred miles away from Linfen, but I could not find one after several days so I went back. Knowing this, Mr. Huang laughed at me, saying: "How can you easily find it since it is such a rare treasure? I have been looking for it for over five decades, but all I find are fake ones with no effect at all."

I think I will never see *Kongqing* (*Azurite*) in my life. Nevertheless, since there are gold mines and copper mines at home and abroad, those miners should have seen it. Even though they may see it, it is still meaningless because they might have already buried it with other waste minerals.

Kongqing (*Azurite*) is not some extinct species; it is our ignorance that regards it as waste.

Every time I arrive at Anguo in Heibei Province, the distributing center of Chinese medicinals, I will notice the couplet on both sides of the hall entrance. It says herbs will become medicines only after they arrive at Anguo. I always stare at this couplet for a while with emotions.

There are so many people gathering there with numerous bags of herbs that may become Chinese medicines. People there often say: "You never know how precious those herbs are until they become medicines."

Is there any country without herbs? Of course herbs do not only grow in China.

However, since Shénnóng (神农) had tasted hundreds of herbs in ancient times, some herbs became Chinese medicines to save lives. Other countries, however, had no similar figures in their history, so they have no idea what are the functions of those herbs. No matter how many exotic flowers and rare herbs they have, they cannot become treasures. If their ancestors had tried similar things as Shénnóng (神农) did, those herbs might have become priceless as well. Not only China but also many other countries have their own herbs, but except China, herbs of other countries are still plants not medicines because there is no Shénnóng (神农) in their countries to taste them.

How many rare treasures like *Kongqing* (*Azurite*) on earth are regarded as waste?

Nowadays, the westernization of TCM seems to study Chinese medicinals in a more scientific approach, but it is actually the study of 'botanical medicines', changing precious 'Chinese medicinals' into 'botanical herbs'.

As I am writing this, I would like to slightly change the meaning of the couplet to "only herbs in China can be called medicines and it is Qi-Huang that endowed them with priceless value". Flowers and herbs growing in China can become precious medicines with high price and realize their true values rather than only for ornamental use for people and the nature. What is more, only those doctors with authentic TCM principles and thoughts can apply these precious herbs to treatment effectively and express the true value of those herbs. This is the significant value of those herbs.

When I saw the 'antique' preserved in Mr. Gao's home, it felt like finding a rare treasure.

Several old people in the neighborhood came to Mr. Gao's home, saying he was less skillful than his father who had great ability in treatment when he was still alive.

Later on, I knew that his family has been famous for TCM surgery for eight generations. Without any professional titles, he treated diseases only relying on what he had learnt from his father. A family working on surgical TCM for generations was so rare that he was the only one I met with so far. In ancient times, surgical TCM doctors were really good at curing carbuncle and tumor (cancer).

I then asked: "have you taught your children about these skills?"

He answered: "no."

I asked: "why not?"

He said disappointedly: "they don't want to learn!"

I said: "why? What an amazing skill!"

He said with a deep sigh: "they think it can't make a living. They are now all Western Medicine doctors in the department of surgery."

I felt so upset to hear that and could not say a word. It seemed that such a precious skill might be lost from then on.

I plodded away and turned around after a long distance, finding Mr. Gao with his grey hair standing in front of his house and looking at our direction. He waved his hands to us and so I waved back, like bidding farewell to an era.

I was not able to calm down after coming back home: if two sons of Mr. Gao could have inherited the medical skills that have lasted for eight generations, how many patients suffering from cancers could be protected from the torture of surgery and radiotherapy and chemotherapy, or could be saved by them?

It turns out be impossible however. What a lost to TCM! "Alas! If he has determined his mind, I am not able to leave him behind no matter how many times I chant *Yangguan Sandie* (translator's note: a poem to express the feeling of farewell)." I cannot help again and again reciting this sentence from Li Qingzhao's poem *In memory of a Clarinetist on Phoenix Terrace.*

I then suddenly remembered that a Polish scientist Copernicus proposed the 'heliocentric theory' due to the fact that he discovered the earth goes around the sun in the late 1500s, overturning the 'geocentric theory' claiming that the sun was supposed to go around the earth; however, in the early 1600s, the Italian Roman inquisition declared the *Revolutions of the Heavenly Bodies* by Copernicus as a banned book; what was worse, they tortured the Italian scientist Galileo who supported the heliocentric theory by interrogation and brutal punishment, and burnt the scientist Bruno who developed and advocated this theory to death. All these were because the truth had to be judged by the inquisition!

Similarly, from Yú Yúnxiù (余云岫) in the 1930s to contemporary advocates against TCM, those people also have played a role as the inquisition, while others who announced to revitalize TCM by westernizing it, measuring and altering it using the standards of modern medicine have deep-rooted complex of 'inquisition' as well. There is only one criterion in their mind to judge — the modern medicine, causing the thorough westernization of TCM.

How inferior they feel about our nation behind the westernization of TCM!

In 2010, I was introduced to a private TCM doctor, Sū Yǒngquán (苏永泉) who is three years older than me. At that time, he lived a block away from the children's hospital in the city. His house was low-rising and crude, but it was full of children and their parents from Guangxi, Wuhan, Shandong, Henan and Beijing who all visited him for treatment. Most of those children were suffering from diseases for a long time without any effective treatment. He had some unique skills that he could cure diseases simply by putting his hands over children's navels without any touch of their skin or the support of medicines. He had already saved many children's lives. Some experts in both Western Medicine and TCM from major hospitals, including the children's hospital asked for his help as well because they would like to protect children from the harm of antibiotics.

How magic his hands are! We felt like old friends at the first meeting and quickly became very close friends. I asked where he had learnt this skill from. He then told his story to me.

He was from Dongmo Village, Ximo Town, Ruicheng County, Shanxi Province. He became a farmer at home before he graduated from high school. When he was 30, he knew that there was a highly skilled doctor in pediatrics called Rèn Huàtiān (任化天) in Dongdizhang Village, Xiezhou Town, Yuncheng City who had unique skills — Tai Ji Massage for infants and children. A lot of visitors came to visit him every day, and local people all knew the saying that 'visit Rèn Huàtiān (任化天) to keep child diseases away.'

Sū Yǒngquán (苏永泉) was very curious about it and decided to acknowledge him as a teacher to learn the unique skill.

However, there was a problem that a mountain was between Su's and Ren's villages. He had to walk over 50 km to visit this doctor. Therefore, he often got up and went back at midnight, walking swiftly or even running to Ren's home dozens of times a year. He never quit no matter how heavily it rained. There were lots of times that he encountered wolves, sometimes even with nine wolves, but he could always run away intelligently.

Having kept doing so, he however could not learn anything from Rèn Huàtiān (任化天) until Ren was moved five years later and decided to teach him everything he had known. Su in this way finally mastered the authentic skills of Tai Ji Massage for infants and children. After learning from Ren, Su cured numerous patients no matter how severely they suffered from infantile pneumonia, high fever and even infantile malnutrition. Wényuān (文渊), the director of Shanxi TCM Authority at that time was quite warm hearted that he organized clinical observation activities and arranged for Su to be in Shanxi University of Traditional Chinese Medicine to systematically summarize the pediatric skill, contributing a lot to the publication of Sū Yǒngquán (苏永泉)'s *Authentic Skill of Tai Ji Massage for Infants and Children* (Sū yǒng quán yīng yòu ér tài jí àn mó zhēn chuán, 苏永泉婴幼儿太极按摩真传). Nowadays, Su has become a famous expert in TCM pediatrics. How magic this therapy is! Since Sū Yǒngquán (苏永泉) is the only person in China or even in the whole world that masters this skill, he is also a rare treasure similar to *Kongqing* (*Azurite*).

In the middle of May, 2012, Sū Yǒngquán (苏永泉) came to me in a hurry. I saw he was very anxious, so I immediately asked what happened. He said that related departments sealed up his clinic and asked him to pay the fine, for the reason that he had no medical diploma but a practice medical license issued by Yuncheng City. He asked for advice from me. I said I did not have any idea since I was only a poor scholar, and I persuaded him to leave this place.

Eventually, he left Taiyuan. Sometimes when I passed by the lane he used to live in, I would notice there were still some parents with children asking about Doctor Su, but nobody ever knew where he went.

I am really concerned that such a rare treasure would vanish. Although he published some books, many secrets of TCM are not able to be expressed through words but to be taught by teachers in person. There is lots of precious experience from Liáng Xiùqīng (梁秀清) that cannot be delivered by words, only parts of which are recorded in books. However, different from 'three-leg toad' and '*Kongqing (Azurite)*' that I only heard of, the 'Tai Ji Massage for infants and children' is the real skill I witness by myself!

The over-concern on the
TCM education

— The discussion on the problem
of authentic TCM

I often go to different universities of TCM due to my job. Every time when talking about the current education of TCM with relevant people, I often hear the similar words: contemporary students in universities of TCM should both learn TCM and Western Medicine, as well as modern science, English and computer skills. It is said that only by mastering interdisciplinary knowledge can they develop the effect of TCM knowledge in a better way. Otherwise, how can they adapt to the need of modern society after graduation? We are now training new TCM doctors rather than authentic TCM doctors in traditional significance.

I always feel disappointed to hear this. The reality shows what they think is totally wrong.

There is no denying that an increasing number of new TCM doctors have been trained based on the above ideas in the past decades and they are on duty in many hospitals now. Two ruthless truths however still exist:

Firstly, the entire TCM medical proficiency declines and the problem of the westernization of TCM is very serious. Many TCM doctors also treat patients relying on their test reports and ask their patients to receive transfusion treatment. It seems that every patient feels that 'it is too hard to find a highly-skilled TCM doctor!'

Secondly, the employment difficulty of graduates from universities of TCM perplexes everyone like a haunted ghost.

Some teachers in universities of TCM directly tell their freshmen: "80% of you will change your career after graduation." How pathetic it is to both those students with dreams and those educators.

It is these inevitable and more obvious contradictions that probably urge some people to put forward the idea of authentic TCM education, which holds a totally opposite view with the training of new TCM doctors, causing an argument of these two sides. Actually, this argument has lasted for quite a long time.

However, I think it is meaningless to argue about the meaning of authentic TCM doctors because there are no 100% authentic things.

As far as I am concerned, the so-called authentic TCM doctor refers to doctors that can make treatments based on the idea of TCM. They may neither systematically learn Western Medicine and modern science nor have any knowledge of foreign languages and computer skills. In other words, the authentic TCM doctor is equal to a conventional TCM doctor.

If universities train such kind of authentic TCM doctors, will they adapt to the development of modern society? It mainly depends on whether the society needs them or not.

For example, Zhāng Zhòngjǐng (张仲景) should be considered the ancestor of authentic TCM doctors. If he would be alive now with his skills written in *Treatise on Cold Damage Diseases* (*Shāng hán lùn,* 伤寒论) and *Synopsis of the Golden Chamber* (*Jīn kuì yào luè,* 金匮要略) and with the principle of 'observe the pulse and symptoms carefully and treat the patient accordingly', can't he cure diseases in modern society? Will he have no patients or have difficulty in employment? I do not think so.

TCM doctors in modern society who can learn well and master parts of the knowledge of Zhāng Zhòngjǐng (张仲景) will cure many severe diseases or become a famous doctor, let alone be proficient in his knowledge. Zhāng Zhòngjǐng (张仲景) himself does not need to treat patients in person at all. People in modern society still respect him as the Medical Sage.

Another example is about the four famous doctors, Xiāo Lóngyǒu (萧龙友), Kǒng Bóhuá (孔伯华), Wāng Féngchūn (汪逢春) and Shī Jīnmò (施今墨) before the founding of the People's Republic of China and the masters Pú Fǔzhōu (蒲辅周) and Yuè Měizhōng (岳美中) after the founding of PR China. They were of course all authentic TCM doctors. If they would be alive now, would they be lack of patients since they do not know how to read test reports? I am afraid not. There would be even more patients visiting them actually.

It is quite simple that no matter how developed the science and technology is in modern society, people will still have a cold after receiving wind pathogen, suffer swelling sensation in hypochondrium after getting angry, suffer reversal cold of hands and feet after yang deficiency, and suffer vexing heat in chest, palms and soles after yin deficiency. Are there any differences between them and people in ancient times? Although they have names and entities now, they can still be diagnosed by the theory of three types of disease cause in TCM. How can eight-principle syndrome differentiation be outdated?

My three teachers were also authentic TCM doctors in the present age. Are they ignored by the need of people in modern society? I do not think this should be concerned.

Liáng Xiùqīng (梁秀清) only graduated from middle school before the founding of PRC and he taught himself TCM under the guidance of his father. In the late 1970s, he lived in a small and remote cottage in Houma Town in Shanxi with no signboard in front of his house when I firstly met him. However, patients visiting him were not only from China but also from Japan, Southeast Asia and other countries. He was quite popular at that time.

In 1986, Zhang Zhennan, the secretary of the county Party committee of his hometown, Julu County, Hebei Province held a special meeting and decided to send people from the organization department to investigate whether he had cured dozens of cancer patients living around Houma. After the investigation, he along side with his family was picked up by a special car to Julu and he became the dean of TCM Tumour Hospital of Julu County that was particularly established for him.

My second teacher is Huáng Jiéxī (黄杰熙) who used to be an ordinary teacher in No. 7 Middle School of Taiyuan. In 1957, he was judged as a member of the Right Wing and was dismissed. Since he lost his source of income, he started to learn TCM to make a living because his grandfather was a TCM doctor.

When the Cultural Revolution started in 1966, he was put into prison because there were so many patients visiting him for treatment, causing traffic jam in Ximi Lane in Taiyuan, making rebels angry.

When I acknowledged him as my teacher in 1986, he was already rehabilitated and reinstated as a teacher. Since he was good at curing severe and stubborn diseases with cheap and normal Chinese medicinals, there were always full of patients in his clinic. He wrote and edited six books, including *Commentary and Notes of Meteria Medica* (*Běn căo wèn dá píng zhù*, 本草问答评注), thoroughly explaining profound theories in simple language without any exaggeration. These six books are not comparable with other ordinary ones, so they receive great reputation both at home and abroad.

My third teacher is Lǐ Kě (李可) who used to be the dean of TCM Hospital of Lingshi County in Shanxi. He learnt TCM in prison by himself. He was like a great general during the clinic treatment. Thousands of patients in danger were saved by him through the use of large dosage of *Fuzi* (*Radix Aconiti Lateralis*), among them over one hundred patients had received the critical condition notice from hospital.

What Lǐ Kě (李可) did breaks the conventional idea that TCM doctors are not able to cure emergency diseases. Therefore, his clinical experience is especially precious.

The publication of *The Collection of Treatment Experience from Emergency, Severe, Rare and Stubborn Diseases by Veteran TCM Doctor Lǐ Kě* (李可) (*Lǐ kě lăo zhōng yī jí wēi zhòng zhèng yí nán bìng jīng yàn zhuān jí*, 李可老中医急危重症疑难病经验专辑) caused great echoes, especially in the TCM field. Numerous people from China and abroad visited him for treatment or medical skills, though he was still a TCM attending doctor in his eighties.

All of the above is just my own experience with inevitable limitations. However, according to the idea of some wise men, it seems that cultivating authentic TCM doctors like Liáng Xiùqīng (梁秀清), Huáng Jiéxī (黄杰熙) and Lǐ Kě (李可) will not adapt to the development of modern society. Aren't they over-concerned? (This article was published in *China News of Traditional Chinese Medicine*, October 11, 2007.)

Where are those fish in the sea?

— The second discussion on the problem of authentic TCM

The issue of authentic TCM is actually the problem of TCM. It is due to the fact that there exists serious westernization of TCM that people put forward the idea of authentic TCM to differentiate it from those who take treatments in the name of TCM while using western medical ideas. In other words, the authentic TCM is the TCM with traditional significance; the word 'authentic' just represents an era of TCM.

I have been keeping in touch with, learning, concentrating on and thinking about TCM for about half a century. Therefore, I would like to share with you my feelings based on my past experience.

I still remember in my childhood there were always some well known veteran TCM doctors in towns and villages who cured many severe and lingering diseases and were highly praised by neighbors.

At that time, famous doctors from both towns and provinces all had high reputations received based on their curative treatments rather than relying on the advertising by newspapers and TV stations or being designated by any governments. They might have no titles such as 'professor', 'director' and 'expert' or received no special allowance from governments, some of whom were even lacking experience, but they were indeed authentic TCM doctors learning from highly-skilled doctors. Everyone including migrant workers clearly knew what unique techniques and specialties they had.

In fact, it was not difficult for people to find a skillful TCM doctor because 'there are plenty of fish in the sea'.

However, since famous doctors in older generations passed away one after another with time passing by, the situation gradually changed.

Nowadays, there are groups of 'professors', 'directors' and 'experts' we can see or read in TV, newspapers and hospitals. Modern news media have changed and improved their advertising strategies and methods; however, disappointingly, the curative effects have also changed as well. I hear less and less information about highly praised treatment skills; instead, more and more people complain it is too hard to find a good TCM doctor.

It is definitely not easy to find a TCM doctor who can treat patients relying on pulse feeling and authentic TCM principles rather than test reports, let alone a famous TCM doctor like before.

I started working at Shanxi Science and Technology Press to be in charge of the publication of books of Chinese medicine in 1984. Due to the fact that I had witnessed and heard a lot of the miracles of TCM as well as my passion and persistence in TCM as a TCM doctor, I determined to take advantage of this position to revitalize TCM.

I have actively arranged the publication of many books of TCM along with my colleagues, traveling to different places in China within fifteen years.

In 1994, the Publishing World magazine released 'famous presses and books listed by readers', among which was the Shanxi Science and Technology Press — a small and unpopular press.

To be honest, however, there are only less than ten books among all TCM books published by the press that have practical value and significance in my opinion. As far as I am concerned, among hundreds of writers of those books I have contacted with, there are only no more than five that can take treatments by TCM thoughts.

How pathetic it is to find out such a result after making so much effort for fifteen years. Where are those fish in the sea?

In 2005, Jason McGavin, then assistant of commercial counselor of Australian Embassy invited me to Austria to see patients.

I said: "I'm afraid not. I don't understand English."

He told me seriously however: "actually we only look for TCM doctors incapable of speaking English for treatment. We think they are authentic TCM doctors!" I was really shocked after hearing that.

At the end of the next year when I finally arrived in Australia, I seemed able to understand it.

I was having a seminar with students from the TCM department of a university that day, and learned that they totally copy the teaching model from China, i.e. the combination of teaching both TCM and Western Medicine. They face the same difficulty in employment after graduation and could not even find an internship. Everybody knows, however, that there are many TCM clinics in Australia. Why can't they find a place for internship?

I consulted a person in charge of Australian Acupuncture and Chinese Medicine Association for this question.

He answered: "they (graduation from TCM universities) know nothing about TCM, so we refuse to have them to do internships in our clinics."

It is known that Australia is the first country except for China that admits the effectiveness of TCM and Chinese medicinals among the world, and the State of Victoria even realizes the legislation of TCM. All TCM doctors in TCM clinics are only allowed to prescribe Chinese medicinals, and they all become authentic TCM doctors.

No wonder they exclaimed: "here comes the real TCM doctor!" when I only shared a little bit of conventional TCM principles and prescriptions experience with them.

Recently, I start to hear of 'real TCM doctors' from foreign peers and 'authentic TCM doctors' from foreigners I keep in touch with.

In 1996, when I went to America, I noticed that the TCM examination in some states surprisingly contained *Pulse Classics* (*Mài Jīng*, 脉经) by Wáng Shūhé (王叔和) which I hadn't seen for a long time.

However, it is hard to imagine that pulse-taking in China only exists in name right now no matter from the viewpoint of education or clinical practice. How could it be possible that western countries regard it important? Would they return to the original nature of TCM while China is welcoming a new era?

At present, I witness the fierce argument whether to train new TCM doctors or authentic TCM doctors for a second time, making me as an ordinary TCM doctor feel very anxious. Therefore, I write the above words based on my experience to more or less inspire others, though may be with little significance. (*China News of Traditional Chinese Medicine*, October 19, 2007)

Appendix

Some hopes on TCM

— After reading '*Where are Those Fish in the Sea?*'

Shí Guóbì (石国璧), the counselor of American Traditional Chinese Medicine Association and Alumni (TCMAA)

After reading the article *Where are Those Fish in the Sea* by Guō Bóxìn (郭博信) released on Page 3 of your newspaper on October 19, I cannot help but think about it. The different situations described at home and abroad entirely respect the truth and are worth having a deep consideration. It is time to take actions for improvement now.

I have been a doctor for 54 years since 1953, during which time I keep learning and thinking of TCM and Western Medicine. After retirement in 1995, I was invited to deliver lectures in America in 1996, and lived in America by chance for more than ten years, within which period I cured many patients that were not able to be cured by many major hospitals in America. For example:

An African-American patient suffering from diabetes had been in an American hospital. His blood glucose was over 600mg/dl and could no longer be decreased after being brought down to 400mg/dl by taking western medicines. He then went to my clinic for TCM treatment.

I found that his pulse was wiry, huge, and powerful on both hands, and his tongue coating was thick and sticky, indicating the internal accumulation of dampness-heat. Therefore, I prescribed him the medicinals with functions of clearing heat and eliminating dampness. After taking several doses, his blood glucose decreased to 150mg/dl from 400mg/dl. He was very pleased.

Another example is a 73-year-old white man having arthralgia. He told me in my clinic that his blood glucose remained steady at approximately 200mg/dl. I therefore added some medicinals based on his original prescription in accordance with syndrome differentiation. A week later, his blood glucose decreased to 73mg/dl from 200mg/dl during treatment for the second time. He could not believe this result initially until he took three more blood glucose tests which all showed 70mg/dl.

He said: "it is hard to imagine that Chinese medicinals have such a great curative effect on diabetes!"

I told him the effect of Chinese medicinals was not on reducing blood glucose but on keeping one's body in balance.

There was an American patient suffering from prostatitis which was of high incidence in America and was deeply studied by American hospitals. This patient was reluctant to receive surgery and failed to have positive effect on treatment in many hospitals in America and many TCM clinics, making him very upset.

His wife was from Taiwan. After hearing the information of my treatment from the radio, she suggested him to pay a visit. Symptoms of this patient included the convulsive pain in testis and in parts of caudal vertebra, aversion to cold, insomnia, a deep, thready, and weak pulse, a light whitish tongue with a thin coating.

After the examination, I found that he suffered the syndrome of kidney yang deficiency and prescribed him *Bawei Dihuang Tang* (*Eight-Ingredient Rehmannia Decoction*). Having taken for six doses, he felt his symptoms were relieved.

After receiving the treatment for over a month, all his symptoms were eliminated. He said with pleasure: "you are the only doctor in this city that can cure prostatitis."

There were also two American Western Medicine doctors asking for treatment from me, one of whom was an expert in internal medicine and had liver cirrhosis. She did not receive curative treatment in Western Medicine, so she would like to try taking Chinese medicinals.

She had abdominal distension and bad appetite with pain in liver. She breathed hard and easily felt exhausted. I found that she had a wiry, thready, and weak pulse, a light whitish tongue with a thin and white coating.

After the examination, I realized that she suffered liver depression and spleen deficiency, and prescribed her medicinals with functions of tonifying qi and invigorating spleen, soothing liver and relieving depression, and activating blood and regulating qi.

Having taken my medicinals for three months, she felt very much relieved and gradually had a good appetite. Her body condition was improved and had better test result.

After taking the medicinals for another three months, she received good result from test report and her esophageal varix was also relieved.

She said happily: "I did not expect that Chinese medicinals could have such a great effect!"

She invited me to treat hepatopathy cooperating with her friends in Western Medicine. Since I just arrived in America at that time with poor English skills, I refused her request.

Another American medical expert had a large clinic where he invited me to pay a visit. He and his wife wanted a baby, but his wife had irregular menstruation and he himself had insufficient number of sperms with poor motility.

I treated both of them for over a year before his wife finally got pregnant and gave birth to a baby when she was 43 years old.

All the above examples indicate that TCM is really a great treasure that has positive effect on both Chinese and western people, of course provided that correct syndrome differentiation and proper treatment were used.

Modern medicine develops very rapidly with high-end technology, but it still cannot replace TCM.

TCM and Chinese medicinals are developing in a fast speed in countries having improved Western Medicine.

Those of us who are abroad have some expectations for colleagues and leaders in the TCM field in China:

(1) TCM and Chinese medicinals are springing up and developing very rapidly in western countries, but related peers are still difficult to make a living mainly due to the fact that foreign administrative directors and Western Medicine doctors have less understanding and approval of TCM, sometimes even producing obstacles on purpose. Some Western Medicine doctors advocate that Chinese medicinals have toxicity and are not safe to be utilized. We have to advocate TCM through practical curative effects and patients. We hope directors and leaders in China can positively communicate with health and administrative departments in other countries to reduce obstacles.

(2) Universities and colleges of TCM are supposed to cultivate advanced talents in TCM and its medicinal fields. They should, in accordance with principles of Hengyang Conference, mainly concentrate on teaching Chinese medicine, followed by Western medicine in order to train 'real TCM doctors' with qualified competence and skills. It is said that

some universities of TCM currently establish Western Medicine major, probably resulting in the TCM colleges existing in name only.

(3) The research direction of TCM and Chinese medicinals should place its basic theory study at a very important position instead of only paying attention to the study of medicinal development. China Academy of Chinese Medical Sciences has been established for over 50 years, and every province has also founded its own research institute of TCM with plenty of staff and investment. However, it is still difficult to explain exact meanings of kidney-yang deficiency, kidney-yin deficiency, spleen-yin deficiency and spleen-yang deficiency in modern language or to define their quality and quantity in standard inspection measures.

(4) The development and research of many Chinese medicinals aim at abandoning TCM and only remaining Chinese medicinals nowadays. There are many anti-inflammatory and antiseptic medicines, anti-rhinitis pills, anti-prostatitis pills, anti-gastritis pills, lipid-lowering pills, glucose-lowering pills and anti-hypertensive pills with no syndrome differentiation when prescribing. In this situation, what on earth is the significance of TCM theories?

I still remember that when I visited Japan few years ago, a Japanese friend told me: "We fail to study Chinese medicinals most of the time."

I said: "The main reason is that you do not combine the research with TCM theories. Only under the guidance of TCM theories can Chinese medicinal application be curative." For example, *Huangqi* (*Radix Astragali seu Hedysari*) will be useful in tonifying qi only when the patient suffers qi deficiency; otherwise, it will be harmful. 'Excessive qi causes fire syndrome', so using *Huangqi* not in the situation of qi deficiency will result in fire syndrome which will produce phlegm. Xú Língtāi (徐灵胎), a mecial scientist in Qing Dynasty once wrote, '*Renshen* (*Radix Ginseng*) can kill people' in one of his articles. *Renshen* (*Radix Ginseng*) is an advanced tonic, but it may also kill people if used in an improper way.

I am not against the study of Chinese medicinals by using modern experiments; however, if they still regulate those medicinals in the same way as western medicines, the phenomenon of abandoning TCM and keeping only Chinese medicinals will occur and TCM will probably be eliminated in the end.

Similarly, if they operate TCM hospitals and universities in the same way as they do to Western Medicine, TCM may have a worrying prospect.

It is the best time to develop Chinese medicine now due to the fact that the State Council and government leaders at all levels pay unprecedented attention to it, creating a great opportunity for the development of Chinese medicine. I hope that leaders in TCM departments can positively recognize problems, seize opportunities and solve problems in order to promote the development of TCM and bring benefit to both Chinese and international people. This is the only expectation I have as a veteran TCM doctor.

(NOTE: the author is a visiting scholar in the US and chief TCM physician who used to be the Deputy Director-General in Gansu Health Department and Dean of Gansu Traditional Chinese Medicine Institute.)

(This article was first published in *China News of Traditional Chinese Medicine*, December 7, 2007)

Several inspirations from TCM study

I am not clever enough so that I dare not slack during my 40-year TCM life, due to which, I have some simple and plain personal understandings to share with beginners as a reference:

I. Reading the classics carefully

TCM classics are the highest wisdom of TCM and need to be studied and experienced repeatedly through clinic practice in the whole life.

For people living in modern society, most of us have never read the Four Books and Five Classics (Sishu Wujing) or receive any education of traditional culture so that we tend to analyze problems more visually and superficially. The vital importance of reading classics is to change our ways of thinking and perspectives in order to learn syndrome differentiation and treatment. In other words, the altitude changes your perspective and the angle changes your attitude.

There are many experts nowadays who frequently who criticize that studying TCM classics is 'ancient renaissance', 'past unitarian' and 'blindly following the past'. Most of these are actually the ignorance and misguidance of TCM.

An entrepreneur once said with emotion: "it's better for people without corporation management experience to not to speak too much. There are so many cases of misleading the younger generation with only one sentence." It is similar in the TCM field. Business people misled by others may suffer bankruptcy but can still make a living in a second time; doctors misled by others however may do harm to numerous people's lives!

TCM classics are ancient which do not stand for being backward but refer to a splendid scientific palace built on general concepts. Confucius said: "I looked up to them, and they seemed to become higher; I tried to penetrate them, and they seemed to become more firm; I looked at them before me, and suddenly they seemed to be behind." (The Analects of Confucius, Chapter 9 (Lún yǔ • Zǐ hàn piān, 论语·子罕篇)) (Translator's note: this quote is from Yen Yuan, an apprentice of Confucius.) The essential factor of leaning TCM well is to believe in TCM classics. Belief does not refer to superstition but means trust and admiration. How can people read classics carefully if they do not believe in them?

Reading carefully refers to the fact that people should not only understand those words superficially but also think of them repeatedly, especially through clinical practice, from which they will gradually comprehend them thoroughly and acquire great thoughts and new ideas. Carefully reading those classics means people should regard learning them as the vital importance: no matter how many kinds of books we read, classics should always be in the first place.

TCM classics are books that will be studied and applied to use endlessly by every TCM doctor in their TCM life. They will not know the meaning of 'reading classics again and again tirelessly to gain more and more detailed knowledge' until they study it intensively.

TCM is so broad and profound that it seems to have no bound or bottom. Despite of this, we still need to study and pursue it within our life. 'It is enough for me to contemplate the mystery of conscious life perpetuating itself through all eternity, to reflect upon the marvelous structure of the universe which we can dimly perceive, and to try humbly to comprehend even an infinitesimal part of the intelligence manifested in nature,' quoted from Albert Einstein.

II. Doing clinical work in a down-to-earth manner

Sūn Sīmiǎo (孙思邈) from Tang Dynasty said: "it seems that there is no incurable disease during the period of learning TCM after three years while there is no useful prescription during three-year clinical practice." This sentence means three-year TCM study only teaches students knowledge and principles recorded in books, making them feel they can handle every disease as long as they master those 'rules'; however, it is with less effect to apply those 'rules' to patients during clinical practice. After doing clinical work for three years, doctors will start to realize there is no cure-in-all prescription without any alterations. Prescription making will not be with proficiency until they make knowledge into practice.

Hú Jūrén (胡居仁) from Ming Dynasty said: "students should underestimate their effort rather than overrate it, laying a solid foundation instead of seeking for high skills. 'Underestimate' and 'solid foundation' here refer to doing clinical work in a down-to-earth manner. 'The superior man wishes to be slow in his speech and earnest in his conduct,' this quote from Confucius should be particularly borne in mind.

Those ridiculous arguments of the westernization of TCM mostly come from pedants who look down upon the clinic and people with irredeemable national inferiority complex.

III. Learning from the seniors in the TCM field with great respect

TCM is an intangible science. Leaning TCM not only relies on the intelligence and memory capacity, but also needs comprehension and experience from teachers. How can I possibly know the profundity of pulse feeling without the help of Liáng Xiùqīng (梁秀清)? How can I know syndrome differentiation and prescription without knowledge from Huáng Jiéxī (黄杰熙)? How can I know how to cure severe and emergency diseases by using large dosage of *Fuzi* (*Radix Aconiti Lateralis*) without learning from Lǐ Kě (李可)? Although I am not smart, I more or less learn from them to save many lives as well as myself. I appreciate their mercy of life-saving grace, so I regard them as my respected teachers. Acknowledging one teacher will help us open one window and gain one skill of saving lives; therefore, the more teachers we learn from, the more skills and enlightenment we can gain. Isn't it true that Yè Tiānshì (叶天士) acknowledged 17 teachers before he was honored as a 'perfect doctor'?

Students should respect their teachers; otherwise, how are they willing to deliver knowledge?

TCM can be taught by oneself, but experience is more important. One can gain double results with half the work under the enlightening and teaching from teachers. It is common that one sentence from a teacher may be more rewarding than doing ten years of reading. Ming Weimin from Ming Dynasty said: "we may waste our time though with great aspiration unless meeting with a good master."

IV. Sincerely sharing medical experience with peers

TCM is so broad and profound that one can only learn a small part of it; therefore, most of doctors will have their advantages and disadvantages. If we can share medical experience with peers sincerely, we can learn from others' advantages to cover our shortages.

My treatment methods and prescriptions are learnt not only from classics and teachers but also from peers. If I did not treat them sincerely, they would not share with me anything.

Hence, I particularly appreciate the wording by Liáng Qǐchāo (梁启超): "I will respect them as my teachers as long as I learn something from their words or sentences." I always respect people as my teachers provided I can learn from their advantages regardless of their qualifications and professional titles. I have even learned a lot from folks.

Gě Hóng (葛洪) from Jin Dynasty once said in *Baopuzi*: "studying alone without any friends will make people lonely and ill-informed; thus, sharing experience with peers will create mutual benefit."

That we should have access to others' advantages and recognize our shortages is the sincere way to make friends. Confucius said: "In a group of three people, there is always something I can learn from." People who can truly obey this will become the 'sage'; by contrast, he or she will be a vulgar one 'if they treat themselves as the best in the group'.

People will acquire reward now or later if they treat others sincerely. 'It is important to both have a good teacher as well as a friend in study'. (*Qián shū·Jiǎng xué* (潜书·讲学) compiled in Ming Dynasty).

V. Being an authentic TCM doctor

I will either choose to be an authentic TCM doctor or totally change my career.

What is exactly an authentic TCM doctor? It refers to a pure and absolute TCM doctor.

This was supposed to be a question too simple to be discussed. There is a saying in villages of Shanxi: "you should concentrate on what you are doing." If you are a Christian, you should focus on reading the Bible; Buddhist should focus on reading the Buddhist Scriptures; TCM doctors should act like a pure TCM doctor. Is there any problem here?

As a TCM doctor, we should not ignore the tradition. If someone starts to follow the fashion and keep pursuing updated modern scientific words after only understanding the knowledge from books without any solid practical foundation, it actually refers to the westernization of TCM rather than learning TCM! In other words, they 'fly to distant places before noticing where their feet stand on' like 'willow dancing without root' and 'petals flowing with river'.

The only reason to be an authentic TCM doctor is to know how to give treatments i.e. be responsible to patients and respectful to lives! There are no other reasons anymore. 'Mastering in one thing is enough even though we are not proficient in others.' (Lù Yóu (陆游) from Song Dynasty, *Jian Nan Poem Manuscript* (*Jiàn nán shī gǎo,* 剑南诗稿)) We should stick to this resolution!

VI. Following the classic principles

We should concentrate on learning each branch of science in order to have some inventions and creations.

TCM is an intangible science which is easy to learn but difficult to master. People learning TCM have to penetrate this path in order to live up to their effort. Returning to tradition is the only solution for TCM.

The simplest way is actually the most correct one. Learning TCM in a too general and too complex way seems to modernize and scientize it but in fact 'leading it too far from the path from the initial', said by Master Hóng Yī (弘一) (*Hanjia Collection* (*Hán jiā jí,* 寒笳集)). All those knowledge are just the tangram and kaleidoscope which is easier to lose than to control. The more complexity they learn, the less judgment they have. How can they save people's lives with only general knowledge?

It will mislead both patients and themselves, and they should feel sorry for ancestors, patients and mankind.

Returning to tradition does not equal to 'sticking to old path with new mode'; instead, it is 'the captivation of the truth' like Isaac Newton.

VII. Progressing step by step

TCM is a science. No science is easy to learn so that people should acquire knowledge and make progress step by step. 'Long distance is covered in small steps (*Dà dài lǐ jì, quàn xué* (大戴礼记·劝学)).' Sun Yat-sen once said: "Knowledge should be acquired gradually rather than by chance (*The Complete Works of Sun Yat-sen* (Sun Yat-sen quán jí, 孙中山全集))." One should make progress step by step like a follower. Progress is not hard to make with a right direction. Where there is a will there is a way.

Although it is difficult to go forward, one should bear in mind that there will always be new brightness waiting at the next stop. What a pleasure it is!

VIII. Working conscientiously in medical practice

Learning TCM well will not only help you save lives and share patients' happiness, but also make you addicted to it. 'The charm from outside may be disgusting after a long time, but the charm of books will be stronger without any disgust (Chéng Xuān (程瑄) from Ming Dynasty, *the Record of Reading* (*Dú shū lù,* 读书录)).'

As for me, learning TCM is an enjoyment. Although I am aged now, 'my will is never old with my age (Lù Yóu (陆游), *Jiannan Poem Manuscript*(*Jiàn nán shī gǎo,* 剑南诗稿)).' I dare not say that 'I still have ambition in such an age', but I am still 'motivated in making effort'.

It seems that people in their sixties should be retired and enjoy their rest of life at home. However, there is no veteran TCM doctor, my teachers included, who chooses to get retired after 60. They are still busy saving lives though with grey hair and teetering steps. Chén Tóngyún (陈彤云), a classmate of my mother-in-law in Fu Jen Catholic University, is still giving treatment in her nineties; TCM masters like

Dèng Tiětāo (邓铁涛) and Zhū Liángchūn (朱良春) still come up with new ideas and efforts for TCM revitalization in their nineties. Xú Língtāi (徐灵胎), a famous doctor in Qing Dynasty, was still invited to give treatment to the emperor when he was 100 years old. He was sent to the palace in a sedan with a coffin. He once said: "I have been busy in TCM treatment in my whole life and I am still closely related to TCM though I am over 100."

This is exactly TCM.

This is what the Qi-Huang spirit is!

Epilogue: The charm of
Traditional Chinese Medicine

Lǐ Kě (李可), my respected teacher, resolutely decided to join the army when he was only 16 before graduating from middle school. When he was 23, however, he was wronged to be sent to jail twice till he was redressed in his fifties. After all, there is no doubt that it is a tragedy in his life.

Nevertheless, having known him for 20 years, I never see him making any complaint; instead, he always smiles when mentioning the past. Why? It is all because of a veteran TCM doctor he knew in the jail that led him to the life of TCM, encouraging him to study TCM in adversity, especially *Treatise on Cold Damage Diseases* (*Shāng hán lùn*, 伤寒论) which deserves life-long study. 'Misfortune might be a blessing in disguise,' quoted from him. He always feels very lucky.

It is ancient TCM that helps a person out of trouble. What charm *Treatise on Cold Damage Diseases* (*Shāng hán lùn*, 伤寒论) has within only forty thousand words!

Similarly, I was also attracted by the same book and changed my career to TCM in mid-age.

I was a graduate majoring in arts at first, but I resolutely decided to learn TCM after working for a short while and have been a TCM doctor for several decades. What is the reason for me to change my career?

Actually it is quite a long story. My hometown is Fengrun County, Hebei Province. I moved to Liangdu Town, Lingshi County, Shanxi Province in 1954 because of my father's job transfer. I never saw my grandfather, but my father often told me that my grandfather had suffered dysphagia (esophagus cancer) in around 1936, causing him to be very skinny due to difficulty in eating. My father then had invited a famous veteran TCM doctor from Tangshan who had prescribed three medicinals and then left immediately after feeling my grandfather's pulse and having a deep consideration. Surprisingly, my grandfather had been cured instantly after taking the medicinals and had never relapsed until he passed away.

My father only remembered that the prescription contains 250g of *radix rehmanniae preparata*, but could not recall the other two medicinals. He always cannot help but praise the superb skills of that TCM doctor.

Afterwards, my father suffered stomachache and was cured after taking three doses of the decoction prescribed by Yuè Měizhōng (岳美中), a doctor in Tangshan.

My father often talked about Yue's voice and expression with pleasure, contributing to a particular familiarity every time when I read books written by Yuè Měizhōng (岳美中) after I have been a TCM doctor.

In 1955, my mother suffered a rare disease that she would suddenly had spasm and groaned with tears and nosal discharge for several hours though she acted normal most of the time. She would have these symptoms once around one to two months.

I was only 12 at that time, so I always felt very scared when my mother fell ill. I can still remember how painful I was in my heart.

My father was so worried that he found doctors everywhere to treat my mother but failed to have any effect after taking excessive western medicines.

My mother had no choice but to find a distantly related uncle in Hebei for help. He was a locally famous doctor in east Hebei at that time; I had heard lots of magical stories of his treatments in my childhood.

After feeling the pulse, the doctor said my mother suffered from the syndrome of internal stirring of liver wind.

My mother said she indeed 'exhaled wind' (probably large amounts of belching) from her mouth after taking the medicinals. Miracle did happen! My mother never relapsed since then.

My mother only remembered the prescription contains a lots of *Shetui* (*Periostracum Serpentis*)(translator note: it's a kind of snakeskin), so she often said it was snakeskin that cured her disease.

Another case is that *The Collection of Treatment Experience from Emergency, Severe, Rare and Stubborn Diseases* by Veteran TCM Doctor Lǐ Kě (李可) (*Lǐ kě lǎo zhōng yī jí wēi zhòng zhèng yí nán bìng jīng yàn zhuān jí*, 李可老中医急危重症疑难病经验专辑) mentioned a patient Wáng Shūchén (王淑臣) who had thyroid cancer metastases. The patient was the mother of Zhāng Yánzōng (张延宗), my classmate in primary school. I remembered in my childhood that she had a bun-sized tumor on her neck. Surprisingly, when I saw her again in the late 1970s, her thick neck turned into a thin one. Having asked her, I realized that she was cured after taking the medicinals prescribed by Lǐ Kě (李可), a TCM doctor in Lingshi Town.

Zhāng Yánzōng (张延宗) told me secretly that the formula also contained scorpion and centipede (there were 12 scorpions and 4 centipedes contained in the prescription). I could not understand in what way scorpion and centipede can cure the disease.

All of the above are magical experience I had about TCM in my youth, but I absolutely did not think about being a TCM doctor myself.

When I graduated from high school in Jiexiu County in 1963, my Chinese teacher Zhāng Féngchūn (张逢春) wrote me a parting poem, the meaning of which is like: A person without any skills is talent-less even though he or she acquires many degrees or titles; we should rather choose to be an eatable rice grain than cast ourselves to be a pretty peony.

I regard this poem as my motto and often recite it to remind myself, from which I benefit a lot. Maybe this also lays a foundation for me to change my career to TCM and to realize my errors when I was lost in the westernization of TCM.

I was admitted to the Department of Chinese Language and Literature in Shanxi University in 1963. During my third year of study, I was elected by classmates to write an article 'Opinions on Contemporary Education Reform', which was highly praised by our principal and was printed to be shown to each department in the school for discussion.

The principal immediately came to our class for investigation and appointed our class as a pilot class of education reform in the university. He often talked with me, and I also regarded him as a supervisor who offered me support and encouragement.

In 1964, I indeed made the first prescription in my whole life.

I was sent to Gongxiwang Village, Nanzhang Town, Zhangzi County, Shanxi Province as a member of Ssu-Ch'ing Working Team that year, where I met a four-year-old boy when I had dinner in a local family. He was full of impetigo on his face, especially on cheeks with pus. I could only recognize his eyes, so I sympathized him very much.

His family said the disease was inborn. Numerous anti-inflammatory drugs he had taken all failed to cure his disease. His parents were so worried that they already had grey hair though in such a young age.

Coincidently, I just saw an empirical formula on *Shanxi Nongmin News* (newspaper of peasants) by chance that could treat diseases similar to the boy's. The formula called the disease as 'fetal toxin'. I copied the formula right away and gave it to the patient's parents.

Nonetheless, around four days later, the father took his son to my home and shouted at me: "His disease got more severe after taking your medicinals!" I noticed that his face condition was more serious than before! I was too astonished and scared to talk and felt so regretful, thinking: why should I have poked my nose into their business since I am not a doctor? I did make a mess!

Peasants were so kind and simple that he did not say anything but walked away with his son in silence.

I then suddenly found that newspaper on the table when I was still out of my mind. I subconsciously read the formula for the second time and then figured out that there was a line of small words beside the formula, saying that this prescription aimed to use poison against poison so that it may worsen the disease at first after taking the medicinals and would cure the disease after keeping taking it.

I was as pleased as grasping the last straw so that I rushed out of the house and ran to the farmer's home. I told the father: "don't worry. The formula is against the pathogen right now. Just keep taking it."

The father took his son to me again after around ten days. He asked his son to kneel down in front of me immediately after they entered in, asking me to be the boy's godfather.

I was so relieved and excited after seeing the boy's face was finally smooth with lovely cheeks.

Afterwards, I thought I should keep the newspaper but I was not able to find it anymore. I still regret about it nowadays. However, I remember clearly that there were also scorpion and centipede in the prescription.

I started to come closer to TCM after experiencing more and more similar magical stories, but still had no idea of 'changing career'.

In June, 1966, the Cultural Revolution erupted. Principal Liú Méi (刘梅) was framed as a member of 'counter-revolution gang'. The university was full of Dazibao (a wall-mounted poster for propaganda) with 'fighting against Liú Méi (刘梅)' written on it.

I therefore organized students to write Dazibao to counter attack back, turning me, a well-known good student in university to a notorious 'royalist'. Such a situation was just like the poem written by Dù Fǔ (杜甫): 'Clouds in the sky change so quickly that sometimes are like white coats while other times are as dark dogs; people are never able to predict what may happen the next day.'

In 1968, I graduated during the time the university was under messy circumstance. Having been 're-educated' by working and training, I was sent to the Publicity Department of Party Committee of Linfen Textile Mill in Shanxi Province in 1971. It was a large-scale factory with over 4000 workers under provincial governance. Since I was hard-working, I was treated with great importance by the deputy secretary in charge of publicity department, Luó Bórěn (罗伯忍), who often praised and encouraged me.

However, during the period when I was sent to the countryside by the governor in 1972, my life was totally changed.

At that time I was sent to Xiyong Village, Xionghuo Commune, Hongdong County, Shanxi Province. One day I had my meal in the house of a retired veteran TCM doctor, Lǐ Sōngrú (李松如) who was over 80 years old with a long beard, just like an authentic veteran TCM doctor. He was concentrating on reading a book with a magnifying glass in his hand. I asked curiously: "What are you reading, sir?"

He smiled and said it was *Treatise on Cold Damage Diseases* (*Shāng hán lùn, 伤寒论*). He then told me with emotion that this book was the one that he had read and used in his whole life but he still could not be able to finish reading it or stop using it.

I was very curious, thinking what kind of book it was that attracted the veteran doctor so much.

Mr. Lǐ Sōngrú (李松如) passed me the thin book. After only reading the preface written by the author Zhāng Zhòngjǐng (张仲景), I was then totally attracted: "It is beyond understanding that intellectuals nowadays don't care medical knowledge which not only can relieve the diseases of the emperor and relatives, but also save the lives of poor, and prolong one's own life. These intellectuals just fight for fame and wealth, and are bent solely on profit. What they have done is only focusing on the immediate interests but totally ignoring the future, which exactly indicates that 'all that glitters is not gold'". He also treats these 'greasiness' as 'walking dead'. I was totally inspired by these words. Sir Zhāng Zhòngjǐng (张仲景) pointed out the method of TCM learning by using such a short phrase 'diligently studying traditional principles and generally adapting to different prescriptions'.

Lǐ Sōngrú (李松如) also told me that people with lofty ideals in ancient times would 'either choose to be an upright official or a skillful doctor' (which I knew later was quoted from Fàn Wénzhèng (范文正), a famous politician and member of literati from the Northern Song Dynasty).

He added: "As a graduate majoring in arts, you are very suitable to learn TCM. People in ancient times often said 'nine of ten Chinese scholars are able to be TCM doctors'. It is also said that 'scholars to learn TCM is as easy as to chop tofu'."

Having listened to his words, I clearly realized that my bachelor degree of arts could lay a foundation for TCM learning. It was in that villa that I as a idolater of Lǔ Xùn (鲁迅) made up my mind to walk on a path totally opposite to his — 'engaging in medicine while giving up literature'.

I started to memorize prescriptions of decoctions, practice acupuncture in person like a primary school student, asking questions and finding solutions from the veteran doctor every day.

Villagers began to look for treatment from me since they knew the veteran doctor took me as his apprentice.

The first time I paid a home visit was to treat a middle-aged peasant who suffered from haemorrhoids swelling and bleeding. There were lots of bloodstain on the bed and bedding. He lay on bed, groaning painfully.

Folks looked at each other speechlessly: they could not afford to receive treatment in the city.

After feeling the pulse, I prescribed 15g of *Danggui Wei* (*the tail of Radix Angelicae Sinensis*), 25g of *Shengma* (*Rhizoma Cimicifugae*), 15g of *Dahuang* (*Radix et Rhizoma Rhei*) and 10g of *Fengmi* (*Mel*).

In fact, this prescription was copied from the first volume of *Shanxi Folk Remedies and Prescriptions* (*Shān xī mín jiān yàn fāng mì fāng,* 山西民间验方秘方). Fortunately, the patient was fully cured after two doses which cost less than 0.40 yuan.

This case caused a sensation. Villagers even from villages nearby also came to me for treatment. Therefore, I had to make treatments while reading books. I was so busy in giving acupuncture treatments and making prescriptions at that time.

Farmers strived to ask me to have dinner in their houses, making me a 'popular star' in their eyes.

I was totally changed when I left the countryside. Despite working on time, I was fully addicted to reading TCM books in my office without caring any irrelevant information. As for my job, I just walked it through. At that time, I was regarded as a geek, arousing my colleagues' dissatisfaction, especially secretary Lu who had highly praised me. No matter how earnest he persuaded me, I would not change my mind. The situation lasted for over four years.

Another person that was disappointed with me was Principal Liú Méi (刘梅) who had supported and encouraged me a lot before.

After the end of the Cultural Revolution, many veteran cadres, like Liú Méi (刘梅), staged a comeback. Since the education system had been suspended for ten years, talents were badly wanted in each relevant organization. Liú Méi (刘梅) then thought of me, asking people around: "Where is Guō Bóxìn (郭博信)? Ask him to come back!" A mentor of mine, Mr. Guo, who worked at the education committee in province at that time, wrote me a letter, appointing me back to a provincial department. However, I rejected their appointment in reply. To be honest, I had already rejected two similar opportunities, in one of which they specially assigned a person to talk to me face to face.

Although those opportunities were very precious for some people, they however had far less attraction to me than *Treatise on Cold Damage Diseases* (*Shāng hán lùn,* 伤寒论). I was absolutely obsessed with it, which could not be understood by others or explained clearly to leaders.

It was either the destiny or my persistence in the TCM impressed the 'God'. In 1976, Secretary Luo who had criticized me for my ignorance of job and had argued with me several times unexpectedly against all the odds granted special favor to send me to the TCM department of Linfen Textile Workers' Hospital to be a TCM doctor!

Although I wore the doctor's white coat, I still had no 'right to prescribe' without a medical degree. Therefore, I had to ask other doctors, no matter western or TCM doctors, to sigh on my prescription before filling it. It was not until 1978 that I was finally admitted to be a certificated TCM physician and had right to prescribe after passing the national unified examination.

I finally achieved my goal to be a perfectly justifiable TCM doctor, so I was full of enthusiasm in working.

Around five years later, I met my respected teacher Liáng Xiùqīng (梁秀清).

Liáng Xiùqīng (梁秀清) was born in Liangzhuang Village, Zhangding Town, Julu County, Heibei Province. His family had been doctors for nine generations. He was tall and thin with a benign face, dressing like a farmer.

Liang only graduated from primary school, but I felt outshone by him though I had an undergraduate degree and medical certificate. There were so many patients coming to him for treatment from distant areas while I as a modern TCM doctor also treated plenty of patients every day because of the brand of our major hospital.

I was as excited as Columbus finding the New World!

Sir Liang treated me as his natural child because of my honest and sincere attitude. He taught me in earnest, asking me to feel the pulse after he did and told me the difference of different pulse condition as well as the relation of pulse and syndrome.

I always concentrated on feeling the pulse and learning TCM, thinking I would be a TCM doctor as Sir Liang.

However, my enthusiasm vanished only after one year. Why? On the one hand, I had to spend lots of time from Linfen to Houma due to long distance; on the other hand, as a civil servant, I did not have much time learning from him since I only visited him every Sunday. More importantly, no matter how hard Sir Liang taught me the skills of pulsing feeling, I always felt confused and could not feel the pulse correctly as he did.

He smiled and held my hands, saying: "look at your fingertips. The skin there is too thick to be sensitive of the pulse."

He then showed me his three fingers, nails of which were all over the fingertips.

"What are fingernails for? For protecting your fingertips," he said.

He often told me about the principles of pulse feeling, most of which were quoted from *Internal Classic* (*Nèi jīng, 内经*) and *Classic of questioning* (*Nàn jīng, 难经*).

He said: "You could not only understand the surface meaning of those books. You have to practice. It is like playing erhu. You never know how to play a whole song until you practice a lot." He also told me that I should do exercise outdoors every early morning, i.e. to concentrate on thinking of my fingertips by closing my eyes till I could have the feeling of some insects moving on my fingers, after which I could start feeling the pulse.

I finally realized after listening to his words: it turned out to be that the simple 'three fingers and one small pillow' contained such profound knowledge! We only knew that there were highly skilled doctors in ancient times while had no idea that how much effort they spent in only practicing pulse feeling.

Therefore, I started to do exercise every morning outdoors. After a long time, I could still not have the feeling just like he described.

I still practiced a lot though, thinking 'everything comes to him who waits'. I had to persist in practicing for I believed 'where there is a will there is a way'!

Afterwards, I heard of a piece of news that made my enthusiasm almost disappeared again.

It was during the conversation after a treatment that Sir Liang told me he was instructed by his father to practice pulse feeling when he was only 8 years old, three years after which he began to learn about prescription. It turned out to be that he learnt TCM from his childhood! I only knew that Beijing Opera and Kong Fu had to be learnt in childhood, but I had never thought that learning TCM was the same as them. How profound TCM is!

I then faced a ruthless truth: I was already over 30. I had spent my entire youthful days in acquiring knowledge not relevant to TCM. In addition, I still had my work to do so that I could only learn TCM on Sundays; since it took a lot of time from my home to Liang's, how much time on earth do I have to learn it? How could I master the essence of TCM in such a situation?

More despairingly, most of famous veteran TCM doctors had passed away. All TCM doctors I visited nearby were 'modern TCM doctors' from medical schools. They felt at ease to make a living in their positions and receive promotions. I visited them one by one and heard the same answer: "Pulse feeling is actually not a matter of concern. What era it is nowadays! Instruments with advanced techniques of course have better results than pulse feeling."

It really made me have neither motivation to make progress nor determination to give up.

In 1983, when I still felt confused and depressed, Xiè Xīliàng (谢锡亮), a veteran doctor in Shanxi acupuncture field was invited by Shanxi Health Department to established the 'advanced class of acupuncture skills in Shanxi Province'. He asked my superior to temporarily transfer me to help him. He invited many teachers to give lectures, one of whom is Fàn Qíyún (范其云), the contemporary editor from the editorial office of medicine and health of Shanxi People's Publishing House.

Fan was a graduate from Fu Jen Catholic University before the founding of the PRC. He also changed his career due to the love of acupuncture.

He found out that I had both the knowledge of literature and medicine that was very suitable for being a medical editor in the press house. Therefore, he immediately reported it to leaders after returning to Taiyuan, and the province sent a transfer order to the organization department of Party Committee in Linfen Textile Mill.

I however did not reject this opportunity like before.

I felt really hesitated: if I receive this offer, it meant I changed my career back and worked on literature again, but I loved my position as a doctor; if not, it was still against my intention to be an ordinary TCM doctor with no proficiency. What should I do?

I met with a crossroad in my life for a second time. I considered for half a year after receiving the offer.

One day however, I suddenly realized that what if traditional veteran TCM doctors like Liáng Xiùqīng (梁秀清) passed away sometime? Who would have the chance to know the magic of TCM? Never! It would totally disappear! The duty in the editorial office of medicine and health care was to publish books of medicine. Even though I could not be a great doctor myself, I would still express my love of TCM by publishing books of TCM doctors, like Liang in order to tell the world what the authentic TCM doctors were.

I started to have the sense of mission. In my opinion, even if I would have been a great doctor, how many lives could I save? It would be much better to tell people what TCM was and to encourage them to learn TCM well, by which more lives would be saved. I would rather sacrifice my prospect for a better result. Having realized it, I resolutely went to the publishing house.

Consequently, I started my career as an editor in 1984 and was crazy in soliciting contributions and editing books of TCM during the next fifteen years.

Once I was elected to be the Editor-in-Chief of the Shanxi Science and Technology Press with additional post as the president of the periodical office of *Traditional Chinese Medicine Research*.

In 1994, the Shanxi Science and Technology Press was the only press of medicines and drugs among all 14 presses out of over 500 in China selected into the 'famous presses and books in the eyes of readers' list published in the ninth volume of *Information of Publishing* hosted by China Research Institute of the Publishing Science. The review goes as follows, 'books of medicine and health care published by this press are very outstanding, including folk prescriptions, remedies, dietary therapy and health care.' I regard this nomination as a reward to my work.

In 1995, Mr. Zhang, the contemporary deputy director of Shanxi News and Publication Bureau in charge of human resources (after transferred to be the secretary of prefectural party committee) would like to appoint me to be the Editor-in-Chief of Shanxi People' Publishing House.

Among in local presses, people's publishing house would always be acknowledged as a leader with a higher administrative level, compared with which, other professional presses are all 'small-scale presses'. Therefore, this kind of appointment was actually a promotion, but I still refused it without any hesitation.

If I transferred to the publishing house, I would have no chance to publish books of TCM, which meant I had to suspend my beloved TCM career.

I was afraid that Director Zhang had never met a subordinate as unappreciative as me. He did not know however I was busy on business trips to solicit contributions and looking for veteran TCM doctors either in remote areas or with titles who were able to cure diseases around China. No matter what professional titles they had, I would always encourage them to write and publish articles as long as I found them. I was busy fighting for my 'TCM career'.

Huáng Jiéxī (黄杰熙) once sent his manuscript to a professional press of medicine in Beijing, but they sent it back to him without a glimpse the next day, the reason being that the manuscript was sent from a middle school in Taiyuan and not from a medical institution.

Huang was then dispirited. Having read his manuscript, I was more than happy and cherished it as a treasure. Why? Although Mr. Huang was a teacher in a middle school, his understanding of TCM was so comprehensive and thorough that I had never seen before.

Hence, I immediately edited and published it, and then offered him a new topic. He then published several other books later.

After I found Mr. Huang, I came to the press at 5 am plus every morning, busy compiling manuscripts and arranging tasks. After other staff all arrived at the press at around 8 am, I would ride to Mr. Huang to learn pulse feeling and prescription making. At about 11am, I returned to my office to finish my tasks. I seldom took a break at home on weekends in order not to affect my daily work by TCM learning.

In 1991, I met Lǐ Kě (李可), the dean of the hospital of TCM in Lingshi Town. The hospital at that time only had several old and low tile-roofed houses. The house was dimly lit. An old man with grey hair and thin cheeks sat in a chair; his eyes however were very sharp and bright, making him look like a holy scholar with outstanding manner.

I felt like I found 'the New World' a second time after only talking for a short while with him. I acknowledged him as my teacher and requested him to write books. For the next ten years, I frequently traveled between Taiyuan and Lingshi.

The Collection of Treatment Experience from Emergency, Severe, Rare and Stubborn Diseases by Veteran TCM Doctor Lǐ Kě (李可) (*Lǐ kě lǎo zhōng yī jí wēi zhòng zhèng yí nán bìng jīng yàn zhuān jí*, 李可老中医急危重症疑难病经验专辑) was published in 2002. I wrote a foreword for the book. Why? As far as I was concerned, the book was so important that it filled a gap of TCM treatment of severe and emergency diseases. Indeed, there was no doubt that every veteran TCM doctor who made a living in

TCM for a life had their own precious experience and advantages, which deserved our study and inheritance.

The importance of Lǐ Kě (李可) is that he had the experience that other veteran doctors did not have. He was brave to fight against the death and concentrated on helping patients; he experienced many special difficulties in his life; he had great love and persistency in TCM; he had incomparable sensitiveness to the highly toxic *Fuzi* (*Radix Aconiti Lateralis*), all of which could not be found in others.

Even till now, I still think that meeting with my respected teacher Lǐ Kě (李可) was the most grateful thing after I took over the charge of the publication of TCM books. After being published, the book has been reprinted for 29 times within ten years and is still one of the bestsellers nowadays.

After I retired in 1998, I established a small platform for myself — a medical clinic. Besides piles of pieces of Chinese medicinals, all I need is 'three fingers and one small pillow'. I started to be an authentic TCM doctor with no burden or hesitation and was fully in charge of the clinic. I set three rules for myself: purchase authentic medicinals regardless of price and cost; use medicinal wild plants rather than cultivated ones; choose medicinals with better quality. Therefore, I not only select medicinals by myself at the medicinal materials market in Anguo, Heibei Province for countless times, but also gather and taste medicinals in person in and out of many provinces. I acknowledge teachers, make friends, give treatments at daytime and read books in the evening till now with great pleasure and no sense of time passing.

The only aim of this was to verify the scientific attribute of TCM through my practice, so I wrote this book. In memory of the past, I had similar feelings as my teacher Li did, i.e. 'it is the most delighted adventure in my life to become a TCM doctor'. I also feel that I could rectify my errors and find the right way back after getting lost in puzzle during the period of learning TCM.

I never encountered the misfortune Mr. Li did and I never had the feeling of 'gaining a blessing from a loss'. It is the charm of TCM that guides me to this path without any hesitation every time I faced a crossroad, and I can also be impressed by the charm every time in practice.

As far as I am concerned, it is not enough to feel the charm of TCM by myself.

In January 1988, many Nobel Prize winners from the world went to Paris for a conference and a surprising announcement was made at the end of the meeting that 'if mankind is to survive, we must go back 25 centuries in time to tap the wisdom of Confucius' (*Canberra Times*, Jan 24, 1988, Australia), reported by a journalist named Patrick Marnham in Paris.

If mankind would like to solve the problem of medical treatment crisis in the 21 century, it also must go back over two thousand years in time to tap the wisdom of TCM created by Chinese ancestors. Is there any other method we can approach? The charm of TCM will be spread to every person in different nations, countries and areas.

At last, I would like to end my book by quoting from Madame Curie, the first woman to win a Nobel Prize, to express my current feeling:

'Looking at the silkworm dedication and hard work, I feel that I and they are very similar. I like them and I always patiently to our own efforts focused on a goal. [...] I know life is short and fragile. I know life leaves nothing. I know other people hold the different views on what I am doing, and I am also not sure whether it conforms to the truth. However, I am still working on it.'(*Madame Curie*, Beijing: The Commercial Press, 1984:265).